Appealing spaces

The ethics of humane networking

The interplay between justice and relational healing in caregiving

Dr Aat van Rhijn
Dr Hanneke Meulink-Korf

Text translated and adapted by Daniël Louw

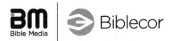

Copyright © 2019 Biblecor
Biblecor is a division of Bible-Media
Private Bag X5, Wellington 7654
Orders: 0860 26 33 42
www.biblemedia.co.za

All rights reserved. No part of this book may be reproduced or distributed
in any form without permission in writing from the publisher.

Unless otherwise stated all Scripture quotations in this publication are from The Holy
Bible, New International Version. Copyright © 1984 International Bible Society.
With permission

Design by Marthie Steenkamp
Set in Minion Pro in 12 pt on 15 pt by Marthie Steenkamp
Cover design by Natascha Olivier
Cover image: Painting by Daniël Louw

First edition, first print 2019

ISBN 978 1 77616 030 3

We believe the right product at the right time in the right hands can make all the difference.

Our aim is to provide young believers, congregation members and leaders of our country with a wide variety of affordable products.

Become part of our team by sponsoring products, giving donations or supporting us financially.

Bible Media Team

Contact us at: 021 864 8268 or info@bmedia.co.za
Banking details: Bible Media, Absa, Wellington | Cheque account: 405 118 1699 | Reference: Surname and cell number

Contents

Preface	9
1. The interplay between relational ethics (Nagy) and conscience (Levinas)	**25**
Detecting the problematic field and preliminary remarks	27
Basic directors and foundational concepts in Nagy's contextual model	31
Further outline of research project and demarcation of research objectives	47
2. Ethical entanglement as paradigm for a foundational contextual therapy: Exposition of Ivan Boszormenyi-Nagy's theory	**53**
Biographic sketch: An introductory outline	54
Nagy's professional decor: Two important partners in the discourse on family therapy (Fairbairn and Bateson)	67
Nosology: The paradigm switch from pathology to mindful understanding of interactional obstacles	78
Towards an "operational anthropology": Probing into human well-being	81
Loyalty: The quest for an ethical approach to existential entanglements within human encounters	83
Justice and social dynamics: The public framework for community and familial well-being (the invisible becomes visible)	94
The interplay: Dialectics – dialogue (*respondeo, ergo sum*)	102
In retrospect: Short concluding remarks on healing and repairing the hurt human justice	116
Nagy in a nutshell: Hope within relational repairing and caring encounters	120
The art of re-balancing: The healing power of "loyal silence" within the spiritual dynamics: Justice – mercy (*ḥēsēd*)	124
3. The ethical dynamics of contextual encounters: On entering the unpredictable space of humane reciprocity	**127**
The interplay between "context/contextual" and human well-being (therapy)	131
The networking framework of heteronomous relationality and the ethics of intersubjective obligations	137
Children as reliable resources of care and reinforcement (*the giving child*)	140

Paradigm switch in psychotherapy: From psychic terminology to legal terminology (*judicial language*) — 143

The interplay: Buber (dialogical encounter) – Nagy (therapeutic context) — 144

The "I-Thou" reciprocity: Interpreting intersubjectivity as the origin of authentic human being — 146

Dialoguing: In search of a common ground for the a priori of relationships — 150

Nagy's appeal on Buber: Basic questions about the status of a "human order of being" and the interplay with "a common order of justice" — 151

Levinas and Buber: The discourse about dialoguing within the ground structure of subject-responsibility — 156

The meta-realm of subjectivity: "Mammon" (*bekol me'odéka*) as an embodied soulful investment in life! — 165

4. "The silent partner" and the founding of subjectivity (the subject) within the theoretic discourse between Nagy and Levinas — 169

The status of the subject: Grounded in ethics — 170

Emmanuel Levinas – biographical sketch — 174

Human subjectivity within the framework of relational ethics — 178

The threat of war and violence: The breakdown of totality (detotalising) — 185

The metaphysical dimension — 189

Habitational enjoyment: Being at home in worldly spaces and embodied encounters — 196

Encountering visage in the quest for meaning (*sens*): The subject in search of his/her master/mistress — 200

Subjectivity as animated mercifulness (Levinas) — 218

Subjectivity within the familial paradigm of intergenerational dynamics: The asymmetry of reciprocity (Nagy) — 223

The quest for humanity within the trace of the Other/other: Two intersecting perspectives – Nagy-and-Levinas — 245

Parallels (*l'un-pour-l'autre*) and differences ("*visage*") — 249

Challenging confrontations: The trace of a peculiar weakness — 252

The ambiguous connection: Transcendence-in-immanence – the enigmatic factor of disturbance (*dérangement*) — 270

Justice within social dynamics: The quest for loyalty and the establishment of a "balance of justice" — 274

On challenging the loyalty of the single individual — 276

Time as discontinuity — 279

Multidirected partiality as condition for therapy and pastoral care — 280

Towards a *meta*-perspective on intersubjectivity: Hospitality as inclusive intercession — 285

5. Retribution, forgiveness and release — 292

- The complexity of forgiveness, revenge and retribution — 293
- The judicial context of "exoneration" — 296
- Exoneration within the realm of contextual therapy (Nagy) — 297
- The ethics of relational loyalty: Exoneration as transformation rather than the generosity of forgiveness — 305
- Exoneration within the dynamics: Guilt – guilt feelings — 308
- The asymmetry and mutuality of existential guilt: The hurt victim — 309
- The fourth dimension: Existential responsibility and "survivor's guilt" — 311
- Forgive as fore-give: The opportunity of compensation and the re-establishment of trust (Hargrave) — 313
- Complexity of exoneration and forgiveness: A kaleidoscope of aspects and perspectives — 318
- Irrevocable time and the impossibility of indifference within the triadic obligation of forgiveness: *Human being – neighbour – God* — 324
- The peculiarity of forgiveness in Levinas' writings: The ethical principle of "one-for-the-other" (*l'un-pour-l'autre*) in an anthropology of forgiveness — 327
- The I and the obstacle of totality: Delayed justice and immature forgiveness — 332
- Endless time and forgiveness as a purified present — 335
- Nagy's re-interpretation of exoneration. Towards an anthropology of accountable responsibility within the tension: Levinas (encountered by/encountering Visage) – Nagy (preceding indebtedness) — 341
- Towards the significance of dialoguing encounters. Concluding remarks on a reinterpretation of exoneration — 348
- Forgiveness and the quest for sacrifice: The liturgy of the sanctification of life — 353

6. Pastoral care within a contextual paradigm: In defence of "gratuitous subjectivity" — 357

- The proprium for pastoral care: The ecclesial space of fellowship — 358
- Care of human souls as care for justice and ethical networking: Towards an "a-theistic freedom" of subjectivity — 365
- Debriefing. The interplay between subjective encounters (facing the other) and ethical entanglements (indebtedness): A way out? — 368
- The mandate of pastoral care: The diaconic outreach of the fellowship of believers (church) to the other/others — 375
- Pastoral care within ethical entanglements and violent aberrations: The challenge of a contextual approach in family care — 381
- Adjournment of violence — 386
- Towards a reformulation of basic concepts: The measure of familial dynamics (directives and norms) — 392

The praxis of pastoral engagement	393
The quest for methodology in pastoral engagements	395
The method of multidirected partiality: Conditional accountable regard	398
Justice as frame of reference in contextual pastoral care	403

Bibliography 414
Glossarial explanation of core concepts 427
Summary 434

PREFACE

Pastoral encounters as appealing spaces of meeting and healing

For a very long time, very specifically during the second half of the 20th century, healing and wholeness in caregiving and counselling were dominated by communication strategies and listening skills designed for psychotherapeutic strategies mostly based on personality theories, intra-psychic dynamics (psychoanalyses) and individualistic "self-realisation" – human self-determination (Sperry 2002:3). Operating with the dominant presupposition that the individual person has the inner-potential to develop self-healing and attain wholeness, healing and human well-being have become a mode of "self-fixation" running the danger to reduce the human self to intra-psychic constructs. However, developments in, for example, family therapy with the emphasis on a systems approach, the paradigmatic scenario started to change from pathological thinking to networking thinking. Human beings are not isolated and merely individualistic islands (encapsulated selves) but dynamic interacting entities operating within interrelational systems and intergenerational networks in time, place and space.

Due to the above-mentioned paradigm shift, three important perspectives become imperative to enhance and broaden the scope of caregiving in the pastoral ministry of the church, namely:
- The impact of dynamic interacting relationships embedded in ethical frameworks;
- The value of a dialogical approach within the ontic dynamics of humane encounters;
- The appeal of the other on human responsibility when one becomes aware that being present with other human beings in time and space,

implies a metaphysical and transcendent horizon of unseen loyalties and needs.

Thus, the reason for a research project focusing on three influential thinkers. Their theories do impact on therapy, the value of human encounters, and the understanding of dialogue and ethics within relational networking.
(a) Ivan Boszormenyi-Nagy, renowned psychiatrist and family therapist, most well-known for being the creator of *Contextual Therapy* and his emphasis on a multi-dimensional approach and relational ethics focusing in particular on the nature and roles of *connectedness, caring*, reciprocity, loyalty, *legacy*, guilt, fairness, accountability, and trustworthiness within and between generations;
(b) Martin Buber with his *philosophy of intersubjective I-Thou encounters* designating a relation between subject and subject, a relation of reciprocity and mutuality; and
(c) Emmanuel Levinas with his theory that ethically we are responsible for one another in a face-to-face encounter; *the revealing other in his/her alterity*, not merely as shock but as primordial phenomenon ("enigma") of gentleness; freedom as framed by transcendence and heteronomy of the other.

With their dissertation, *De Context en de Ander: Nagy Herlezen in het Spoor van Levinas met het Oog op Pastoraat,* published in 1997, Aat van Rhijn and Hanneke Meulink-Korf embarked on a research project to enrich practical theology and the understanding of the challenges of the Christian congregation within the interplay between theology and the human sciences. Thus, the decision to translate the dissertation in order to broaden the theoretical and paradigmatic framework of the pastoral ministry.

The focus of the research project is on three important dimensions in caregiving, namely (a) the relational framework of human encounters; (b) the impact of space as an ontic structure of existential networking and (c) compassionate caring, as well as the ministerial responsibility for the suffering other and diaconic outreach to people in their frailty and quest for meaningful and humane encounters.

To translate an academic dissertation into caregiving language in order to enhance theory formation in pastoral encounters, was a challenging endeavour. Important decisions had to be taken. Information applicable for academic purposes had to be reduced. In order to attend to the logical flow of the argument and the connection between paragraphs and chapters, research material had to be reorganised while chapters and sections had to be provided with headings that did not appear in the original document. Thus, the reason for reworking and reformulation in order to contribute to a publication that could be used by scholars and readers interested in a multi-approach to healing, human well-being and spiritual wholeness (see Louw 2016).

Spiritual wholeness: On seeing the bigger picture of life

With "spiritual" is not meant a religious abstraction and disembodied "soul" open to sheer speculation or dualistic schisms between the material world and the immaterial dimension of life. With "spiritual" is meant frameworks of meaning that is captured in symbols or metaphors in order to guide human actions in terms of ideas, convictions and belief systems. In this sense "spiritual" describes the telic dimension in embodied manifestations and the significance of being in terms of norms, values, virtue, culture and custom. In religious terminology it refers to the transcendent dimension of life and how the understanding of divine powers and God-images influences conceptualisation and philosophies of life.

The quest for a kind of "spiritual wholeness" is the attempt to understand how different perspectives on life and different interpretations of the religion determine our mode of being, attitude, aptitude and disposition. Spiritual wholeness wrestles with the quest for human identity, human rights and human dignity. Thus, the reason why an integrative approach to the meaning of life should empower human beings to discover goals that enhance the quality of our being human and inspire human beings to make decisive decisions regarding responsible behaviour and ethical frameworks that instil sustainable hope, celebrating thankfulness and everlasting joy.

For spiritual wholeness one should start "seeing" the bigger picture of life (the role of destiny, calling and vocation). Integration of life experiences revolves around a moral framework or belief system or philosophy of life (constructive life views; the idea behind the conative; the driving forces in behaviour). On becoming "whole" in a praxis of hope care, presupposes a moral character.

"Moral character that integrates a plurality of attitudes and virtues such as: capacity for wonder and respect in the face of the stranger; sensitivity and receptivity; courage to risk and to be surprised; freedom to be vulnerable and open to learning and growth; disposition to recognize, accept, and honour those deemed to be different; hospitality grounded in compassion, humility, and generosity; passion to care and creative energy to transform the inherent violence of separation, prejudice and the alienation into a way of being with (empathy) and for (sympathy) the other as neighbour and partner in care and healing" (Schipani & Bueckert 2009:317).

"Soul" as a qualitative and relational concept: Habitus

Spiritual wholeness presupposes a very specific approach to anthropology in pastoral caregiving. It operates on the basis of the following presupposition regarding the meaning of "soul" in "soul care" (*cura animarum*):

"Soul is not a thing, but a quality or a dimension of experiencing life and ourselves. It has to do with depth, values, relatedness, heart and personal substance" (Moore 1992:5).[1] In this regard, soul as *habitus*, as a qualitative and systemic relational concept, and as the enfleshment of the wisdom or *phronesis* of God, and of vital virtues (normative frameworks and ethical propositions) represents the spiritual realm of a praxis of hope. Instead of personality or the general notion of an individual person, the notion of attitude and disposition reflects better the dynamics of *nephesh* (human life as a qualitative concept in Old Testament thinking operationalised in compassion and sacrificial love), and its connection to the organic dynamics of life, relationships and the qualitative stance of positioning within a systems understanding of our being human (pastoral anthropology) in caregiving.

Wholeness in hope care is about peace (*shalom*); wholeness implies different perspectives on the meaning and destiny of life. Wholeness is never completed and static; it incorporates a very specific spiritual endeavour namely to promote unconditional love, grace and reconciliation in attitudes by means of wisdom thinking. Spiritual wholeness represents the ethos of sacrificial love and this exhibited in a position of sharing, enriching and reaching out to

---

1 See in this regard the argument in Nauer 2005:471 for *cura animarum* and its connectedness to *nēphēsh*. Humans don't have *nēphēsh*, they are *nēphēsh* (2005:472). We are in our totality soul, in all relations. See also Louw 2016:58-86.

others in need. Friedman supports this emphasis on position in his book on the healing of family processes. "The most important ramification of homeostasis for family theory is its emphasis on position rather than personality when explaining the emergence of a symptom" (Friedman 1985:24).

Systemic and networking thinking in healing endeavours

With reference to Boszormenyi-Nagy's terminology, networking is shaped by what he calls the *intrinsic transgenerational tribunal* as extension of the dyadic parent-child-ledger. The implication of such a systemic network, framed by ethics, is the introduction of an inclusive consequential criterion in processes of healing that spans countless generations in the survival of the human species.

With a systems approach is meant an understanding of our being human within the dynamic networking of relationships. This dynamic refers to the importance of attitude, space, value, meaning, experience, relationships, and, what Ivan Boszormenyi-Nagy, called "context". In the words of Friedman (1985:24), the emphasis is on position rather than personality. Problems are therefore not necessarily located in the symptomatic patient but often in the structure of the system (1985:19). In a nutshell: "The components do not function according to their 'nature' but according to their position in the network" (Friedman 1985:15).

The paradigm shift, from individualistic self-help to interrelational healing and mutual caring, brought about a shift from "self" to "context". Thus, the relevant research question is how to link the dynamics of context to the healing of human beings. Is it possible to see space and the encounter with the other as a therapeutic environment to foster human well-being, to contribute to human dignity and to link therapy to the ethical notion of justice and an ethos of loyalty?

Basic paradigmatic issues in theory formation for pastoral caregiving

In this respect, the publication deals with the following paradigmatic issues: (a) encountering as the art of relational "*presencing*"; (b) the systemic networking of intersubjective, relational networking and dynamic contexts and the impact thereof on dialogue and identity; (c) the human quest for meaning within the past-present-future chain of intergenerational connections; (d) the countenance of "facing faces" – the other, and (e) space as the hermeneutics of life within pastoral and compassionate engagements (diaconic outreach).

Encountering: The art of relational "presencing"

Entering the delicate and frail space of another human being, is the most precious gift of humane human encounters. And that is precisely what the Christian tradition of *cura animarum* (care and cure of human souls) is about.

Encountering is about the networking space of relational "presencing". "Presencing" is an ontic category with effect in time, space and place.

With *presencing*[2] is meant a kind of encounter wherein past, present and future intersect so that sensing (experience) and present moment (state of being) coincide in such a way that a linear understanding of time makes place for circularity and a spiral interpretation. Presencing is about the "opening of the human mind" (significant reflection) and the "opening of the heart" (wisdom). It implies the paradigm shift from analytical causative thinking to integrative circular thinking. In Old Testament thinking, presencing refers to the notion of fellowship with God – *coram Deo*. Presencing is also not a neutral category but implies normative issues and ethical responsibility.

In terms of the thinking of Ivan Boszormenyi-Nagy, one can emphatically state that being with the other, should be an expression of fairness, integrity and dignity. At stake are two components of healing, namely compassionate being-with and the maintenance of a kind of ledger that refers to loyalty and justice.

In terms of Emmanuel Levinas' "metaphysical mystique", presencing in humane encounters is about transcending: The mystical, even meta-physical

---

2   For the use of the concept "presencing", see its meaning within the parameters of the interplay between a pastoral, psychological and spiritual approach in coaching; "… presencing shifts the place of perception to the source of an emerging future whole – to a future possibility that is seeking to emerge" (Kempen 2015:140). "*Presencing* is a blended word combining *sensing* (feeling the future possibility) and *presence* (the state of being in the present moment)" (Kempen 2015:140). "The boundaries between three types of presence collapse: the presence of the past (current field), the presence of the future (the emerging field of the future), and the presence of one's authentic Self. When this co-presence, or merging of the three types of presence, begins to resonate, we experience a profound shift, a change of the place from which we operate" (Kempen 2015:140-141).

superseding of human transience (Emmanuel Levinas). Presencing, thus, describes an existential ontology of meeting of one another; interpersonal engaging as the dynamics of mutual exchange (Martin Buber).

Within a psychotherapeutic understanding of the interactional dynamics between human beings, encounter was mostly interpreted in terms of what one can call the listening skills and communication techniques of "counselling". However, counselling in healing endeavours entails more than merely psychotherapeutic techniques of talk therapy; it is about existential networking within the happenstances of life-promoting humane encounters. In fact, one is exposed not merely to one self (who am I?). One is challenged by the other in terms of loyalty and ethical imperatives. Loyalty not merely towards the person, but to all others, present, absent and to be born. Thus, the emphasis on the ethical dimension of networking, talking and conversing (Ivan Boszormenyi-Nagy and Emmanuel Levinas); on interrelational networking and systemic interaction: the realm of existential contexts.

Relational dynamics as systemic networking: Contextualising context

Nagy's emphasis on "context" can be viewed as a breakthrough in psychotherapeutic thinking. He shifted the theoretical paradigm, with the aid of Buber's relational and dialogical model, into the direction of the other human sciences. Psychotherapy should acknowledge the fact that it is in essence a human science, and that it should, thus, contribute to the promotion of the quality of our being human in this world.

Contextuality is therefore embedded in a dialogical setting of interdisciplinary interaction. The human psyche should be viewed as a social, historical and intergenerational networking entity.

With "context" in healing encounters is meant: The dual exchange of giving and receiving. It describes the ethical dynamics of relational interaction within social settings, indicating the quality of intersubjectivity. With personal context (subjective dynamics) is meant: The current relational networking of a person, including both past relationships as well as future relationships.

In this networking and systemic sense, context describes patterns of paradigmatic frameworks of meaning, interactional networking of intersubjective relationships; concrete existential happenstances of life; local embeddedness in place as demarcated by culture, customs, convictions, belief systems and philosophical worldviews.

Context even transcends the limitation of concrete places and physical boundaries. Context is part of the "transcendent realm" of life wherein the quest for meaning surfaces: Where to? Wherefore?

Meaning within intergenerational networking

The questions *where to* and *wherefore* point to what the sociologist Peter Berger (1992:121) calls: The quest for "signals of transcendence". We each have a desire, or need, for something greater than ourselves; some bigger purpose or *meaning* in life. "In openness to the signals of transcendence the true proportions of our experience are rediscovered. This is the comic relief of redemption; it makes it possible for us to laugh and to play with a new fullness." Signals of transcendence create spiritual spaces for processes of hoping when life seems to be merely the tragedy of a cul de sac.

In humane encounters, one is confronted by the significance of human existence as well as with a chain of intergenerational networking. Loyalty summons one to promote human dignity; it unmasks one's deepest intentions; it awakens conscience and is in a very pregnant sense a test for ethos and compassionate being-with the other. In this sense, loyalty is both an ontic and qualitative phenomenon. It determines the quality of human interaction and mutual communication. It defines spaces and places of meeting. Therefore, guilt and the insight of injustice could play a detrimental role in processes of healing.

Existential guilt implies that being human within intersubjectivity always presupposes that guilt is an inevitable ingredient of our relationship with the other. The further implication for therapy and counselling is that the other human being is co-present within the space of encounter, healing and helping; the other is always present in the counselling room of the therapist.

As an event of countenance, meeting the other is challenging; it makes an appeal to the quality of our being-with the other, namely diaconic outreach to people within the realm of frailty and suffering. But meeting also creates significant experiences of sheer joy and intimate embracement.

In fact, in the I-Thou embracement (Martin Buber) one is shaped as a co-creator of meaning: The significance of mutuality and relational interaction. And this is the challenge of the book: How to conceptualise the meeting space of human and pastoral encounters so that life and human beings could be healed?

The dimension of encountering within humane meetings: Facing faces as "envisioned visage" and "encountered countenance"

Meeting another human being implies more than merely making contact. As said, meeting is about encountering. It implies mutuality, exchange, influence; it is about the risk of entering the unique space of the other; it is about an exposure to the dynamic interaction between "you" and "me". It describes an existential event wherein all the realities of life are incorporated: Our fears and anxieties; our wrestling with despair and the hope to discover meaning in life; our awareness of guilt and guilt feelings; our vulnerability, loneliness, frailty. In this kind of encounter, one puts one's being at risk because the other is more than a mirror. The other is about the mystical experience that human beings coexist together in time, place, space and context. Encountering the other is the shocking discovery: I am there with the other: Facing the other within the mirror of many unseen faces.

It is indeed difficult to translate what is meant by "visage" in Emmanuel Levinas' thinking. One needs to reckon with the fact that visage is not merely a physical phenomenon that can be experienced in the appearance of the other. The face of the other (*le visage d'Autrui*) functions as the opening of a spatial encounter wherein accountability as an ethical category emerges as an appeal. In the face-to-face encounter, responsibility in its most original form of response, or language-response, arises. The ethics of re-*spond*-able responsibility, and the appealing otherness of the other, emerges in face-to-face, humane encounters.

The other is to a large extent a transcendent figure and *meta*-physical element in human encounters; the other is an ontic structure in all encounters, not determined by context, but by an ontic rootedness within a network of being. In its appearance, the other makes an appeal on my being human. The other does not fit into any system; even not in love relationships and family systems. The other is a unique particularity: *The appearance of the other creates a kind of disturbance and uneasiness* (epiphany). The other transcends the limitation of relationships and social systems. As such, the other makes the notion of justice urgent. Therefore, the priority of ethics in a philosophy of responsibility.

Central in Nagy's approach are the concepts of accountability and responsibility as explanatory framework for the understanding of justice.

Although not being a philosopher per se, accountability and responsibility within the order of justice determine the basic methodology of Nagy.

In order to promote humanity, human beings should act in an accountable and re-*spond*-able way. Respond-ability and responsibility become pivotal in the structuring of pastoral encounters. Thus, the role of Levinas' thinking in spatial encounters.

The central question is the quest for, and possibility of, responsibility for the other. Responsibility is not a kind of contract emerging from the dynamics of mutuality. Correspondence, not mutuality makes human beings responsible. It is the unique existence of the other (*autrei*) that makes an appeal on my being human and summons me to a qualitative mode of responsibility. Responsibility, thus, becomes in Levinas' thinking a distinguishing mark and sign (*insigne*) that comes into being when the existential quest for humanity appears and the significance of being is at stake. In this respect, responsibility cannot be reduced to a stage model within a developmental understanding of subjectivity. Responsibility is neither merely psychological, sociological nor historical. It is a characteristic of being, and therefore an ontic and being category.

Furthermore, meeting as encounter implies facing the other/others: countenance and visage. It is, thus, about the creative and moulding experience of "contextual existence" as "facing faces". By the latter is meant: To enter the vivid corporate space of personal being-with; of interactional exchange and relational networking wherein human beings are confronted by the reality of many layers of meaning and paradigmatic frameworks.

In space many interactional patterns of meaning open vistas and horizons of options and possibilities that can contribute to either an enriching in-depth sense of human dignity or a painful experience of rejection and abandonment. Space in connection to place is in a phenomenological and existential sense: contextual.

In the encounter there are many "faces" so to speak. But "face" is not merely about the form and physicality. Face is part of embodiment and the impact of spatial positioning. Face is about facing one another – it describes a mode of facial disposition; countenance as relational encounter; countenance as the opening up of one's being-there for the other. As an existential phenomenon, the notion of "face" in Levinas' thinking could perhaps be better described as "countenance"[3].

Countenance creates healing spaces wherein not merely physical appearance determines the quality of our being human, but even the "unseen faces" of many others. In this sense, countenance functions like a visage: a vision and vista of all the pre-faces of the past, the existing "faces" in the present, and the possible "faces" in future. Countenance is embedded in a chain of intergenerational networking. Countenance is not about individuals, but about the appeal of many "others" (the living, the dead, the unborn future generation). Others function like "facial mirrors" wherein one is confronted with oneself; with one's own life and quest for meaning; with one's very unique normative system and set of values. Thus, the reason why countenance and encountering are never "neutral".

Countenance in human encounters operates on two levels:
(a) On the level of aesthetics: the quest for meaning, significance and identity. Thus, the challenge in healing endeavours, and therapeutic interventions to deal with the human quest for dignity.
(b) On the level of ethics: ethos (disposition) and ethics (normative framework of life). Thus, the challenge in "counselling interaction" to supersede the level of merely personality theories or psychic turmoil. The challenge is to enter into the imperative dimension of justice and human rights: The appealing space of ethical endeavours and the summoning of humane encounters.

The point is that human encounters should never be disconnected from the awareness of the interaction between countenance (the other as a givenness: being-there) and space (as an invitation to encounter and to position oneself within relational dynamics).

Appealing spaces: The hermeneutics of life

In terms of hermeneutics, meaning is about the art of interpretation and the attempt to comprehend our daily experiences of life. "Meaning is the web of

---

3   By "face" Levinas means the human face (or in French, *visage*), but not thought of or experienced as a physical or aesthetic object. Rather, the first, usual, unreflective encounter with the face is as the living presence of another person and, therefore, as something experienced socially and ethically.

connections, understanding, and interpretations that helps us comprehend our experience and formulate plans directing our energies to the achievement of our desired future. Meaning provides us with the sense that our lives matter, that they make sense, and that they are more than the sum of our seconds, days, and years" (Steger 2012:165).

It can be argued that position can be rendered as more fundamental in anthropology than psychological categories such as personhood, personality and individual characteristics/traits; it is even more comprehensive than the notion of "psyche" and "soul". All of these play a role in processes of meaning-giving. However, fundamental is the question how one positions oneself (the existential dynamics of disposition and attitude) within the many ambiguities, discrepancies and paradoxes in life. Position is about meaningful orientation within space and place.

A surprising fact is that the Greeks had already discovered the importance of space and place for our being human. The ancient Greek term *chora* means space or place.[4] Bollnow (2011:28) refers to Aristotle who examined in detail the problem of space as linked to place (*topos*) and time (*chronos*). What is important for our reflection on the connection between space and meaning is the fact that the value of space depends on position (Bollnow 2011:29). Both place (*topos*) and space (*chora*) are interrelated. The Aristotelian concept of space therefore indicates place (*topos*), location and position. Everything in space has its natural place. Stemming from the verb "*choreo*", space as an existential category means primarily to give room, more generally, to give way, to shrink back, and particular to vessels: to hold something, to have room to receive something (Bollnow 2011:30).

Space is indeed a many-layered concept. Due to the fact that I want to connect a systems understanding of the value and meaning of our being human to space as a category of position, orientation and the soulfulness of life, I shall thus concentrate on space as dwelling place in our spiritual search and quest for meaning; *space then as an existential category*, that is, "*experienced space*" (Bollnow 2011:216). Space in the true sense is what Bollnow (2011:43) pointed out: only needed by the human person.

In an existential orientation, it is important that space should refer to

---

[4] For this interpretation, see the discussion of Økland (2004:154) on the meaning of *chōra* and the current debate in French philosophy, for example, Derrida.

the *intimacy of dwelling*. As a human being, we dwell in this world. Dwelling then refers to a form of "trusting-understanding bond" (Bollnow 2011:261). "Everywhere it is a question of designating a particular intimacy of the relationship, with which something mental or intellectual is to some extent merged into something spatial" (Bollnow 2011:263).

Human spatiality as a mode of dwelling in this world presupposes *human embodiment*. The only way in which a human soul can dwell is via and through the human body. One, thus, occupies space and has space. As Merleau-Ponty pointed out: The human being is admitted to the spatial world through my body; "the world is given to me à travers mon corps, in a sense right through my body, which itself is something spatially extended and whose various sense organs are already separated from each other by spatial distances" (Merleau-Ponty in Bollnow 2011:269). Incarnation is therefore to be at home in one's body within the dwelling space of trusting relationships.

Space as a resort for dwelling, and a starting point for wandering, a place to rest as well as a region to be transcended, presupposes a free space, a kind of "home" – exposure to comfort and compassion. This is the reason why hope as a mode of trusting should be connected to space. Hope then as new state of being (the bright side of trust and affirmation) within the shadow side and cold atmospheric quadrant of homelessness. In space, we should be protected. Bachelard (in Bollnow 2011:281) says, "Space, vast space, is the friend of being."

Space and countenance and human encounter are closely connected to the hermeneutics of being-there together. Countenance is *visuel* and opts as a chiffre of life.

Karl Jaspers introduced the notion of chiffre to the art of interpretation. *Chiffre* is about signs, which signify "transcendence", that which supersedes the senses and points to a beyond or metaphysical realm. *Chiffre* is inherent to our being and functions as the speech (*Sprache*)[5] of reality that makes "transcendence" visible (*schaubar*) and significant (*deutbar*) (Jaspers

---

5   See the following differentiation between signs as pointers to something else, symbols as making something else present as visible, and *chiffre* as the language or speech of a spiritual realm, the transcendent in life: "Zeichen sei definierbare Bedeutung eines Anderen, als solches auch unmittelbar Zugänglichen; Symbol sei die Gegenwart eines Anderen in anschaulicher Fülle, in der das Bedeuten und das Bedeutete untrennbar eines, das Symbolisierte nur im Symbol erst selber da ist; Chiffre sei Sprache als Transzendenten, das nur durch Sprache, nicht durch die Identität von Sache und Symbol, im Symbol zugänglich ist" (Jaspers 1962:157).

1932:146-148). Through the notion of *chiffre*, the art of interpretation should take account of the fact that the whole of life and the cosmos are transparent for the ultimate, for a meaning that supersedes the senses and creates a kind of significance. For that matter, even art functions as a form of *chiffre*[6] (Jaspers 1932:136); it attaches vision and significance to things. Thus, the reason why reality is fundamentally a "spiritual entity" (*geistige Realität*) (Jaspers 1962:163). Life is actually an art describing a journey of spiritual poetics.

The philosopher Wilhelm Dilthey called the spiritual poetics in art "imaginative poetry" (Dilthey 1961:82). Imaginative poetry creates an awareness of transcendence and links experience to the symbolic meaning of life; it requires a kind of spiritual hermeneutics in order to discover meaning in life. Hermeneutics (Dilthey 1976:248-249) could therefore be described as the "art of understanding"; it detects meaning as a relational category inherent in life; it comprehends life and the connections between part and whole (Hodges 1944:20). In this regard hermeneutics functions as a kind of spiritual poetics that helps human beings to become aware of the fact that life is structured by *chiffre*, by visionary thinking and creative ideas; spiritual hermeneutics is an invitation to vision (*visuel*) – it shows us more than we had suspected in familiar things, and increases our power of discernment, understanding and imagination.

Transcendence: The mystical yearning for more and visionary thinking

In this respect hope and visionary thinking are connected to *chiffre* (symbolic language of transcendence), signs signifying a sense of yearning for more ... for that which surpasses all sensory observation. They operate like peepholes within an in-between, namely of that which transcends, supersedes or befalls our being human. The in-between of life is the realm of the sublime, despite the threat of the ridiculous. Framed by the mystery of the unseen, the sublime unfolds in our daily existence as the surprise of some awful transcendent awareness. Brute realism is then countered by awesome amazement (*verwondering*): The yearning for meaning and spiritual vision. Aesthetics and inspiration frame the praxis of practical thinking, thus the aesthetics

---

6 "Aber auch die Kunst, wo sie eigentlich ist, ist nicht unverbindlich. Sie spricht vielmehr selbst als Chiffre" (Jaspers 1932:136).

of creative vision; inspiration as the *poesis* of the human soul; the awesome horror of the sublime.

The mysterious experience that one is overwhelmed by surprise and awe, the fact that seeing and living entails much more than observation by the senses, bring about a kind of existential amazement; it creates an awareness and discovery that things change and that the essence of being can also be different (*anders-syn*); thus, experiences of wonder. Suddenly there is the passion to know and to transcend the factuality of phenomena.

C Verhoeven, in his book *Inleiding tot de verwondering* (1971), refers to this kind of knowing as a constructive kind of knowledge wherein panic and passion become combined, leading to a deeper and fundamental sense of wisdom (1971:12). Wonder/*Verwondering* is the starting point of wisdom thinking (*sophia* = love for wisdom); it creates the knowing mode of philosophical reflection. Philosophy is therefore the radicalisation of wonder (1971:13); it creates a longing (hunkering) and hunger for vision and hope. In awe and wonder, one becomes unoccupied and overwhelmed by a sense of void: there must be more in life than insignificance and nullity. This sense of more-in-life is closely connected to the human attempt to create frameworks of understanding in order to comprehend the essence of being and life: life views (*Weltanschaung*).

In countenance and human encounter, healing and human well-being are constantly dependent of the question: How do we "see" ourselves, and how do the other view us. The other becomes the "eye" of the "I", and, in this sense, is always appealing; that is, inviting the "I" to reposition oneself, to rediscover identity and re-orientate oneself in time, place and space.

In his book *Seeing things*, Stephen Pattison sums up the predicament of people living in an age of what might be characterised as "visual overload" or hyper-visuality: "We have so much but see so little" (Pattison 2007:1). We are living in a visual culture overloaded with images. Images rain upon us in all spheres of life. "With the extension of sight by microscopic, telescopic, electronic, digital and other means symbolised by instruments such as electron microscopes, scanners, cameras and photographs, we are all too aware of living in a world structured round sight and the visual" (Pattison 2007:3).

"If the scopic regime of the 'arrogant eye' is to be rejected in favour of fostering more intimate fellowship with visual artefacts, then an alternative approach is required that allows the emergence of a more intimate, loving gaze" (Pattison 2007:19). Moreover, in religion this *loving gaze* is closely related to an iconic view on life. And it is due to this loving gaze, that pastoral care as the enfleshment of the *passio Dei* and the exhibition for compassionate being-with comes into play.

It is indeed a fact that Christianity contributed to the split between the realms of the animate and inanimate (Pattison 2007:17). In the contemporary Western intellectual world, images are subordinated to words. "Thus, logocentric culture needs to overcome its scopophobia if it is to appreciate the importance of visual objects and artefacts" (Pattison 2007:20). It is indeed a challenge to a spiritual and loving, hopeful gaze, to become engaged with the embodied materiality of objects, thus the need for a metaphoric approach (Pattison 2013).

And this is what this book is about: Encounters as the embodied speech of other-exposure, and the diaconic demonstration of loving "seeing" and compassionate "being-with". Encounters as spaces of healing demarcated by the ontic category of justice; the ethos of loyalty; the disposition of responsibility and re-*spond*-ability, the notion of accountability; the mutual exchange of giving-and-receiving and the alarming *presencing* of countenance: Facing the faces of many others in time and space. Thus, the challenging endeavour of appealing spaces, dialoguing encounters and therapeutic caregiving.

The reader has to "face" the following intriguing questions: Can encounters become healing spaces for humane interaction in order to foster human dignity, even for the extensive interconnectedness of intergenerational trajectories? Is it indeed possible that diaconic engagements can instil justice and renew human beings, and that pastoral caregiving can, within the mode of compassionate being-with, framed by the ethics of loyalty and the ethos of sensitive listening, bring about change and transformation?

But (and this is the basic precondition for healing interventions) caregiving should rediscover the challenging position and appealing space of the other/Other; the other/Other as disturbing countenance and conscience for authentic humane encounters.

Daniël Louw
Stellenbosch
March 2019

CHAPTER 1

The interplay between relational ethics (Nagy) and conscience (Levinas)

The practical engagement with pastoral care, psychotherapy and education could be viewed as incentives for this study. The unique space of subjectivity within the dynamics of relational networking, brought the researchers in connection with the psycho-psychiatric reflections of the Hungarian–American therapist Ivan Boszormenyi-Nagy[1]). Although not necessarily a religious thinker, and not per se associated with theology, the link between life issues and the dynamics of human intersubjectivity, creates new avenues for the praxis of caregiving. It brings about new perspectives for family therapy as well.

The notion of "contextuality" underlines anew the importance of *responsible dialogue* in a re-interpretation of intergenerational interaction. Due to several relational infringements, the quest for an ethical approach to a "*psychology of relationships*" (Nagy & Krasner BGT, 1986:xii) surfaced. To address the phenomenon of estrangement in familial interaction (Nagy & Ulrich 1981), the link between context and therapy becomes paramount. In the prologue to *Between Give and Take,* Nagy (inspired by the I-Thou approach of Martin Buber) mentioned the urgent need for a paradigm shift: From an "existential-psychodynamic approach" to a "systemic-transactional" definition of family therapy.

Nagy can be called the founding father of "contextual therapy". Fundamental is the human quest for trustworthiness, a humane world wherein one can gain confidence and trust. Thus, the importance of relational interaction,

---

1   Referred to as Nagy in the document.

specifically the dynamics of intergenerational relationships, and the impact of the ethical dimension of life on the quality of intersubjectivity. For Nagy, trustworthiness and the mutuality of generational interaction, are paramount. To be human, implies an interconnectedness with previous and coming generations (offspring). The latter is decisive for a qualitative understanding of life and future human orientation. Thus, the reason why Nagy can be viewed as a kind of "family therapist"[2].

The notion of the ethical framework of being, is not always welcomed and accepted by the more disciplinary psychotherapeutic discourses. The emphasis on the relational-ethical dimension is neither self-evident. Even in pastoral caregiving, researchers tend to avoid the topic. Thus, the attempt to explore the link between ethics and mercy – the sensitivity of being-with and being-for-the-other. Eventually, one becomes challenged by fellow human beings on the fundamental quest for justice.

In this respect, Emmanuel Levinas is becoming an important research partner. During the research project, Meulink-Korf and Van Rhijn became convinced of the relevancy of Levinas' fundamental presupposition, namely that the human self-awareness is immediately interconnected with the penetrating sensitivity of conscience. The moment I become aware of myself, I am confronted with my own, natural tendency to perform injustice; I become aware of the damage and destruction (infringement) I inflict on the other due to the dubious character of my ego-structure (Levinas MG:41). The ethical dimension is not external to the structure of being, but the primary structure of our being human.

Ethics should therefore not be founded by the affective dimension and needs determined by the individual psyche; it is not the manifestation of the will to survive (conative dimension). For Levinas, ethics is prior to ontic matters. In fact, it penetrates the essence of being and operates within the realm of philosophical mindfulness and reflection on ontic matters. It also includes reflection regarding human responsibility and our understanding of God.

The assumption that ethics is more primordial than ontology, is indeed a very challenging thesis.

---

2   David Ulrich and Nagy wrote together an article wherein inter alia the concept of "rejunction" (to establish new connections; responsible dialogue, especially with family members from whom one became isolated) is designed and worked out.

Thus, the core problem of the research: What is the relationship between the research of Nagy on psychotherapy and Levinas' descriptions of intersubjective responsibility within the encounter with the other? How could Nagy's therapeutic approach to relational dynamics be merged with the rather complexity of forgiveness as developed by Levinas, and his emphasis on the metaphysical desire (*désir métaphysique*); the significant and relational quest for the "humane other". Both Nagy and Levinas are heuristic in their attempt to detect the meaning of true humanity. Both share the interest to reflect on the "motivational layer" of our being human (Nagy). The intriguing question is: But what is the source for humane, authentic being and responsible concern (Levinas), despite different theoretical and disciplinary points of departure?

Detecting the problematic field and preliminary remarks

The attempt to link the two thinkers with one another is not evident. Nagy's focus is what he calls "contextual therapy". The term suggests a kind of social context necessary for making a therapeutic diagnosis. Psychotherapeutic interventions are embedded in social environments and are dependent on intersubjectivity and relational networking. The latter is framed by an ethical dimension and operates within the realm of meaningful actions of helping and healing.

Levinas' approach is totally different and from a more ontological angle. Levinas does not specifically refer to context. The other is to a large extent not determined by context, but by an ontic rootedness within a network of being. The other as countenance appears within encounters, and, in its appearance makes an appeal on my being human. The other does not fit into any system; even not in love relationships and family systems. The other is a unique particularity: *The appearance of the other creates a kind of disturbance and uneasiness*. The other transcends the limitation of relationships and social systems. As such, the other makes the notion of justice urgent. Therefore, the priority of ethics in a philosophy of responsibility. In order to promote humanity, human beings should act in an accountable and re-*spond*-able way.

The significance of "context" in Nagy's approach is quite unique. Primarily, Nagy wants to qualify context from the experience of justice in human encounters. In an interview, Nagy maintained that, within the dimension of a relational ethics, justice becomes a very important criterion for the qualification of the relationship. He renders justice as the driving force in relationships (Van Heusden 1983:140-144). Central in Nagy's approach are the concepts of accountability and responsibility as explanatory framework for the understanding of justice. Although not being a philosopher per se, accountability and responsibility within the order of justice determine the basic methodology of Nagy.

Levinas' emphasis is slightly different. The central question is the quest for, and possibility of, responsibility for the other. Responsibility is not a kind of contract emerging from the dynamics of mutuality. Correspondence, not mutuality makes human beings responsible. It is the unique existence of the other (*autrei*) that makes an appeal on my being human and summons me to a qualitative mode of responsibility. Responsibility, thus, becomes in Levinas' thinking a distinguishing mark and sign (*insigne*) that comes into being when the existential quest for humanity appears and the significance of being is at stake. In this respect, responsibility cannot be reduced to a stage model within a developmental understanding of subjectivity. Responsibility is neither merely psychological, sociological nor historical. It is a characteristic of being, and therefore an ontic and being category.

In a very special way, Nagy's understanding of the ethical dimension of intersubjectivity, is largely influenced by Martin Buber's "philosophy of I – Thou". The basis for Nagy's anthropology and theory on human relationships, is the dialogical principle of mutuality. Because Levinas' philosophy of co-humanity, and the humane value of the other, are not shaped by Buber's dialogical principle, the controversy between the two thinkers resides in the fact that the otherness of the other is an ontic premise and not the outcome of responsibility, shaped by a relational and mutual dynamics.

In order to summarise the argument, one can say that Levinas' thesis for the appearance of the "face of the other" (visage) as a kind of relational disturbance and shock in the event of encounters, posits an ontic category sui generis. Therefore, the difference with Martin Buber, and the reason why the researchers cannot follow Nagy's advocacy for a therapeutic approach based solely on Buber's dialogical principle of mutuality. Furthermore, it is for the understanding of Nagy's therapeutic engagement, decisive to accept the assumption that every human being is embedded in a fundamental in-debtedness towards past and future generations.

The eventual scope of the research project is the field of pastoral care. Both the practice, as well as the mandate and legitimacy of pastoral care, are objects of research. Within the scope of the basic argument, it is important to understand that both points of departure in Nagy's and Levinas' models are fundamental for theory formation in pastoral care. Thus, the underscript in the title of the book: *The interplay between ethics and relational healing in caregiving.*

Within the Christian tradition of pastoral care, caregiving had been described and qualified by the traditional term of "soul care" (*cura animarum*: care/cure of human souls). It was used for the office of care and the endeavour of hospitality in the church. Therefore, a rereading of Nagy within the paradigm of Levinas, presupposes the realm of pastoral care and the diaconic outreach of ministry. A contextual approach to the dynamics of relationship could benefit an interdisciplinary discourse between psychotherapy and pastoral care.

Nagy's emphasis on "context" can be viewed as a breakthrough in psychotherapeutic thinking. He shifted the theoretic paradigm, with the aid of Buber's relational and dialogical model, into the direction of the other human sciences. Psychotherapy should acknowledge the fact that it is in essence a human science, and that it should, thus, contribute to the promotion of the quality of our being human in this world.

The point of departure for the theoretical basis of pastoral care is the following: In our actions and performances, caregiving takes place within the relational dynamics of what is now called "*presencing*": Entering the presence of God and living within the acute awareness of a continuous encounter with God: *coram Deo*. The Old Testament's imperative for a compassionate concern for the other, the acute awareness of neighbourly love as co-humanity, should be viewed as a kind of commandment for the enhancement of humane living and the quality of all modes of human relationships (Deurloo 1967:103, 95). This humane emphasis and commandment for the quality of co-humanity could be rendered as a directive and guideline for all kinds of human relationships.

The following assumption will function as the undergirding presupposition for dealing with the interplay between psychotherapy and pastoral care: There exists a vivid tension between the human sciences and theology.

CHAPTER 1

According to Karl Barth, theology is "*theantropology*", and not "onto-theology" (Levinas AZ:14).

The researchers are convinced that the skilfulness of pastoral caregivers is dependent on thorough knowledge regarding the dynamics of human relationships. The latter should be directed by the principle of co-existence within the presence of the living God (*coram Deo*). The dynamics of human relationships (personal and interpersonal) cannot be divided into two separate categories, namely pastoral care and its sole focus on a sphere of life reserved mainly for God alone, and psychotherapy operating in a sphere of human life, isolated from the presence of God – the dynamics of life as the sole domain of psychotherapy. The interplay between psychotherapy and pastoral care is dependent on the question how both sciences operate together in an inclusive approach, keeping their intradisciplinary discourse open and fruitful for one another (an interdisciplinary discourse). This is the reason why the research project wants to reread Nagy in the light of Levinas. It wants to enhance the quality of pastoral care. The mutuality and interplay should be an indication of the biblical principle of merciful grace, pity and compassion (hèsèd), as enfleshed in the dynamics of human relationships. Due to grace and benevolence, we owe one another mercy. Therefore, the importance of hospitality and forgiveness in a diaconic outreach to the vulnerability of the other.

In order to re-interpret Nagy's exposition of the ethical dimension within contextuality, one must gain clarity on what is meant by this dimension. Especially, if it should be interpreted as a sign, trace, pointing to the dynamics of "*coram deo*". *Coram Deo* should be explained in a very explicit way, namely as a kind of wisdom-truth within the arena of many different opinions and approaches. *Coram Deo* should, thus, signify a condition and constituency of our being human that inflicts a sense of existential disturbance. It should not be limited to the confines of a positivistic understanding of science. On the other hand, it should be relevant; that is, it should operate as a directive within many scientific discourses. It should stimulate the interplay between pastoral caregiver and psychotherapist.

Furthermore, *coram Deo* should become a creative event of encounter in order to foster that kind of discomfort and disturbance that open up new avenues of reinterpreting the past from the perspective of the future. Both psychotherapist and pastoral caregiver are engaged in events of disquiet uneasiness – a kind of "spiritual and relational turbulence". It should create a sense of eschatological discomfort, or utopic conscience (*utopie de la conscience*) – a not-yet of conscience (Levinas DQVI:132). This interesting dynamic occurs within the sound interdisciplinary tension between theology and the other sciences.

Theologians will, thus, be exposed to this interdisciplinary tension when Nagy is reread within the confines of Levinas' thinking. It is the sincere hope of the researchers that the dynamics between context and the particularity of the other could help pastoral care to operate in a much more fruitful and appropriate way.

In order to make a pastoral assessment of Nagy's contextual approach, it is important to give attention to some of the most basic concepts in Nagy's reflection on therapy. These concepts play a fundamental role in his argumentation and theoretical outline. Thus, the need for a thorough attention and further reflection on the core issues that helped to shape Nagy's theory on contextual human well-being.

Basic directors and foundational concepts in Nagy's contextual model

The following conceptional issues shape Nagy's approach and theoretical thinking:
(a) An intergenerational vision on merit, guilt and injustice.
(b) Guilt, conscience, and accountability.
(c) Loyalty and justice.
(d) The entitlement of giving – receiving within the confines of human needs.

(a) An intergenerational vision on merit, guilt and injustice (Exod 34; Ezek 18)

One is often not aware of the fact that problems in the life of adults do have consequences for children and consecutive generations. It is indeed interesting that in Exodus 34:4-7 it is mentioned that wickedness, rebellion and sin will be punished by the Lord. Destructive behaviour and disobedience are so serious, that Exodus 34:7 warns that God punishes the children and their children for the sin of the fathers to the third and fourth generation.

It is indeed a hermeneutical and exegetical question whether one should read the text from a causal and linear perspective, or from the interplay between God's design for live (the Torah) and irresponsible behaviour and disobedience to the law. In Exodus 20:6 the intention of the text is clearer. In a profound way, it states that punishment is related to the third and fourth generation of those who hate God, and therefore deliberately reject the confines of the ten commandments. The punishment is not automatic and fatalistic. Throughout the pericope it is the steadfastness of God's love, mercy and grace (God's *ḥēsēd*) that determines the admonishment of punishment. The confrontation is against the injustice and wickedness (*awon*) of the fathers as continued by consecutive generations. This interpretation is supported by Ezekiel 18:2-3. The saying and proverb in Israel refer to the fact that the fathers ate sour grapes, therefore the reason why the teeth of the children were set on edge. However, due to the covenantal grace of God, it is not anymore necessary to quote this proverb. The point is: "The soul who sins is the one who will be punished and die" (Ezek 18:3-4).

The argument is that guilt, due to irresponsible behaviour and disobedience against the directions of the law, should be punished. The punishment is not unqualified; it is qualified by God's mercy. This fact is underlined by Levinas' remark that God's mercy is more fundamental than his disciplinary admonishment. For the rabbis in the Jewish tradition (see rabbi Chananja), the mercy of God is much stronger than his strictness. The reasoning and calculation of grace imply that the victory over evil, and the establishment of what is good for life, is never in vain for believers who adhere to a kind of "moral optimism" (Levinas AV:129-130).

The notion of intergenerational transmission and the connection with difficult life issues, guilt and traumatic experiences wherein human beings are exposed to injustice, gained attention, even in the human sciences and psychotherapeutic research (see Giat Roberto 1992; De Levita 1994; Lindt 1993). It surfaces also in literature on pastoral caregiving and psychotherapeutic approaches (Edwin Friedman 1985; Patton 1985). However, the notion of intergenerational transmission is complex. It could leave the impression of pathological helplessness; a kind of psychological fatalism and victim-passivity.

The threat of pathological helplessness is often a real danger in professional models of helping and healing. See in this regard, the struggle of *proto-professionalism*[3] in dealing with intergenerational transfer, moral and reflective judgement (Brinkgreve 1984:17-24).

Nagy's approach is different. Intergenerational transmission is not about fate, but about relational dynamics and the quest for convalescence and healing (human well-being). For Nagy, injustice must be restored. In this respect, it is paramount to give attention to injustice inflicted by "forefathers" and others. The forefathers then as a kind of "relational resource" for consecutive generations.

Nagy links intergenerational transmission to the notion of "revolving slate"; that is, a mode of relational consequence wherein restorative revenge eventually creates "new victims". However, the problem is that innocent victims could be treated in the long run as original and causal culprits. Nagy, therefore, introduces the ethos of accountability and responsibility. He maintains his assumption, namely that personal accountability should be rendered as a guideline for caring and relational integrity. The latter forms the cornerstone of trustworthiness and individual health (Nagy & Krasner BGT:62).

This cornerstone is the basis for his clinical work, theory formation and conceptualisation. Individual uniqueness and personhood are framed by the dynamics of a relational reality (Nagy & Krasner BGT:7-8). This dynamic consists of four dimensions[4]:

1. Information as related to human embodiment and concrete social settings.
2. Processes within the psychic make-up of the person.
3. Transactional patterns of networking.
4. The dimension of relational ethics; "the ethics of due consideration and merited trust".

---

3   The concept refers to the application of insights and knowledge within daily events over a period of time. Since medical information became more public, patients enter the counselling room of doctors with more knowledge about their clinical condition. In a more general sense, "proto-professionalization" refers to the process of how professionalization occurred across the continuum of medical education. Knowledge is acquired after a prolonged period of experience (and reflection on experience). In such a process, experience becomes part of the professional's evolving knowledge and skills base. The prior period is then termed as one of "proto-professionalism". Proto-professionalism includes moral and psycho-social development and critical reflection. It even contributes to the development of meta-skills.

4   Concerning a fifth dimension of ontic dependence. See Ducommun-Nagy 2008. This addition came after the present research project.

Nagy's epistemology is shaped by an understanding of these different dimensions of the relational reality of life. In fact, they create "useful assumptions" about relationships. The further spinoff is that they become basic presuppositions that contribute to the overcoming of different kinds of psychological reductionisms (absolute modes of psychic determinism as linked to classification strategies and causal explanatory theories in psychotherapy). They can even help to supersede the fatalistic nihilism and "power confrontation" of Jean-Paul Sartre (Nagy & Krasner BGT:32).

The bottom line in therapy is: The vicious cycle of failure, and imperfect shortcomings, must be overcome. In this respect, Martin Buber's *I-Thou approach* was most helpful in Nagy's attempt to formulate theses four "useful assumptions" (Nagy *Interview* 1992). They even helped to move from a pathology paradigm to an ethical paradigm in addressing life issues that eventually determine human well-being.

In 1985, Nagy wrote: "Contextual therapists had to rely on a concept, borrowed from Buber, "the justice of the human order", as a quasi-objective criterion of interpersonal fairness" (Nagy F:306).

(b) Guilt, conscience and accountability (About existential guilt within the dynamics of intersubjectivity)

Life is framed by guilt and guilt feelings. Very specifically this is the case when one deals with relational infringements. In T. S. Eliot's play *"The cocktail party"*, the psychiatrist Dr Reilly, said to Celia Coplestone: "You suffer from a sense of sin, Miss Coplestone? This is most unusual …"

Early in 1957, Martin Buber delivered several papers before colleagues at the *Washington School for Psychiatry*. He was fortunate to meet Carl Rogers. Gradually it became evident that Buber's conceptualisation of the interaction between "I and Thou" differs largely from Rogers' "client-centered therapy" with his emphasis on empathetic listening. While Rogers emphasised empathetic mutuality and transfer, Buber maintained that the therapeutic relationship between therapist and client is non-reciprocal (Buber 1965a; Buber 1988). The reason? Accountability is a fundamental feature of being and in the first place not an outcome of the dynamics of relationships. Guilt should be rendered as personal and connected to individual responsibility. Guilt operates within the existential realities of life.

Buber's paper on *Guilt and Guilt Feelings* (Buber SuSg:475-502), played a fundamental role in Nagy's understanding of the interplay between guilt and guilt feelings. It is therefore paramount to give a summary of the content of Buber's paper.

In this paper (SuSg), Buber distinguishes between intrapersonal images of guilt and the interpersonal, existential reality of guilt.

For Buber, guilt is real due to personal responsibility. It is an existential reality and not the outcome of external factors, isolated from individual accountability and concrete situations. In the Freudian tradition, guilt is linked to the transgression of a family taboo, or external rules set by society. Due to orders and regulations of our being human in the world, existential guilt sets in when humans violate rules established by the bigger society, and worldly stipulations for structuring human orientation in life. In general, these orders and stipulations are acknowledged as directions for personal existential orientation, as well as guidelines for human behaviour in wider social networks. This is why, for example, a medical doctor caring for a patient, needs to enter the existential and social realm of guilt when dealing with a patient's experience and memory of guilt (Buber SeSg:216).

The core argument is that at the heart of guilt is the acknowledgement and existential awareness of "I", "the other", or "many others". Therefore, the reason why guilt is an existential and relational reality within concrete life settings.

The problem with many psychotherapeutic approaches in their focus on the intrapersonal realm, is that the paradigm of psychic images of guilt becomes so predominant, that the events that contributed to existing images and perceptions of guilt, are becoming irrelevant and underplayed. Guilt then becomes a merely reduced psychological perception (Buber SeSg:212). In the case of Freud's more ego-approach (Freudian materialism), and Jung's transcendental religious awareness (*pan-psychism*), guilt becomes a hiatus in the processes of individualisation. Guilt is then reduced to the realm of the human I, exclusively related to him/herself. However, if psychotherapy has to adhere to the true character of the discipline of healing and helping, it is paramount to surpass the narrow confines of intrapsychic processes. The focus should rather become our being human as related to the other within the "I-Thou dynamics of life" and existential networking (Buber SeSg:213).

Buber differentiates between the judicial sphere (the domain of the judge), the sphere of our conscience (the domain of the healer and psychotherapist), and the sphere of faith (the domain of the spirit – spiritual realm). Each of the three spheres requires a three-fold operation.
(a) For the judicial sphere: Acknowledgement; exercising of punishment; reparation and compensation.
(b) For the sphere of human conscience: Self-illumination and clarity; perseverance in conscientiousness; reconciliation.
(c) For the spiritual realm of faith: Confession of sin; remorse; penance.

For Buber, the sphere of the conscious and the realm of faith are intertwined. He gives thorough attention to the sphere of the conscious. Perseverance in consciousness defines Buber as the input to persevere. In the discovery that being is exposed to the humble awareness, and humiliating knowledge, that the person in the now of events is identical with the former human I, perseverance becomes decisive in order to deal appropriately with existential guilt (Buber SeSg:224).

In the case of existential guilt, the damage cannot really be compensated for. Compensation does not extinguish guilt and the consequences of transgressions. The implication is that the person to whom I am guilty should rather be encountered by me, within the clarity of my self-illumination (insightful self-understanding). Although the latter is extremely difficult, and limited for human beings, existential guilt becomes operationalised when it is confessed to the other. In this way, the "guilty I" becomes involved in the attempt to help the other as good as possible. At stake, is then the question how to deal with the consequences of my guilty actions, as well as how to overcome them in a meaningful manner (Buber SeSg:234). Reconciliation sets in, when the confession of guilt is not meant to maintain or restore a good self-image, or just to get rid of guilt feelings, but when it is the eventual outcome of an internalised (not merely arbitrary) new establishment of authentic human being (a new, existential realisation of "I").

Being guilty is a human ability. This is possible due to the fact that, according to Buber, our being human in this world is embedded in an ontic and inter-subjective structure, a human order of co-existence. We are embedded in a "human order of being". The impact of this ontic structuredness is twofold: We can contribute to the upholding and establishment of this human order of being or violate this order. Guilt is therefore always personal and cannot be reduced to guilt feelings resulting from the impact of powerful external taboos on transgressions.

Buber defines conscience as a kind of radical discernment. It is about the ability and disposition of human beings to discern (in the light of previous and future attitudes in life – *habitus*) between good and that which is to be disapproved and inappropriate for our being human (Buber SeSg:222). Consciousness is not the introjection of an external authority, but a personal established mode of being, based upon the unique human ability to distance oneself from one's *self* in order to attain clearer self-reflection and self-acknowledgement. This existential consciousness even implies the ability to establish oneself or to reject oneself (critical self-denouncement).

Conscience is the order of being within the realm of personal selfhood; it indicates a mode of being wherein a person fully accepts accountability for the essence of our being human in this world. Our being human as an ontic category, cannot be isolated from the order of being. It takes place constantly within an awareness of personal responsibility. Accountability is connected to self-insight and self-illumination, thus, the emphasis on a vital spirit and the courage to be. Without self-knowledge, as related to personal consciousness, a juridical acknowledgement of guilt is irrelevant and without meaning. Even religious confessions of sin are becoming merely pathetic stammering. Nobody will respond and listen to these meaningless sounds.

The point is, that a juridical acknowledgement of guilt, presupposes insight in the character of guilt. It demands a kind of struggle with the question whether one is guilty or not. The quest is about the tension: Innocence or responsibility.

This struggle is illustrated by Franz Kafka's novel *The Trial* (*Der Prozess*), written between 1914 and 1915. It tells the story of a man (Josef K) arrested and prosecuted by a remote, inaccessible authority. The nature of the crime is never revealed to Joseph K. Life then becomes a struggle to resolve the mystery of being judged; it becomes an existential struggle to vindicate oneself. Despite the confrontation with a priest in a dark and empty cathedral, the discussion leads to nowhere without any answer to the intriguing questions: Who is right? Who is wrong? Without the proof of guilt and clarity on the question of innocence, life becomes in vain. In the encounter with a faceless fate, one is doomed to failure (Kafka 1982:213). What is depicted in this novel, is that futility is a general and universal phenomenon. Life is a kind of trial in search of justice. It is impossible to avoid this search and quest for justice within the basic, daily struggle for coming to terms with guilt.

With reference to Martin Buber's term "the human order of being", judgement is a kind of existential layer within human relationships. Humans cannot avoid the interplay between guilt, punishment and innocence. Especially when one is engaged in the dynamics of human relationships. Even in religious thinking, lurks the connection between guilt and eventual, eschatological judgement and punishment.

The implication of Buber's term "the human order of being", is for Nagy threefold.

- Existential guilt implies that being human within intersubjectivity always presupposes that guilt is an inevitable ingredient of our relationship with the other. The further implication for therapy and counselling is that the other human being is co-present within the space of encounter, healing and helping; the other is always present in the counselling room of the therapist.
- The realisation of personal guilt and how acts of transgression impact on the "human order of being" (contributing to existential hurt), presuppose also the possibility of healing and growth. Acknowledgement of guilt and insight in the character of the transgression contribute to human well-being.
- The concept of the "justice of the order of being", can be associated with Nagy's notion of a "transgenerational tribune". The latter could even be called a kind of "secularised eschatology".

Nagy proposes the term "... *intrinsic transgenerational tribunal* as extension of the dyadic parent-child-ledger into an inclusive consequential criterion that spans countless generations in the survival of the human species" (Nagy F:308). The criteria for judgement are difficult to predict. Not even from religious, cultural or superego morality of any type. "Only an ongoing monitoring of factual consequences for the other determines the impact on the, always multilateral, balance of interpersonal fairness" (Nagy F:309).

It becomes an intriguing question how and by whom should the consequences for the other being be monitored and safeguarded? This is indeed a fundamental question in cases where the other is not remote but living very close to oneself.

"The requirements of species survival constitute the reality of transgenerational solidarity. As an invisible third party, this solidarity participates in family relationships, especially in intergenerational ones. The rules of its intrinsic covenant provide the ethical guidelines for close relationships" (Nagy F:307-308).

The presence of a kind of participating, invisible third party, is not an object to be depicted and verified. The invisible third party disappears and vanishes beyond the horizon of the visible – the more of life. Life implies both anticipation and a dimension that surpass the realm of direct observation. In this respect, it seems as if Nagy transcends the parameters of his own discipline. It even points in the direction of an indirect attempt to maintain the notion of hope in healing; hope as an option to repair the hurt human justice (Nagy & Spark IL:53).

The more one scrutinizes Nagy's terminology, the more one becomes aware of the fact that his terminology is embedded in intersubjectivity. His terminology refers to thinking about human relationships from a very specific perspective, namely an ethical perspective.

This ethical perspective promotes an understanding of our being human wherein accountability and responsibility are embedded in a sense of networking belongingness; that is, to be connected to the other. It describes interpersonal loyalty with special and important others, for example, parents within an intergenerational framework. The further implication is that accountability and loyalty emanate from the bigger inter-subjective order, an order which can be described as humane, just and righteous.

It is indeed an appropriate question whether the notion of order is not a paradox when it is linked to human dignity and righteousness. The notion of "human order" is to a large extent relative, especially when it refers to a cultural context. It becomes more complicated when order is about an ontic condition; a kind of existential structure of our being in this world. Even if this ontic structure is embedded in justice.

The idea of such a moral (justice of the human order) and ontic embeddedness correlates with Buber's thinking. Levinas (NP:47) refers to this notion of an ontic order in Buber's I-Thou approach, as not a clear and sound voice; it seems a bit creaky to him.

The notions of order and existential structures are even difficult to maintain in Nagy's approach. However, Nagy does not mean with "order" a kind of subordination or relativism. In fact, Nagy is in search of categories that are not delimited by intrapsychic structures or forces of power. When it is about the dynamics of human relationships, a righteous and humane order should be interpreted within the inter-subjective interplay between guilt and guilt feelings. "Justice of human order" is not to be interpreted literally. That is specifically the case in Buber's model (AJ Flink in conversation with VR/MK). "The-order-of-being" (Buber 1988:126), "an order of a human world" (Buber 1988:117), and "the human order of being" (Buber 1988:122) are used to indicate that being guilty, and the awareness of guilt, are characteristic of our being human in the world. "Man is the being who is capable of becoming guilty and is capable of illuminating his/her guilt" (Buber 1988:136). It is from this background that Nagy derives his term "justice of the human order".

"Justice of a human order" within a clinical context, as well as in theory formation, is for Nagy "intrinsic ethics". Every kind of therapeutic theory should try to deal with a panoramic overview in order to promote change and empower human beings. Thus, the reason why Alan Gurman (in Giat Roberto 1992:ix) remarks as follows: "Like gases, transgenerational models […] seem […] to expand to fill any space available." Every kind of therapeutic theory is directed by basic assumptions and indicators for the praxis of human encounters. One cannot avoid ethical impulses (Th De Boer in Bleijendaal 1991:131).

Hypothesis

The hypothesis of the research project is that Nagy's reflection on justice, and its ethical implication for a transgenerational model, shape a kind of anthropology wherein accountability and responsibility are predetermined by the problematic dilemma of freedom and the predicament of not being free. This is the reason why a rereading of Nagy within the framework of Levinas' philosophy can help psychotherapy to undergo a paradigm switch from intrapsychic inclusiveness to relational networking and contextual interaction. Therefore, in terms of Levinas' terminology, responsibility does not emanate from a totalitarian, dominating structure (manipulative power play). One mode of totalitarian manipulation is morality based upon the abuse of power. Another mode is general ideas extrapolated into ideology. Ideas then become an ideological force that is compulsory for every concrete human situation. In the same way, the notion of "intergenerational structures" and "family systems" have been abused by many ideological views on family care.

Responsibility as re-*spond*-ability is determined not by ontology but by the other/others: One is challenged to establish trustworthiness due to a foundational indebtedness wherein not only past relationships play a decisive role, but also the not-yet of future coming generations. Intergenerationality is shaped by the duality of justice-injustice within the dynamics of multidirected partiality. Thus, the assumption that the practice of pastoral encounters (the ministerial framework of service) can benefit, and even be enhanced, by an ethical framework wherin the command (the torah) summons one to helping and healing interactions; that is, to reach out to the weak and vulnerable other (*diakonia*). Pastoral endeavours are therefore directed primarily by pity and ḥēsēd.

Core research questions

We arrive now at the stage to pose the important question: What is meant by an "ethical dimension" in Nagy's theory for intergenerational therapy? Is Nagy's approach not a subtle form of reduction; that is, reducing ethics to facts, intrapsychic dynamics and dominating transactions? Is his "relational ethics" not a new mode of ideological enslavement? The danger lurks that morality can become a systemic force that change human beings into victims: The human being as dupe. Even the other as threatened dupe.

(c) About loyalty and righteousness

On the first page of *Invisible Loyalties*, Nagy and Spark write: "We can terminate any relationship except the one based on parenting; in reality, we cannot select our parents or children" (IL:xiii). It is difficult to deny the previous assumption. However, what one needs to understand is that, for Nagy and Krasner, the core issue in parenthood and the relational dynamics between siblings, is the notion of *fairness*. Fairness as expression of righteousness does not happen automatically. Fairness presupposes a personal conscience and is impossible without the correlate: Justice in society. Fairness is not a genetic issue (determined by "blood") but founded by ethics.

Fairness is in the last instance not determined by familial and parental roots. Nagy once referred to the interplay between roots and relationships within the context of legacies (Nagy F:217-219). This, however, does not imply that a sense of genetic rootedness determines the character of fairness. It is interesting that even Levinas maintained more or less the same position. For Levinas (TO:202), human beings are not static as trees rooted in the earth. Human beings are different. Human beings can migrate and start with a new beginning elsewhere.

Fairness is rooted in righteousness and not in the "blood of nature" so to speak. References to a kind of "innate tendency to care" (Nagy & Krasner BGT:78) do not mean that fairness as expression of loyalty and generosity (Nagy & Krasner BGT:278), is a kind of "general" and "natural" parental ability for care and the upbringing of a child. In their reference to injustice and unfair exploitation of children (Nagy & Krasner BGT:301), it is stated that fairness is not instigated by a natural biological capacity how to treat children. Children do have a right to a sustainable caring environment based on justice and loyalty. They are in need of a humane infrastructure that safeguards a caring space for responsible human development. In this regard, one can speak of a "natural" and inherent right of little children to be cared for (Van Heusden & Van den Eerenbeemt 1992:55).

With "nature" is then meant a humane space for a humane mode of upbringing. Within a systems approach, "nature" refers to the characteristics of a systemic energy that causes change due to the dynamics inherent to the inter-relational coherence and closeness of the system (See Verbeek 1977:16-18). Positions within intersubjective exchange of meaning determine the humane quality of the system (Friedman 1985).

The position of children within the dynamics of the family system, makes an appeal on parental care and responsibility. The appeal of the child makes the parent responsible. Parents need to have a capacity for care in order to provide a "reservoir" of loyalty and trustworthiness. Children appeal to this reservoir, even in cases when parents do not act in a trustworthy way. This is the reason why the family system requires a sustainable, positive process of caregiving.

One needs to acknowledge that Nagy's emphasis on the irrevocable character of familial connections, could eventually imply an amalgamation between what is "natural" and what is "normative". "Natural" is not necessarily "ethical". The appeal on loyalty and righteousness (the quest for an ethical based concern in Nagy's thinking) does not originate from within the system, but from the "outside", namely from the humane other and order of justice.

With reference to Levinas (TO:179-180), our "natural embeddedness" in this world, should become a humane and hospitable environment. In this regard, it is *the other* that contributes to a kind of humanisation of our being in this world. The spirituality of humanism is determined by the other in the symbolic figure and presence of widows, orphans and strangers (outsiders). "I am the powerful in relation with the other" (Th De Boer in Duyndam, Foreword 1984). I should, thus, act accordingly: humane.

We now need to pose the important question: What is the connection between loyalty and trustworthiness with regard to the other (the vulnerable other/others) in Nagy's thinking?

Loyalty: The complexity of a selection criterion

"Loyalty" is Nagy's term for selecting the one above the other, due to the fact that I owe the other my trustworthiness. In this sense, acknowledgement of accountability as debt, becomes a relational endeavour.

Loyalty is essentially a complex category. It brings about a conflict of interest; it implies a kind of "loyalty conflict". It describes a situation wherein one is situated within a polar field of forces, namely the rivalship between explicit objects that make an appeal upon one's loyalty (a multitude of loyalty-objects). Within a selection process, a decision has to be taken. To be righteous within a competing system of demands, and to respond to everyone's need simultaneously, are virtually impossible. What is most needed within the multitude of demands, is "a constructive discriminating factor". However, one still needs to accept the fact that righteousness is complex. Even constructive expectations can become exploited. For example, "the fundamental primary obligation of repaying with gratitude to those who gave us our lives" (Nagy F:127), can be exploited by parents. Thus, the reason why even inappropriate modes of parenthood can contribute to injustice.

As said, loyalty often implies conflict of interests and, thus, creates the possibility of injustice. This threat of injustice comes into play when the situation of the other (the outsider over against the interests of the insiders – loyalty to the people belonging to the so-called "in-group") must be taken into consideration simultaneously. Injustice sets in when loyalty to the in-group is becoming so paramount that the other disappear from the radar of the subject. Group loyalty in such a case subjugates personal responsibility.

Experiences of loyalty become fatal when relational connections are not guided by the principle of righteousness and justice. In societies where the notion of righteousness is in place and the core principle is not disruption, but fairness, there is order. In social settings, where the violation of regulations becomes normative, the chaos of injustice sets in. When violation and transgression of rules become accepted societal rules, righteousness cannot flourish. Righteousness and loyalty are fed by narratives in society which reflect personal accountability. Loyalty connects and promotes responsibility. Fundamental for the establishment of loyalty in society, are the coming together of personal and social narratives that are, at the same time, exponents of personal responsibility.

Changes within the intimate space of personal relationships affect the dynamics of social contexts. Personal change instigates social change. It is indeed true that we are desperately in need for a better world and just society with a more humane face. But then, in order to promote social justice, loyal interaction, and intersubjective loyalty, intergenerational relationships should be improved.

Exoneration: The quest to be delivered from guilt

Within the attempt to establish a safe and trustworthy world, Nagy introduces the juridical term of "exoneration". In order to deal later on with the connection between revenge, forgiveness and release from guilt, the notion of exoneration should be discussed. Important in this regard, is that, within the encounter between the debtor (the guilty one) and creditor (prosecutor), the notion of release/deliverance should be introduced. It describes the quest of being set free, built upon the cornerstones of fairness and reasonableness. Important to discuss, are the conditions for "exoneration" within intergenerational dynamics. Both the people who need to be released, as well as the people who suffer due to the irresponsible behaviour from the side of the perpetrator, should find protection, indemnity and release. For Nagy the sufferers are not merely the next generation, but also the society at large.

(d) The entitlement of giving within the confines of human needs (Nagy's understanding of subjectivity)

Receiving can be viewed as an entitlement of humane living. For example, one of the basic needs in care, is to receive help. To receive help and empathy are indeed important endeavours in order to gain human dignity and self-understanding. But valid care and education are also about the need and art of giving. One cannot ignore the need and even right, entitlement, to give. One of the basics in the art of giving, is about observing the other from the perspective of merciful listening. It is about the skill of how to understand the real needs of the other from the viewpoint of the other.

To reckon with the "need of the other", opens up exciting perspectives for parenthood. In education, the art of how to bring up a child, the skill of giving, can play a vital role. As said, in giving all the needs, psychological, physical and spiritual, are important. Acknowledgement of needs encompasses the rights and responsibility of the other. In this regard, Nagy's notion of entitlement (justified appeal and appropriate ability) comes into play. Even his advocacy for "on becoming a parent"; that is, "*parentification*", the process of growing into the art of being a caring parent should be read and understand in connection with the art of giving. The notion of "*parentification*" in the process of guiding children into adulthood, is not about a destructive process (a pathological mode of parenthood), but a constructive investment in the developmental growth into maturity. However, in this process of becoming a parent and guiding of children into the responsibility of being an adult, Nagy also warns against the possible dangers of destructive modes of parenting (Nagy & Krasner BGT:65). He refers to "destructive idealising"; that is, the danger that parents work with inappropriate images (distorted perceptions) that do not fit the reality and personality of the child. These images can become hampering factors because they operate with criteria that convey the message: "I am not good enough", thus, contributing to experiences of failure.

The reference to the risk of parenting and the possible danger of pathological modes of parenthood, underline the fact that personal behaviour (my actions) has got a huge impact on the identity and dignity of the other. In this regard, Levinas' thinking is even more radical than Nagy's remarks on becoming a parent within the parent-child interaction. Thus, Levinas' very bold statement that when the needs of the other are at stake, the only person to inform and instruct me, is the other(him/herself).

The other functions as a crack in the totality of a closed system. The other breaks through forms and functions as a "hole in the world". In this sense the other becomes a metaphor for the predicament of the outsider, the naked, the poor, the stranger, the orphan and the widow (Levinas 1987:44). The other is a wakeup call to reinstall justice and trustworthiness in the world.

Conscience and the awakening of the predicament of the other, are essentially determined by the other. In fact, the other functions as a kind of awakening, conscience and awareness. The other conveys the message that there is still time to act differently; even to postpone the betrayal of the other, namely, to do nothing. Not responding to the appeal of the other in caring engagements, exposes human beings to a kind of existential betrayal; that is, not to respond, not to act appropriately. Therefore, sloth and inertia can be viewed as hampering factors in the quality of our being human. Inertia can be called the great law of living in a prosperity cult and the impact of the global threat of massification. But the human-factor, within the demand for justice, can loom up in it, yes, even disturbs it.

Human beings are indeed able to disturb and combat the implications of inertia (Levinas 1987:155). The latter creates the scandal of our being human; it represents an "existential illness" (pathology of being). On the other hand, the scandal of our being human can indeed be transformed into the establishment of good; evil can be penetrated by appropriate, righteous actions.

The point in Nagy's affinity for Levinas' thinking, is the existential truth that nobody derives his or her identity (existential truth) from within him/herself. In the event of receiving identity, lurks the grace of being. Thus, the existential challenge: To perform righteousness in hospitable co-existence with the other. The other grants us identity. In this way, every human being contributes to the trustworthiness of being in this world.

The basic assumption is that within the parameters of righteousness and trustworthiness, Nagy wants to introduce the notion of subjectivity, namely, subjectivity as personal trustworthiness and entitlement to give and to help. The right to give creates a motivational layer in which hope resides for repairing the hurt human justice (Nagy & Spark IL:53). Thus, the assumption that Levinas' advocacy for the other, namely the other as a wakeup call to disturb the betrayal of fellow human beings due to inertia, challenges Nagy to maintain a kind of restorative hope. Through conscience and forgiveness, betrayal of the other (Levinas) can be disturbed (time as inertia) and even postponed. In this regard, forgiveness becomes an operational constituent in time. This disturbance can be linked to Levinas' postulate (saying – *le dire*) of responsibility. The latter implies an exposure to an obligation and ethic of care for which no one can replace the unique "me", thus, the poignant notion of "I-am-unique" (subjectivity).

Further outline of research project and demarcation of research objectives

Immediately, the link with Emmanuel Levinas' thinking, challenges the authors with the difficult task to interpret and understand his approach (De Boer 1976:7). It is about an endeavour to give voice to Levinas' phenomenological description and hermeneutics of lived experience in this world. The link with Levinas is therefore not about merely a re-interpretation. It is about probing into the meaning of the face-to-face encounter with the disturbing other; it wants to reflect on the intersubjective relation at its precognitive core; viz., being called by another and responding to that other.

The second aim of the study is to interpret and to reinterpret Nagy's theory pertaining the ethical dimension in relational dynamics. Via Levinas' emphasis on ethic care, the research wants to detect whether Nagy's thinking has indeed an ethical quality that impacts on our human orientation within contexts.

What is the quality of the ethical discourse within Nagy's theoretical-objectifying discourse?

Undergirding presupposition of study

The undergirding presupposition is that the ethical components in Nagy's theory formation, point in the direction of a kind of crack (Levinas) in our exposure to fate. Ethic care establishes a new beginning. The ethical predisposition is in fact a critical factor that penetrates the natural, social and psychological order of being. This presupposition is more or less in line with previous research done by the authors themselves (Meulink-Korf & Van Rhijn 1990:145).

The research is not focused on methodological issues and technicalities concerning the character of contextual therapy. *The focus is much more on the anthropological basis of Nagy's approach, than on methodology and techniques for psychotherapy*. The latter cannot be ignored. However, to derive from Nagy's theoretical reflection and clinical work one specific method, will be too difficult. More fundamental is to probe into the paradigms that infer interaction and engagements with clients (Hutschemaeckers 1996:14-27).

Furthermore, the challenge is to re-interpret Nagy, and to subject his thinking to a kind of "over-determination" (Levinas), namely, to indicate how ontological concepts are transferred into ethical categories; from being, into the dimension which gives meaning to "being" (Levinas 1994:351-356). Levinas means with such an "over-determination" a kind of superlative – a double emphasis, namely, when one meaning is perforated so that one can connect this meaning to a deeper layer of meaning, contributing at the same time to in-depth understanding. The transfer is not to a different category, but to a deeper level of significance. The focus then becomes that specific dimension of life that constitutes the meaning of essential and authentic being. The ethical perspective must, thus, be illuminated in order to highlight concepts like entitlement, exoneration, subject and subjectivity/intersubjectivity, accountability and responsibility.

On detecting the ethical perspective

Fundamental in the research project, is to detect the meaning of the ethical perspective in the work of Nagy. What is becoming evident, is that an ethical perspective is not about a genetic factor or kind of *naturalistic fallacy* (See the analytic philosophy of GE Moore.) In philosophical ethics, the term "naturalistic fallacy" refers to the attempt to deal with a normative term (for example "good") and try to define it by referring merely to non-normative descriptions. Moore argues that it would be fallacious to explain the good, reductively in terms of natural properties such as "pleasant" or "desirable" (Moore in De Boer 1976:23).

Nagy and Levinas: Two different paradigms within the quest for a new "grammar" in theory formation for pastoral care

Without any doubt, the discourse with both Nagy and Levinas is complex. The reason for this theoretical complexity is that there exists indeed a tension between the different paradigmatic backgrounds of theoretical reflections, and the theological framework of the researchers. Nagy and Levinas represent different disciplines. Within theology the notion of "God" cannot be extrapolated to the level of objectification as, for example, in religious studies. The presupposition is that faith in God, (God as determinant factor in theological reflection), functions as a kind of pre-subject in all thinking about our being human, as well as in the quest for humane meaning and identity in everyday life (worldly relationships).

It is important to channel the hermeneutics of intersubjectivity, as well as the encounter with the other, into theoretical reflections that will be applicable to the profession of healing, helping and caregiving. The intention is to make an interdisciplinary discourse relevant for both caregivers as well as researchers operating from different paradigmatic backgrounds of reflection. This is the reason why the interaction with Nagy is paramount. It also provides pastoral care with a new grammar and language. This will be reflected in the argumentation throughout this book.

The reading of Nagy through the lens of Levinas, brings one into contact with philosophical resources. Levinas will help the reader to reflect on empirical data, and the contribution of the human sciences to the praxis of helping and healing. Thus, the reason why the discipline of practical theology can gain exciting new perspective in the formulating of theory for ministry and the relational dynamics in Christian communities of faith. Congregational studies and pastoral care have a lot to learn from human sciences.

The fact that Nagy does not directly refer to the notion "God", is not a hampering factor in the research project. As therapist his choice is to remain silent because theology is not his specific field of research (see in this regard Buber SeSg:222, 234-235). However, it does not prevent the researchers to keep in mind the dimension of the totally, ultimate Other. God as the ultimate, transcendent Other, is not object of analytical and positivistic reflection. Albeit, the longing for that which surpasses the subject (the transcendent realm and spirituality of faith) is still meaningful when it comes to reflection on theory formation for pastoral care (see the last chapter). The space of being present within the presence of God (the transcendent Other; the visage/countenance in the event of facing the Other) refers to the category of communion (fellowship) with the divine factor in life. That is very specifically the case in the Old Testament. Visiting (exploring) this spiritual space in the research on pastoral care, is important in order to determine the contribution of pastoral care to the profession of helping and healing.

CHAPTER 1

The choice for a pastoral and theological approach, defines the basic paradigm for doing care. The *proprium* of pastoral theology is not merely about connecting life stories to the biblical narrative. The disciplinary challenge is to connect caregiving to a passionate understanding of the meaning of spiritual *presencing*[5], namely what is the impact of facing the Other on the character of helping and healing within the space of human encounters. The core question is not how to speak of God within empirical and therapeutic contexts. The challenge is how to address human vulnerability from the perspective of encountering the frail other; what is the impact of facing the Other, on therapeutic interventions? How is the human realm of intersubjectivity, and the social reality of relational networking, addressed and articulated when one applies categories from Nagy's thinking? The latter will be discussed and re-interpreted with the help of Levinas' thinking on the character of ethic care.

Chapter II will focus on an explanation of Nagy's approach. The notions of "context" and "ethical dimension" in intersubjective interactions, need to be investigated further. That will be done by means of a discourse with Martin Buber's I-Thou philosophy (Chapter III). Nagy's publications *Between Give and Take* (1986, with Barbara Krasner) and *Foundations of Contextual Therapy* (1987) will play a fundamental role in this chapter. Levinas' criticism of Buber will be most helpful indeed.

Chapter IV is about a systematic exposition of Levinas' philosophy regarding the human subject and the notion of subjectivity. Important is his assumption that appropriate change starts in the first place with the subject and not with the dynamics of relationships. Change occurs when the subject starts to act differently. In this respect, the importance of ethics comes into play. The undergirding assumption is that Nagy's conceptualisation of subject, and its connecting to the ethical dimension of life, need a thorough investigation in order to get clarity on the connection between ethics and a contextual approach in psychotherapy. A critical interaction and outline of Levinas' phenomenological description of intersubjective responsibility, will further help to understand the philosophical paradigm behind contextual therapy.

Chapter V will be an attempt to apply the data of chapter IV to the concrete context of exoneration. Attention will be given to exoneration as an

---

5   The action or process of summoning up the presence of something; the action of making present.

ethical endeavour; that is, an attempt to move from guilt into the establishment of a new and fresh start in human relationships. Texts wherein Levinas reflects on "forgiveness" (Levinas TO), will be scrutinized thoroughly.

The intriguing question will be addressed, namely whether exoneration emerges from the meta-realm of psychology, or from the authentic dimension (origin) of ethics; ethics as primary ontic structure of being (the subject dimension of being human).

Chapter VI will focus on concluding remarks. An attempt will be launched to identify some basic indicators for further reflection in pastoral caregiving. It will be necessary to take concrete social contexts into consideration, reckoning simultaneously with the peculiar phenomenon of interactive "disturbing human encounters" within alarming happenstances of life.

References to case studies in the text will be dealt with confidentiality so that data cannot disclose the identity of clients. Some of the case studies will refer to settings of helping wherein supervisors and pastoral counsellors played a role. Others will be derived from contact sessions with people skilled in a contextual approach. Although the method of case study analyses is always exposed to the danger of research manipulation (the researcher deals with the information as illustration of what he/she already has in mind with the conclusion and research findings – the hypothesis is then valid in terms of what the researcher already assumed), the intention of the researchers is not to fall prey to such a "scientific trap". What the project has in mind is to use the unique information of case studies to critically assess the validity of a theory. In this study, the validity of contextuality for the practice of human encounters, needs to be assessed critically. The research data should help the researchers to re-interpret an existing theory and not merely to justify already formulated assumptions (Goud 1992a:174).

The project is about a literature research as well. Therefore, references to poetry and novels. The latter are to be viewed as valid sources for research regarding the meaning of human relationships.

Without any doubt, the method of exegesis will play an important role when biblical texts will be scrutinised and subjected to the hermeneutics of interpretation. The data from exegesis will function like spotlights on a stage. Spotlights emerge from a non-horizontal perspective and create interesting contrasts on the stage; that is, the contrast and interplay between light and shadow. One then enters the space of creative silence. An audible silence that sets the decor for words and talking. One can even say that the biblical text functions in critical research like a spotlight, emerging from the meta-realm of spiritual narratives about our being human; it illuminates storytelling within vivid contexts of encounters with the frailty of life. In this way, the biblical text opens up a kaleidoscope of interpretations for communion, social encounters, and the meaning of human existence in temporary contexts. The exegetic material does not want to "proof" or "verify" data. It only functions as a kind of meta-text, pointing into the direction of the ultimate; a kind of "signal of transcendence" (deprived from artificial myths) (Levinas in Écriture et Sainteté 1989).

The further assumption is that the biblical text can assist the researchers in their attempt to trace back the meaning of concepts related to the realm of spirituality. Such an approach will be most helpful to get clarity on the basic argumentation and logic throughout the document. These biblical interludes will be integrated in the ground text by means of appropriate headings that contribute to the argumentation and outline of the chapter and topic of research.

CHAPTER 2

Ethical entanglement as paradigm for a foundational contextual therapy: Exposition of Ivan Boszormenyi-Nagy's theory

Nagy's basic point of departure for his reflection on contextual therapy is the following: Our being human is fundamentally shaped and determined by intersubjectivity within the networking dynamics of interacting relationships. Being human implies relationality. This intersubjective networking of relational dynamics involutes as a complex system of ethical interaction. Our human reality is essentially constituted by a web of ethical concerns. Therefore, for Nagy the core challenge is to deal with the consequences of ethical entanglements for psychotherapy. The operationalisation of ethical involution for therapy, directs fundamentally his research on the contextualisation of helping and healing interventions. It determines the goal, as well as the selection criteria for a foundational contextual therapy.

Nagy's approach is eclectic and based on the presupposition that juridical-ethical language provides a paradigmatic background for the operationalisation and hermeneutics of concepts like "familial loyalty", "invisible loyalties", "the impact of the other", "entitlement", "balanced fairness" within the interplay between "give and take", and "contextual therapy".

Nagy's thinking oscillates between different approaches. From Freud, existential philosophy, biochemistry, neo-Freudian theories, systems theories, to Martin Buber's I-Thou model. It is therefore virtually impossible to typify his work. It cannot be captured in one system or structure. His approach reveals a dynamic process of development. Nagy wrote about his approach as follows: "From clinical explanation to conceptual framework" (Nagy & Krasner BGT:33-36).

The development of Nagy's thinking will be discussed in three sections. The sections are about a thematic description and not a chronological outline.

(1) *A biographic sketch.* The intention is to show how his own struggle about coming to terms with ethical challenges, influenced his thinking. In 1987 (F:100) he wrote: "Ethical entanglements of our lives are a key dynamic". The intention is not to use biographical material in order to explain his approach in terms of a causative approach. One cannot reduce his work to a description of basic concepts. Even not from the interpretation of colleagues. "The ethical interest did not come from religion or from one of these philosophers, it came from hard thinking about what works in therapy" (Nagy *Interview* 1995).

(2) *The intrapersonal and interpersonal dynamics of a therapeutic encounter.* The discussion will try to highlight the impact of Ronald Fairbairn and Gregory Bateson on two basic characteristic features in contextual and intersubjective approach.

(3) *The paradigm switch: Nosology.* In the light of the previous mentioned two features, the following question surfaces: Within this intra- and interpersonal dynamics, what exactly is the impact on a human's personal orientation in life? How do human beings respond to the challenges created by these intra- and interpersonal dynamics? What is the basic paradigm for his interpretation of therapy? In order to address these questions, a section of the chapter will deal with concepts like "loyalty" and "righteousness". It will be important to indicate how these concepts impact on anthropology: The understanding of our being human within the dynamics of relationships.

Biographic sketch: An introductory outline

Ivan Boszormenyi-Nagy was born in Budapest (1920). He came from a quite wealthy family and was the youngest in the sibling order. He was brought up in the Roman Catholic tradition. His father was a judge and was instrumental in his upbringing. His father's strict commitment to "fair relating" played a directing role in his search for capturing the essence of therapy (F 1987). He described his mother as a "lady".

On a question regarding the impact of the Roman Catholic Church on his upbringing and development, he responded as follows: "I grew up in an atmosphere of tremendous respect for Christianity, but whether that was influencing my thinking aside from some aesthetics ... yes, my religion was an aesthetic one" (Nagy *Interview* 1995). Later in adolescence, he so to speak "abdicated" from the church. That declares more or less his religious affiliation. His father was an erudite and more interested in the philosophers of the enlightenment than in religion itself. This background played a larger role in Nagy's philosophical development than the religious background of his forefathers and Roman Catholic orthodoxy. In his education he discovered Plato, Socrates and even became interested in the pre-Socratic period.

In 1944 he started his studies in medicine (Budapest). He became exposed to the struggle of psychiatric patients. He was deeply affected by the suffering of these patients, especially the injustice they were often exposed to (Nagy *Interview* 1995). It seemed that most of times it was impossible to help these patients. For Nagy it was unfair: "We should try to help them" (*Interview* 1995). The worse scenario was that psychiatric patients were treated by medical doctors and professionals in helping and healing as "objects of pessimistic ignorance and abandonment" (Nagy *AFTA Newsletter* 1995-1996:32). The tragic fate of these seriously confused patients became a main topic throughout his life. He actually wept about the fact that they receive no compassionate attention. They were released from state hospitals and clinics and, thus, neglected. Eventually they became homeless outsiders of society (*AFTA Newsletter* 1995).

The impact of these neglected people on his thinking, was that it helped him to revisit inappropriate classifications in psychiatry.

Influences during his study period

During his clinical -medical training, Nagy was exposed to the German idealism of inter alia Fichte and Hegel. Even the existential philosophy of Heidegger, Jaspers and Sartre shaped his thinking (Nagy BGT:x). With reference to psycho-dynamic influences, Freud, as well as the psychoanalyst Sándor Ferenczi (1873-1933), played a role (Bettelheim 1956:44). Despite these influences, one should not underestimate important differences. In a letter (1974) to Maurice Friedman, Nagy wrote, "Freud fought against his humanistic personal urges through his scientism, and he abhorred Ferenczi's relational emphasis on therapeutic methods" (Friedman 1992b:170). However, Friedman acknowledged: "Yet we cannot imagine Freud working year after year with people and dealing with them only as objects".

Gradually Freud's model made an appeal on Nagy's thinking. Even Freud's depiction of religion as a kind of illusion. It was especially the psycho-dynamic aspect of psychoanalysis that influenced Nagy. Albeit, Nagy never referred to Freud's Oedipus-concept as such.

The political situation of Hungary (1920-1945)

The political dynamics during Nagy's youth were extremely complex. Hungary was treated as one of the instigators of World War I. There were conflicting struggles between Hungary, the new state of Czechoslovakia, Romania and Burgenland. Hungary even became involved in World War II as ally of Hitler over against the Allied Powers. Eventually, Hitler occupied Hungary and many Hungarian Jews were persecuted and murdered.

Nagy and his brother joined the anti-German resistance movement. Nevertheless, they survived the Nazi regime. Hungary lost its independence and became exposed to the anti-Semitic campaigns of Stalinism.

It was under these complex and painful political conflicts that Nagy had to complete his studies in psychiatry.

After 1945: Nagy's interest in biochemistry

After World War II, it was not so much the relationship between psychology, philosophy and psychiatry that interested Nagy. He became involved in the relevancy of biochemistry for psychiatry. "Since even Freud's genius could not offer sufficient psychological clues about psychosis, […] I turned to biochemical ways of investigation" (F:xiii). In an interview (Nagy *Interview* 1995), he clearly stated that after finishing his psychiatric training, he indulged himself in chemistry and physics at the university, while at the same time being a psychiatrist. Besides Freud, Adler and Jung, he became interested in existential psychology as influenced by Jaspers and Binswanger.

The impact of war on his thinking became evident when Nagy gradually realised that the correlation between human behaviour and physical disorders is in the long run deeply affected by what human beings inflict on one another and on themselves. Due to the complexity of disorders, Nagy was during the time of his training convinced that the natural sciences, specifically biochemistry, can shed more light on healing and helping interventions. "... as more knowledge developed more chances of being helpful also developed; [...] that this may be a place where a little bit of more knowledge could make a lot of difference" (*Interview* 1995).

In 1947 Nagy completed his education as psychiatrist. Although he did not receive training or any supervision in psychoanalysis, he indeed studied the literature (Van Heusden & Van den Eerenbeemt 1992:18).

After his studies he was appointed as assistant professor. During this very difficult time of restoration in Hungary, he was spell bounded by the courage and heroism of cardinal József Mindszenty. This cardinal became an icon of hope and spiritual boldness.

Emigration

In 1948 he fled to the West. He was cared for in an international refugee camp in Salzburg, Austria. He started to work there as a neuropsychiatric physician. Eventually he emigrated to the United States of America in order to continue his studies in biochemistry. At that time, he realised that he has become an emigrant-refugee. Migration will be shaping the whole of his being. Although he never explicitly referred to his existential experiences, one can perhaps toy with the idea that it had directly or indirectly an impact on concepts like "intergenerational loyalty" and "transgenerational solidarity". On becoming a family therapist, he wrote: "I must have wanted to fight the dark forces which captivate us in pathological relationship patterns". He also added: "It is difficult for me to make a comparative evaluation of my [...] family experiences as distinguished from those of other people" (Nagy F:119).

The relationship between generations, especially between father and child, became evident for Nagy as he journeyed through life. "My father will always remain my father, even though he is dead and his burial ground is thousands of miles away. He and I are two consecutive links in a genetic chain with a life span of millions of years" (Nagy & Spark IL:3).

In the eighties, Nagy conveyed in a workshop, how the illness of his mother brought him to the intriguing question whether he should stay in the USA or not. After he received the message of her terminal condition, he became acutely aware of his agony: Should he stay or return to Hungary? Eventually he realised that an answer to his predicament is contextual, because it is determined by very specific human relationships. He decided to visit his dying mother instead of proceeding with classes and lectures. Although his mother was attached to his elderly brother, she conveyed to him that she was very proud of him. Eventually, the existential reality of intergenerational dynamics determined his decision.

Nagy's occupation in the USA: Exploring the biochemical model and further developments

His wish was fulfilled when he started a career as psychiatrist at the *Illinois Neuropsychiatric Institute* in Chicago. It gave him the opportunity to proceed with his research on biochemistry and the impact thereof on neurosis. It is also here that a previous supervisor from Budapest, Prof Kalman Gyarfas, became director of the *Chicago State Hospital*. He was a specialist in relational psychiatry. Gyarfas played a fundamental role in stimulating Nagy to further his research in the interplay between intra- and interpersonal dynamics in psychotherapy, as well as the advantages of such a paradigm for psychiatric patients (Nagy F:xiii; Nagy & Krasner BGT:x).

Despite initial hardships and even disappointments with experimental work, he proceeded with his research in a laboratory. Eventually, he could not find substantial evidence for his hypothesis. Very disappointedly he made the following discovery: "I found that the one statistically consistent enzymatic deviation finding was probably due to the dietary composition of meals in one hospital" (Nagy F:xiii). One needs to reckon that during the time of his research, especially during the forties and fifties, there was little psycho-pharmaceutical medication available for treating psychiatric patients.

Already in Budapest, he started with his research on the identification of a biochemical key towards neurotic behaviour. Even now in Chicago he could not find such a biochemical factor. He remarked: "… that the contemporary tools of enzyme biochemistry were no closer to the understanding of psychosis than previous efforts at neuro-histology had been. Nor did the fascinating development of psychopharmacology in the mid-1950s appear to be capable of producing the answer" (BGT:x). Despite setbacks, he still clung to the hypothesis that there could be a link between personal disorientation and neurosis due to genetic factors, injuries during birth and generational connectedness. He desperately did not give up, because in the background of his mind were the many people who could not be helped by psychotherapy and, thus, suffered due to unfair stigmatisation and isolation. He never gave up on the following assumption: "The question about bodily and environmental causal factors is not an either-or proposition. Instead, the correct question should sound: How much of the determination comes from either two areas?" (F:4).

Despite any immediate support, he proceeded with his research. Perhaps, it could be that Kalman Gyarfas motivated him to carry on with research on the connection between psychic disorientation and relational setbacks. Gradually his emphasis shifted from the search for physical causes that could be treated, to the consequences within the dynamics of inter- and intrapersonal relationships. The question became: How to handle the effect on the relational dynamics and what eventually makes therapy work? The dimension of prevention became paramount (Nagy F:286-330). The focal point became not to prevent the birth of a handicapped person, but on the conditions to prevent the consequences of becoming an eventual source, or even new source, for pathology. His focus became the question how to help patients carrying the burden of entanglement; even, how to distribute their dealing with consequences in a fair way. He became concerned with how to help children not to become victims of their predicaments and the danger of becoming emotionally deprived and exploited. The call and challenge in therapy became: Prevention at all costs.

Proceeding to a new horizon

For Nagy, the USA created new challenges. Many acknowledged psychiatrists, psychologists and anthropologists from Europe settled in the USA. They rendered a new depth and different dimension to research in helping, healing and caring. From a psychoanalytical angle, Wilhelm Reich, Karen Horney, Frieda Fromm-Reichmann, Erich Fromm, Erik Homburger Erikson started with new projects. He became acquainted with representors from Gestalt psychology. He encountered the (work of) founding fathers like: Max Wertheimer, Kurt Koffka, Wolfgang Köhler, Kurt Goldstein, and after World War II: Fritz and Laura Perls, the anthropologist Gregory Bateson, as well as the psychiatrists Viktor Frankl, Bruno Bettelheim, Kalman Gyarfas and many others.

It is so difficult to except one researcher (see Van Galen Last 1975:6). There was actually a whole network of researchers who were interested in Freud's work with neurotic patients. They tried to apply his theories to treatment of patients suffering from psychotic neurosis. They started to explore the possible interconnectedness between the social, cultural context and its impact on the intrapsychic structure of human disorientation. In this regard, the names of Horney, Fromm and Melanie Klein surface. The name of Adler could also be mentioned. He lived for a while in the USA. Gradually the insight developed that human beings are products of the relational networking dynamics within society.

It was Maxwell Jones who came across the notion of a "therapeutic community". Together with Gregory Bateson, researchers started to speak of behaviour as the outcome of adequate or inadequate relational networking and communication. Healing should therefore be linked to what one can call a therapeutic community (Maxwell Jones). The capacity and possibilities of human behaviour and freedom reside eventually in the quality of communication.

In 1957 Nagy moved to Philadelphia. He became part of a team of researchers in psychiatry and psychology. He started to work in the therapeutic department of the *Eastern Pennsylvania Psychiatric Institute* (EPPI), and, together with several others, they referred to their approach as "*intensive family therapy*".

In search of new formulations

The focal point of his research turned more and more in the direction of the connection between depth psychology and the impact of new relationships on human behaviour. In this respect, the research of Martin Buber (the interplay between guilt and guilt feelings within the dynamics of I-Thou) and Ronald Fairbairn (object relational theory) made an impact on Nagy's reflection. The psyche is in essence a relational entity (Nagy F:236, 257, 271). This assumption is not far from Erik Erikson's developmental approach. Human identity develops within paradoxical opposites. For example, within the opposites of basic trust versus mistrust.

Together with other family therapists like Nathan Ackerman, Lyman Wynne, Murray Bowen, Virginia Satir and Carl Whitaker, Nagy's research started to concentrate on parent-patient treatment within contexts (Nagy & Krasner BGT:xi); "… the real hope for progress came from the involvement of close relatives in weekly therapeutic community meetings" (F:xvi). He became convinced of family interaction as a source for healing; "… even the (bizarre), withdrawn patient became a meaningful even vital member of the family"

(Nagy F:xvi). Later on in 1962, he promoted buddy-groups in clinical work with patients (see Foudraine 1971:242). Nevertheless, he always came back to the basics of family therapy.

The role of family members became an important source of change and healing. The emphasis is not any more so much on "the identified patient", the family interaction, the paradigm of the extended family or the impact of societal structures. Core issue became the notion of responsibility and the question: But who will take care of the consequences? The problem in the relationship between therapist, patient and family is formulated as follows: "I propose that interpersonal consequence is the most important aspect of close relating and that is the basis of both relational and therapeutic ethics" (Nagy F:287). The further implication of a relational approach is that a linear-causative approach and attempt to identify and blame the "evil culprit", were proofed to be totally inappropriate, even invalid. The shift was towards the impact of interpersonal dynamics.

The task of a caretaker and helper is not anymore about a "retributive function" that resides under the domain of judgemental judging (Nagy & Spark IL:74). Family therapists are definitely not "agents of the police bureau" (see Berns 1979:242). More and more Nagy resisted any form of exploitation and manipulation by traditional family systems and oppressive powers within the confines of the conservative social establishment. "Rather than monothetically advocating destruction of social structure, we believe that a more mature dialectical view suggests a systematic search for a fair balance between the individual's autonomous rights and his investments in the social system he is part of" (Nagy & Spark IL:380).

Integration of systemic and individual views

For Nagy it became evident that an integration between the insights of psychodynamic psychotherapy (the intrapersonal dynamics) on the one hand, and on the other hand family therapy (a systemic approach focused on interpersonal dynamics), is paramount for a coherent approach to therapy. Relational ethics, a theory of justice and the implication of the ethical dimension for therapy cannot be developed without meaningful integration.

He did not want to alienate himself from a medical-therapeutic model. He maintained the thesis that a correlation exists between mental illness and intracellular metabolism (Nagy F:3-7). A medical-therapeutic approach is still valid. "Only a combined knowledge of the extents of both inherited flexibility of the organism, and of the total influence of its environment, would enable us to predict the actual level of healthy mental functioning in a given individual" (Nagy F:5).

Gradually Nagy's psychiatric unit started to become quite influential. It developed into an important training centre for psychiatry. He established contacts with schools, churches and started with projects in deprived neighbourhoods. "This enabled the project to become one of the first known family therapy programs" (Nagy & Spark BGT:xi). The impetus for his model has become the societal background of ripped-off, overburdened, abandoned nuclear families. "We submit that the family is trying to exist in the vacuum that was left when the connection between visible relationships and intergenerational rootedness broke down and the ethical implications of that connection were lost" (Nagy & Ulrich 1981:161; see also Giat Roberto 1992:42).

His research extended to "out-patients programs". Attention was also given to projects in the more slum areas of Philadelphia. His findings during this period were published in a handbook on intensive family therapy (1965). He advocated for a more qualified engagement of society and support to families in order to cope with the pressure coming from the "outside" (Nagy & Framo 1965:141).

During 1957-1974, Nagy had also frequent contact with the German psychiatrist and psychotherapist Helm Stierlin. He started to admire German philosophy, and even motivated Stierlin to reflect on the connection between ethics and generations. In 1967 he lectured on invitation in the Netherlands – "… the first active country in family therapy outside the United States" (Nagy & Spark BGT:x).

The focus on generations in family therapy helped him to start reflecting on the dynamics of interculturality and its impact on intergenerational connections. Intergenerational connections are deeply dependent on the notion of "invisible loyalty".

Invisible Loyalties

In 1973 his book *Invisible Loyalties – Reciprocity in Intergenerational Family Therapy* was published by Harper & Row in New York. It can be rendered as his first major publication. Instead of "intensive family therapy", the term "intergenerational family therapy" was used.

He wrote the book together with Geraldine Spark. The sub-title could easily leave the impression that the book was merely about "reciprocity in intergenerational family therapy". However, it was also about a design for a relational theory and operational anthropology.

The human I and the other, are connected towards one another by means of a dialectical reciprocity. The human I and the other become, thus, partners in an ongoing dialogue. Immediately one can trace back the influence of Martin Buber's I-Thou. Nagy and Spark translated this "I-Thou dynamics" into an intergenerational interconnectedness with the emphasis on sustainability and loyalty. The interesting fact is that the emphasis is no longer so much on pathology, but more on the impact of loyalty conflicts within the framework of intergenerational dynamics. The infringement of loyalty can even become an obstacle in the attempt to gain freedom and to enjoy life. Without loyalty it is difficult to come to terms not only with family members, but also other people in society.

Conflict between parents, and differences in bringing up children, can lead to what Nagy and Spark call *"split loyalty"*. Children develop symptom behaviour when loyalty is disturbed due to different approaches and demands from parents to their children. Loyalty makes it imperative to search for criteria how to distinguish between justice and injustice within intergenerational relationships and relational conflicts. Especially, in cases where one person in the family system is favoured at the expense of the other. It underlines the fact that loyalty is in fact not merely an emotional issue (an affect). It is in essence an ontic factuality of our existential orientation in the world and relational networking.

The reason why Nagy turned to the notion of loyalty, is to shed more light on interconnectedness in familial relationships. Familial relationships must become a source of support and healing; it should prevent the networking dynamics of becoming rigid systems. Infringements can become obstacles, preventing the development of free choices and suppressing individual freedom. Both the dynamics of a vertical loyalty, as well as a horizontal loyalty, should contribute to constructive intersubjectivity and promote familial communication.

A family is an open and free system within the context of culture and the social environment; "... it can be confirmed that the idea of the isolated or totally independent nuclear family is a myth" (Nagy IL:216). Family is an open system and continuously connected to social and intergenerational issues. In this regard, the connection between a core family and the families of origin, are intertwined. Family presupposes the connection with the extended family, past and future members. This presupposition is important for the establishment of family therapy within the framework of a contextual approach.

Between Give and Take

Nagy's book *Invisible Loyalties* was very well received (Rutter 1992). His second book, *Between Give and Take* (written together with Barbara Krasner)[1], focused on dialogue in contextual therapy. They explored the legitimacy of Buber's relational model for healing of familial interaction and communication. They also referred to the important work of Maurice Friedman – a skilled researcher on Buber's philosophy of reciprocity. In 1992 Friedman dedicated his book *Religion and Psychology* to Hans Trüb (1889-1949 Switzerland), as well as to Nagy and Krasner: "... in whose theory and practice of therapy the meeting between religion and psychology has become real and fruitful" (Friedman 1992b:0).

The title refers to "give" and "take". It seems as if it is possible in human life to maintain a kind of equilibrium between give and take (Meulink-Korf & Van Rhijn 1991:12). However, the interplay between give and take is not about a balance of equilibrium. It is about the ethical dimension and the establishment of justice, thus, the importance of the notion of *entitlement*. It means that a human being is in terms of an existential perspective, endowed to live in a space of grace and justice. When a child is born, it is the human right of that child (the child is entitled to be treated with human dignity) to be brought up in a caring space and safe, trustworthy environment. All the needs of that child should be attended to and be nourished.

Entitlement is also focused on the art of being a parent; that is, the dynamics of parenthood. The child has also a helping and healing role to play. The child is entitled to contribute to the quality of the relationship (*earning of entitlement*). The implication is the application of the notion of familial merit,

---

[1] Dutch translation, Haarlem 1994.

"*merited trust*". The further presupposition is that "merited trust" will enhance the quality of other relationships. It can also contribute to the developing of a sense of confidence, trustworthiness, responsibility and freedom. Merit trust promotes "constructive entitlement". When a child is brought up in an unsafe environment, the implication is that in adulthood the child could have been deprived of entitlement. However, that is not the case. On the contrary, the deprived child becomes even more "entitled".

In *Between Give and Take*, Nagy and Krasner (BGT:416) warn that entitlement can become a kind of indictment and invoice to be settled. The innocent other creates a bill to be attended to – *destructive entitlement*, and, thus, the need of vindication and retribution. The point is, destructive intergenerational repetition of injustice should be prevented. It makes an appeal on sources for support, change and healing.

Nagy finds the source for helping and support in the notion of relationality as embedded in reciprocity and the mutual interplay between give and take. It is about a *balance of fairness*, and not about an artificial equilibrium, or the threat: All or nothing (Nagy & Krasner TGN:122). Dialogue implies more than dialectics. Dialogue is embedded in an ethos of "*equitability*", displaying the mutuality of reasonableness and moderation, despite the hampering factor of asymmetric imbalances.

Foundations of Contextual Therapy

After the publication of *Between Give and Take*, a selection of important articles was published with the title: *Foundations of Contextual Therapy* (1987, 337 pages). The selection was done together with Catherine Ducommun. Nagy rendered this publication as fundamental for the understanding of his theory on intergenerational dynamics. The last three articles explain a central topic in his contextual therapy, namely "*transgenerational solidarity*".

The reason why this publication is fundamental for the understanding of "contextual therapy", resides in the fact that Nagy always wanted to contribute to creating a humane future for coming generations. There must be a future – a kind of *intergenerational futurology* founded on the ethos of *transgenerational solidarity* (Once called by Nagy a mode of *indirect theology*; see Nagy F:292-318). At stake, in intergenerational dynamics, is the inevitable presence of an "*invisible third party*". This third party creates a kind of transgenerational tribunal. It refers to people coming after the present "we", and the connection to their children. This present "we-and-their-children" deposits a heritage that eventually will determine the humane space of coming generations. The concern for the invisible third party has, inter alia, in mind environmental problems and the position of marginalised groups in society, deprived from their basic human rights[2]. Without any doubt, social injustice will have an impact on future generations.

Nagy's thinking is about pioneering an uncharted context. In this regard, his friend Stierlin referred in an introduction to his collected papers (F 1987), to the impact of Nagy's very challenging theories: "… the very fact that Ivan Boszormenyi-Nagy so often shows himself to be ahead of his times or is setting himself apart from the mainstream cannot but make him a controversial figure" (F:ix). The focus on the rights of minorities, and oppressed groups in the twentieth century, was not always welcomed and embraced in international and political circles. Stierlin referred to the position of Hungary at that time in Europe. "Within the European community of nations, Hungary represents a prototypical small nation culture. It could only survive by, on the one hand, opening up to diverse cultural influences, while, on the other, asserting and preserving its own unique features. This seemed possible only on the basis of a strong group loyalty and cultural vitality. Here I see one of the sources of Ivan Boszormenyi's *lifelong concern with the underdog* […], the interests of […] *those who have no voice*" (Nagy F:vii; see also *Interview* VR/MK 1995).

When Nagy was asked about his concern for the underdog and attempt to voice the voiceless, Nagy actually rejected this kind of formulation as sheer ridicule: "… it is power language". He responded as follows: "The issue is that it is unfair that we cannot help them. Once they have no voice there is a powerful relation in mind. […] You may have a voice and still be treated unfairly. It is not the same thing (*Interview* 1995).

In a nutshell: To capture the dynamics of Nagy's contextual therapy is a complex endeavour. His legacy can be summarised in the following statement: "… to help free posterity from crippling habits, traditions and delegations of previous generations" (Nagy & Krasner BGT:418).

---

[2] See the position of minority groups in the Netherlands, and the current migration crisis all over the globe.

Nagy's professional decor: Two important partners in the discourse on family therapy (Fairbairn and Bateson)

Introduction

The previous outline was an attempt to understand Nagy's theory against the personal and biographical data of his migrating journey from Hungary to the USA, and the impact thereof on establishing his professional career as intergenerational family therapist. The next paragraph is about a description of the professional décor for the development of Nagy as psychotherapist and family therapist. It is about the development of his model of "relational reality", concerning the intraspsychic (second dimension) and the notion of the interaction between people (the third dimension of intersubjectivity). The fourth dimension deals with the notion of relational ethics.

With reference to the dimension of relationality, one important partner in the discourse on intergenerational dynamics, is Martin Buber. Nagy and Krasner remarked: "His (Fairbairn) psychological view of individual depth dynamics seems to be analogous to and compatible with Buber's existential-ethical view of dialogue as the foundation of human being and becoming. Both perspectives can help therapists better understand the *relativistic basis* of the human mind as well as of human relatedness. The parallel between the two frameworks served as an early foundation for contextual therapy" (BGT 1986:26)[3].

Passion for the other: Ronald Fairbairn

It was the British psychoanalyst Ronald Fairbairn (1889-1964) who laid the foundation for further reflection on family and relational therapy. In this regard, the impact on Nagy's intergenerational and contextual therapy needs thorough attention.

Fairbairn's publication in 1952 (*Psychoanalytic Studies of the Personality*) posed the thesis that the human urge (passion, drift) is not displayed in a desolate and vacant space. The human existential drift is not merely a blunt instinct. It is primarily an existential feature directed towards the other. With

---

3 In chapter III attention will be given to the fourth dimension: relational ethics. In this section the focus is on psychotherapy and its connection with family therapy. Thus, the rationale for Ronald Fairbairn's and Gregory Bateson's scientific approaches. In the professional discourse on psychotherapy, the thinking of Fairbairn is often more prominent than Bateson's model.

passion and drift are not meant merely psychic energy. Drift is an indication of the interconnectedness between form and content within the dynamics of the human self. In this regard, the article of Fairbairn (1952) on the movement from instinct to self, is scientifically speaking quite remarkable.

More and more the notion of the psychic presentation of the other as object of drift and passionate projection, gained momentum in analytical theories. In this respect, the name of Sándor Ferenczi and Melanie Klein should be mentioned. But it is Fairbairn and his colleague Harry Guntrip, that contributed to the conventionalisation of object-relational theories. Very specifically, its impact on theory formation for analytical reflection and the inner-directedness of the human self on the other. It was Fairbairn who initiated the formulation of an object-relational based personality theory, and, thus, contributed to the establishment of the so called "British School"[4].

In the classic analytical approach, the emphasis in psychological research was most of times the intrapsychic structures of the human self. The dynamics of the intrapsychic structure was compiled by the three basic dimensions of the human person: Ego (principle of reality); id (lust as connected to pure energy) and super-ego (principle of direction, normativity, conscience and ideals of I-projection). From all of these three, the id was the most powerful. All human action and reflection are primarily determined by "pleasure seeking". In the process of psychic development, direct desires become suppressed and exchanged for others in events of existential orientation.

The super-ego plays an important role in object relational theories. Images of parents are internalised by children in the super-ego. It is here where the child establishes appropriate or inappropriate relationships with the external other – the parents. Intrapsychic healing is then determined by the notion of internal insight or psychic awareness. Insight in own intrapsychic genealogy brings about healing.

The peculiar paradigm of Fairbairn:
Splitting within "internal relating"

With reference to the notion of intrapsychic dynamics, Fairbairn brought about an important paradigm shift. His basic thesis can be captured as follows: "Libido is not primarily pleasure-seeking, but object-seeking" (Fairbairn

---

4 See in this regard, the work of Laura Giat Roberto's *Transgenerational Therapies*, New York 1992.

1992:137). The other as object of human urge and desire, is rendered as an entity, responding to vivid existential desires and phantasies. The thesis is that relational dynamics and processes of interaction are more fundamental than intrapsychic processes. What becomes evident is that the structure of being is intrinsically directed and steered by relational dynamics. In this dynamic, object relations play a primary role. According to Nagy and Krasner (BGT:162): "… an internal self or 'ego' is intrinsically matched with an internal partner or 'object'."

Fairbairn differs from Freud in the sense that the "central ego" and the two auxiliary ego's (the "libidinal ego" and "internal saboteur") are both object-related and different. Besides an "exciting object" that provides positive satisfaction to the "libidinal ego", there is the "resisting object" that is involved in the establishment of pain and anger. The "resisting object" inflicts internal messages to the "internal saboteur".

The difference with earlier and classical models is that relations are not external supplements to our being human. Fairbairn renders relations as intrinsic structures of human orientation. Relational dynamics should therefore play a fundamental role in psychology. In an existential orientation, "ego" and "object" (the other) are mutually interdependent within the dynamics of an internal dialogue between the human I and the internal object. The human spirit and psyche are being shaped by a relational structure. Structure and content cannot be separated. For example, psychological needs become identified in relationship with the other (the parental "care-taker"). Thus, the internal message: I need your warmth! I am cross with you! Needs exist within the context of a relational structure, and not vice versa.

The dynamic between needs (desires, drift) and object is not always clear. It remains a question in Fairbairn's object-relational theory model whether he made a clean break with the drift-structure model. The question is whether the libidinal attitude determines the object-relationship, or vice versa. It is the contention of Greenberg & Mitchell (in Rouppe van der Voort 1991:157) that in Fairbairn's thinking the object-relationship determines the libidinal attitude. However, it remains a question whether it is the other-as-object (of personal needs and desires), or the "external other" that determines the object-relations.

Albeit, in Fairbairn's model individual psychic needs are central, irrespective of the question whether the needs are created by the subject or external factors. The point is: The fundamental need for satisfactory object-relations is essentially important for meaningful actions performed by the subject. However, it cannot be ignored that many pre-school children are exposed to the frustration of unfulfilled needs and experiences. It is evident that the caring-object cannot fulfil all the needs of children. Thus, the reason why Fairbairn (1992:109) emphatically states: Every human being is exposed to a state of ambivalence towards objects in early life. According to Fairbairn, at any rate, some measure of splitting of the ego is invariably present at the deepest mental level. *The basic position of the psyche is invariable a schizoid position* (Fairbairn 1992:8). This schizoid condition brings about an awareness of "splitting".

For example, bad experiences with important others (parents) in early youth become split from the external parent. Within the inner dynamics, the split experience is established as object of the supportive or helping ego. This dynamic is not established on the level of consciousness. Within the subconscious it is stored. The value of splitting is that negative experiences not necessarily contribute to messages of disturbing disorders. Fairbairn refers to cases where children, abused and maltreated by their parents, still feel related to the "bad father" or "threatening mother". The parent who inflicted the maltreatment eventually becomes split. Splitting of bad or inappropriate experiences become controllable due to specifically this inner capacity to split. The split experiences are eventually stored in the inner structure of the saboteur. However, the interesting fact is that the saboteur does not necessarily disturb the libidinal ego fed by previous satisfactorily experiences. Therefore, the realm of internal ambivalences. The fact is, internal ambivalences eventually influence external relationships.

The advantage of *"internal relating"*, is that it provides specific borders in relationships; that is, it can help to provide safety measurements in order to protect vulnerable victims. For example, it can help to protect the abused child from the abusing mother/father. The identified patient (the child as unwanted object; unsatisfying object) is prevented from going back to the identified bad parent. In this respect, Fairbairn refers to the "salvation from bondage to one's internal bad objects" (Fairbairn 1992:156; see also Nagy & Krasner BGT:230).

The appealing aspect of Fairbairn's intra-relational theory is that the subject's inner dynamics affects, even shapes, the concrete other. The other is not a brute substance or thing. The other can respond. Between other and subject and vice versa, change and healing can set in. The healing is about the possibility of fruitful compromises. It is possible to re-evaluate the other in order to become "good enough". One can derive from this mutual inter- and intra-dynamics, that healing is established by means of negotiation, bargaining and fruitful discussions. This approach is quite practical and pragmatic. It links ethical issues with the inter- and intra-dynamics of our being human. The basic principles and paradigms of this relational model can then be applied to therapy within relational contexts and processes of interaction in care for families.

The fact that the other is shaped by intrasubjectivity, causes to a certain extent concern in other models of therapy.[5] Meulink-Korf and Van Rhijn, point out that in this model lurks the real danger that the other could be shaped by the more personal and egocentric investments of the subject so that the other eventually becomes a by-product of narcissistic needs, desires and expectations. On the other hand, one needs to take cognisance of the fact that Fairbairn did not ignore the unique identity of the other. The other has got a separate inner structure, thus, the challenge to incorporate the other as a partner in compromising dialogues. In this mutuality, both the subject and other are in processes of becoming. In the relationship, the personal reality becomes, as it develops in the relationship, what neither of them would have become apart from the relationship (Guntrip 1992:63).

Nagy was quite impressed by the advantages of compromising dialogues and the relational mutuality between subject and the other. "It is exploitative to relate to a person as if he or she were simply an externalization of one's relational partner" (Nagy & Krasner BGT:162). Nagy realised that this relational mutuality should imply ethical implications. "The emergence of an existentially more appropriate relational dialectic had to wait until the theoreticians of the family therapy field came onto the scene to explore and concern themselves with multi-person relational balances and accounts. The consideration of the existential totality of relationships introduces a focus on ethical, rather than psychological issues" (IL:168). Due to continuous observations, Nagy revised the Freudian proposition and saying (motto or adagium): "*Where the id exists* (lust as connected to pure energy), *the*

---

5   See differences between Nagy and John Bowlby (Browning 1990:9). See also the difference between Fairbairn and Klein's drift-structure model and connection with Freud (Rouppe Van der Voort 1991:61).

human I should become", into: *"Where the id exists (the tendency to objectify all non-!), you (the other) should become"* (Van Rhijn and Meulink-Korf in an unpublished paper).

Fairbairn's approach had a bridging function in the discourse on relational dynamics. The bridging function resides in two aspects: It connected the psychoanalytical approach with relational thinking. The second: Nagy started to apply Fairbairn's theory in therapy to people suffering from severe psychotic delusions, and as a result of this practical involvement, Nagy became exposed to the advantages of a systems approach in therapy (Nagy F:xv; Nagy & Krasner BGT:380). Nagy also realised that individual depth-analyses can be merged with the existential ethics of Martin Buber. Furthermore, he started to realise that dialogue is fundamental for appropriate human existence and meaningful development (Nagy & Krasner TGN:42-43).

One can conclude and say that the classic psychiatric approach and psychological paradigms were shifted from an exclusive and often strict biomedical focus on pathology (the person as patient; as object), to the intersubjective model within the mutual exchange of relational dynamics (the person as dialogical entity, as subject).

Gregory Bateson: The interactional and systemic approach – the logic of mindfulness

In the classic model for psychiatric treatment of schizophrenia and psychoses, the presupposition was that these phenomena could be explained by means of a causal approach and the identification of an internal disturbing instigator and reason. The cause should be traced back within the internal personal structure of the so called "identified patient". Something is wrong "in" the person and should be discovered and identified. The implication was that the causative factor was linked with constitutional factuality, deviations in biochemical processes, or within the functions of the brain. Possible causes are also linked to weaknesses in the ego-structure due to inappropriate adjustments to demands coming from the external environment.

An important paradigm shift took place when researchers started to link diagnosis of schizophrenia and psychosis to behavioural adjustment. Behaviour was seen as a mode of communication of a living organism in interaction with other living organisms. Living organisms create together a vivid "eco-system". Communication is therefore in essence about *interaction*.

The interactional dynamic constitutes between living organisms, patterns of behavioural responses. Every particular element within this interactive system contributes to meaning within the systemic pattern of the whole.

If one starts to call the behavioural dynamics of one element a *text*, it becomes possible to call this systemic wholeness and interrelatedness: *Context*. In this sense, context plays an important role, because if confers meaning to the responses of one element within the event of significant communication and mutual interaction.

This paradigm of communication, understood as an interactional "eco-system", has links with the notion of cybernetics (Norbert Wiener). Cybernetics is about the study of communication systems in machines and technology. Applied to the human being, it helped to understand the complex system of communication in the human brain and neuro system of the body. Communication is viewed as a whole living organism of messages, regularities and the deciphering of significant systems. The essential goal of the broad field of cybernetics is to understand and define the functions and processes of systems that have goals, and that participate in circular, causal chains moving from action to sensing, to comparison with desired goals, and again to action. Feedback in relational interaction becomes central in communication models. Due to these new developments, it is now possible to apply this communication model to family therapy.

The family should, thus, be viewed as a vivid, organic system. A living system is characterised by specific patterns of interaction and transactions between sub-systems within the organic whole of processes of relational networking. Within the mutual reciprocity of positive and negative feedback, a directive, steering function (cybernetic function) is established. With a directive, steering function is meant: The mode by which the system regulates, controls and maintains itself. During a long and continual process of "trial" and "error", patterns of interaction and transaction are established. One can call these established patterns of interaction and transaction, the systemic memory of the organic whole.

Applied to the relational dynamics in family systems, it becomes virtually impossible to maintain that behaviour of one individual is the cause of the behaviour of the other. Every member affects all of the others, and vice versa. The system operates circularly.

CHAPTER 2

It was the cultural anthropologist, Gregory Bateson (1904-1980), together with a team in Palo Alto (California), who developed in the early fifties the systems model. The ecology of the human mind is, thus, constituted by a systemic whole of interactional and transactional patterns of communication. A kaleidoscope of sources was researched. However, an important breakthrough in the comprehensive research project of Palo Alto, was the introduction of Bertrand Russell's theory on *logical types*. This theory is about elements within a collection or corpus. This corpus is from a higher, kind of mega-order. It is, thus, imperative to differentiate between the elements that are collected in this corpus. **Y**, the constituting factor in the collection, can never be the same as one of the elements (**x**). One element cannot be simultaneously part of two different collections (classes) of a "logical type".

In a nutshell, Russell's theory on logical types boils down to the fact that the collection (class), cannot be the element itself. Not one element belonging to a specific collection (class), represents the whole of the collection. The reason: Terminology coined to name the class, belongs to a different level of abstraction than terminology used to identify the elements.

In the light of the previous outline, Bateson and his team developed the hypothesis that when, within the field of communication in close modes of human relationships, the discontinuity between collection (class) and elements is not negated or totally absent, a paradoxical situation (with pathological consequences) is established.

In systems theory, one needs to understand that living systems are organically based and organised in terms of the principle of order. This order or structure is not a subdivision or component of the system itself. The order is from a higher level so that the sum total of the parts creates on a meta-level the abstraction of whole. The order determines the meaning of the system without being part of the system itself, or even the consisting components.

The intriguing question now: Who or what guarantees the order so that it is intact and stays a living organic system?

This question is applicable for understanding the dynamics of a culture, a society or family. In situations of transition (the transformation of society, birth, or dying of a family member), this question becomes poignant. Because transitions are about settings of destabilisation. For example, when one member of the system (a sub-system) presents him/herself as guarantee of the order, the chance is great that the exposure to destabilisation becomes an emotional confusion. Because the dominating factor of the system cannot be a component of the system itself. The process of differentiation (the changing factor) cannot be the instigator of the differentiation. Applied to family systems, the implication is that in a situation of destabilisation, the ordering of the system in itself becomes threatened, and is, thus, to be addressed. Anybody that tries to maintain at this stage the old order, or even try to restore it, takes the risk of becoming a victim of the confusion between class and element. The danger is then, that even others can become confused as well. The further implication is, that in a superficial analysis of the situation, the categories that are implemented to define the problematic area in the system, are reduced and narrowed to the possibility of developing polar tensions: Power – inability (powerlessness); top-dog – under-dog; dominance – oppression; pact – coalition; therapist (professional) – client (ignorant).

Initially, Bateson calls the principle that orders the human system, without being part of the system itself, "*ethos*". Later, Bateson revisited this formulation. The concept "ethos" sounds like some-*thing*. "I handled the word as if it were a category of behaviour or a sort of factor which shaped behaviour" (Bateson 1972:82). He started to consider the word "*dimension*" (Bateson 1972:83).

Nagy was not directly aware of this change. He used instead the terms "*loyalty*" and "*justice*" as principles of ordering. Later on, he changed it to "*dimension of relational ethics*".

In 1956 the Palo Alto group of researchers published a ground-breaking article which became well-known: *Towards a Theory of Schizophrenia*. In this article the notion of "*double bind*" was introduced. "*Double binding*" refers to the communication of apparent contradictory messages. This is frequently the case in families with people suffering from schizophrenia. It could also be presented in other families as well.

In order to pinpoint pathology, the Palo Alto group wrote, "Although in formal logic there is an attempt to maintain the discontinuity between a class and its members, we argue that in the psychology of real communications this discontinuity is continually and inevitably breached, and that a priori we must expect a pathology to occur in the human organism when certain formal patterns of the breaching occur in the communication between mother and child. We shall argue that this pathology at its extreme will have symptoms whose formal characteristics would lead the pathology to be classified as a schizophrenia" (Bateson 1972:202-203).

The core problem in "double binding" is the exposure to systemic confusion. The communication system becomes illogical with contradictory messages. The logical confusion eventually becomes a fixed pattern.

For example: Parents with an over concern for their children, often send confusing messages. "Peter, you should like playing outside; it should be nice for you; well, all children naturally like to play outside".

This is an example of "paradoxical instruction". It is closely related to what can be called "logic-mathematical confusion". It represents a kind of "double binding". Something is asserted; the assertion is about the character of the assertion itself (in the mode of an instruction). However, the assertion becomes a combination of messages that exclude one another in a contradicting manner.

Nagy was in the first place not interested in the "logical-mathematical" aspects of the confusion. His focus is much more on the ethical consequences. In fact, every aspect in the communication between parents and their children, every component, has got ethical implications. Interaction is ethically speaking not neutral. More fundamental is the challenge to define relationships in terms of loyalty and justice. From an ethical perspective, the notion of "double binding" is a threatening issue, and, thus, essentially ethical.

Paradoxical messages affect both the parent and the child. Even the position of a child within the complexity of family systems is paradoxical. A child is to a large extent in fact "my child". On the other hand, a child is never the property of a parent. It becomes evident why some caregivers often deliberately start to use paradoxical messages. They call it "anti-paradoxical" messages in order to defuse the paradoxical situation when communication got stuck (*anti-paradoxical intervention*).

The point is: Confusion in the communication system infiltrates the realm of authenticity and trust. Therapists should therefore realise that paradoxical messages do have ethical consequences and should be addressed in therapy. It is therefore imperative to change the communication rules of the social system, specifically, the quality of the interaction in the family system. Thus, the reason why family therapy should be promoted. It is therefore paramount to move from an individualist approach to a systems approach in order to scrutinize the patterns of interaction. In order to operationalise this theory, the following slogan can be applied as motivational directive: *Systemic healing by means of change in the communication dynamics.* Therapists need to probe into the more fundamental dynamics of the system. They should move from the visible to the more meta-level of systems communication. "Superficial interactions among family members, especially if a dyad is considered in isolation, may be gravely misleading" (Nagy & Spark IL:11). Perhaps the reason why Nagy did not display any affinity for "paradoxical intervention" and, thus, opted for an ethical approach. At stake, is the criterion of relational trustworthiness in therapeutic interventions.

The fact that Bateson introduced a holistic approach to family therapy and theory formation, is most helpful. Systems communication implies connecting patterns (Bateson 1980). Patterns follow a logical order. Communication between an organism and its environment is so to speak "mindful". Mindfulness implies logic. The challenge for Nagy is to link mindfulness to ethics.

Nagy: A heuristic search (dogged perseverance) and paradigmatic change – from "sick patient" to collusive resistance in the family

Like a hunting dog (dogged perseverance), Nagy (F:viii) persevered in his attempt to trace down the core factor for disturbances in neurological and relational networking. What causes mental illness?

In his heuristic search, he had to shift from a biochemical model with its assumption that a biological substratum dictates genetically the changes of an organism to survive, to a social-cultural and systemic relational model; from an exclusive pathological model to an ethical approach. An exclusive approach does not suffice; an either-or proposition is inappropriate. (Nagy F:3). The fact is, in order to survive, the organism has to deal with the impact of the social environment. "It can be assumed that each of us presents a certain amount of this potential strength toward our social environment at the beginning of our interpersonal functioning" (Nagy F:4).

Nagy's work with patients suffering from schizophrenia (bizarre symptomatic behaviour) helped him to shift from merely the "sick patient" to a more systemic approach. In fact, the hampering factor points to resistance to change as residing in the context of family relationships. Both patient and family members are involved in a kind of "collusive resistance". Later, Nagy changed resistance into obstacle. "We prefer to use the word "obstacle" to convey relational or collusive resistance to the therapeutic process" (Nagy & Krasner BGT:419).

Nagy concluded that an explanatory model, operating on the basis of the identification of causal factors, can become a nightmare. Causal explanations only induce more guilt. The focus on the "identified patient" only strengthens the option of blame shifting. In the meantime, the family system is a chaotic confusion of different intentions operating on the level of the subsystem.

What became clear is the following: A multi-approach is evident. One needs an integral and holistic model. "We know a great deal about how unconscious motivations operate in deep psychotherapy and psychoanalysis, but except for the Oedipal triadic situation *there is no consistent theory to explain the deeper, subjective psychology of group interaction*" (Nagy F:18; ital VR/MK). Instead of the explanation and classification of neurotic behaviour and "schizophrenic symptoms", psychotherapy needs a new "logos" pertaining being sick and a "patient". For family therapy a new kind of "*nosology*" becomes imperative. "Such a nosology requires terms based on a psychology which transcends concentration on determinants within the individual patient to include an operational consideration of the unconscious, hidden motivations in the other, presumably healthy members of the patient's family, motivations which act as external determinants of the patient's behaviour" (Nagy F:23).

In a very close reading of the previous paragraph, it becomes crystal clear that Nagy embarked on a quite different programme. He introduced a nosology that does not ignore the intrapersonal determinants of being sick. However, his nosology is an attempt to transcend the notion of individual pathology into the paradigm of systems pathology. Nosology is an attempt to coin language that includes in therapy the so-called healthy family members within the level of the sub-system.

Nosology: The paradigm switch from pathology to mindful understanding of interactional obstacles

It seems as if "nosology" is merely another medical term to concentrate on the sick patient. But this is not the case. Nagy wants to move away from a pathological approach. The focus is definitely not on the sick person but on obstacles within the patterns of interaction. Nosology is about a "logos" probing into the deeper level of subsystems wherein the unconscious motives of other family members lurk and should, thus, be articulated; it demarcates the realm of insightful and mindful understanding of fundamental interactional obstacles.

One should view a family as a system. The implication is that the disturbance or sickness is in fact a symptom of disturbances on the deeper level of the systemic interactions between elements in the subsystem. The symptomatic behaviour of the sick person is systemic. The diagnosis should release the patient from blame (identified patient) and move away from a classification approach that tends to reduce the area of obstacles to the pathology of "sick roles"; that is, the attempt to point out the so-called culprit – "identified patient" or "scapegoat". The shift towards the "sick system" is the advantage of a systems-theoretical-oriented therapeutic model.

With this model, Nagy does not intend to minimise the notion of personal accountability and the role of individual, personal behaviour. On the other hand, the intention is not to reduce the patient or family members to objectified systemic factors. A human system is more than the sum total of personal entities. It is right here that the notion of multidirected partiality comes into play. "Transactional patterning remains a formal and shallow therapeutic framework if it fails to allow for the simultaneous coexistence of several individuals' rights and motives" (Nagy & Krasner BGT:32).

At this stage the critical question should be posed: Does a nosology exclude personal elements of responsibility, guilt and conscience?

In being sick, several issues are at stake. For example, in suffering and the human quest for meaning, human rights and the subtle dimension of motivation play a role indeed. The idea is not that nosology wants to reduce conditions of sickness to merely the realm of systemic disturbances. Nosology is rather the attempt to probe deeper into the dynamic patterns of interaction in order to contribute to a holistic approach. In theory formation one should reckon with the fact that nosology is a scientific mode of dealing with the humane dimension of our being human within the dynamics of inter-relationality; a "*noso*-logos" is an aspect of "*anthropo*-logos".

For Nagy as clinician and therapist, the emphasis is on an *operational anthropology* that supports him to understand and to deal with what is indeed at stake when a person suffers on a psychic level within the interconnectedness of close relationships. An operational anthropology enables Nagy to prevent inhumane, inappropriate and unnecessary suffering. In a nutshell, it can alleviate acute distress in suffering.

In conclusion: The following could be viewed as core directives in a hermeneutical approach and the attempt to interpret and understand Nagy's thinking;

- Nagy did not use the term "operational anthropology". He did not want to design a comprehensive systematic anthropology. He often maintained: "I am a therapist; I'm not a philosopher". His intention is to make therapy work within the existential and relational dynamics of life. In terms of his insight regarding the dynamics of intersubjectivity, he only wanted to be a responsible and effective psychotherapist. Anthropology is a pragmatic issue and not an abstract theory; it should enhance the quality of life and alleviate the suffering of human beings.
- The use of the concept "psychic" is to differentiate human suffering from the more general concept of somatic suffering. It indicates that suffering is for Nagy an existential and personal predicament within the dynamics of systemic interaction: Suffering is not general and abstract, it is concrete, particular and personal.
- Not all forms of suffering are necessary and legitimate. Some forms of suffering are improper, inappropriate and even unnecessary. Whether that is the case cannot be argued in abstract theoretical reflection. It is the patient as subject who has to decide whether the suffering is inauthentic or not. However, there is one form of suffering that is inauthentic; i. e. when the subject is reduced to a merely mechanistic object of his/her suffering (merely a medical or psychiatric case). When one is not deprived of the opportunity to say: "It is I who suffer; I am the subject of my suffering", a subtle form of human dignity is still in place. However, when one is reduced to a helpless, poor object (as in many cases of severe depression), suffering is becoming inauthentic and a subtle form of inhumane violation[6].

---

6   Paul's understanding of suffering as a kind of sorrow and grief according to God's intervention (*kata theon*), should not be interpreted as a kind of mechanistic objectification but as a subjective challenge, namely as a deliberate decision to take on suffering as a "spiritual task", especially in cases where it concerns injustice and the discriminating suffering of the other. Healing in this case is not a psychotherapeutic venture but a spiritual and pastoral endeavour.

- The society should become aware of its responsibility to prevent unnecessary forms of suffering. The society and immediate community should provide appropriate structures and modes of supportive helping and appropriate healing. "It can be predicted that the "therapy" of the family can succeed only if society does not place an insurmountable demand upon family life and parental role" (Nagy & Framo 1965:141).

Towards an "operational anthropology": Probing into human well-being

The unarticulated motivation for Nagy in his search for an appropriate theory for helping, caring and healing, is the quest for an anthropology that deals with the core or key elements for promoting the quality of our being human (Nagy in an interview; Van der Pas 1982:29-34).

The notion of an "operational anthropology", is about the challenge how to apply the concepts "loyalty" and "justice" to a relational and ethical model for contextual therapy. To meet the challenge, fundamental questions regarding the foundational structures of our being human (foundational structures for a psychotherapeutic anthropology) should be addressed. Within the interplay between dialectics and dialogue, Nagy's relational theory deals with a kaleidoscope of concepts and anthropological dimensions, all scattered throughout many of his writings in an unsystematised manner.

Very early in his career, in training sessions for family therapists (Leidse Cursus 1967:39), he referred to the notion: *unit of meaning*. He understood under *unit of meaning*, a pre-conceptual and unarticulated structuring of relationships within the interaction between people. This *unit of meaning*[7] includes motivation (the conative dimension), affection (emotional dimension) and rational capacities (cognitive dimension). These dimensions are displayed within the systemic dynamics of dialogue; a dialogue that takes subjectivity seriously and tries to focus continuously on the particularity of the individual as well.

---

7   In later publications, Nagy did not come back to the notion: "unit of meaning". Initially, this notion refers to Nagy's attempt to deal with relationality as a systemic entity. It should not be interpreted exclusively as an intrapsychic component of our being human.

Since Nagy never wrote systematically about an anthropology for contextual psychotherapy, one has to deal with dispersed perspectives as developed in some of Nagy's most basic publications. One must deal with different concepts and try to detect their meaning within relational interaction. This will be the challenge in an anthropological approach determined predominantly by an ethical paradigm. This paradigm revolves around the following basic concepts: "loyalty" and "justice".

An operational anthropology consists of the following dynamic relational components that together create a humane and dialogical space for caring encounters:

- *Invisible loyalty.* Loyalty as an ethical concern, is most of times invisible and indirectly implied in some dialectic dynamics. In *Hospital Organization and Family-Oriented Psychotherapy of Schizophrenia* (Nagy F:9), Nagy posed the thesis: Loyalty is the key factor in the attempt to understand psychotic and schizophrenic behaviour. The notion of "invisible loyalty" helped him to trace back a meaningful and significant factor in the apparent meaningless behaviour of patients. Loyalty is also applicable to the dynamics of individual psychological behaviour. It even serves as coherence factor in the systemic dynamics of social interaction (Nagy F:xix).

  Other concepts, related to loyalty, are: "obligation", "indebtedness" and "split loyalty".

- *Justice within the interaction of social dynamics (social justice).* The emphasis on ethics in anthropology, deals inter alia with the dialectic interplay between "balance and imbalance" in relationships. This interplay articulates the complexity of justice as key factor in our being human. Other concepts that play a fundamental role are: Guilt and obligation; ledger; merited trust; entitlement; reciprocity; revolving slate; the third other; retributive and distributive justice.

- *The paradigm shift:* From dialectics to dialogue (The dialectic theory of relationships). According to Nagy (Nagy & Spark IL:19), "… the dialectical approach defines the individual as partner to a dialogue, that is, in a dynamic exchange with his counterpart: the other or non-self." In this context, the interplay between dialectics and dialogue comes into play again. Other concepts that demarcate the realm of dialogue, are: Mutuality, individuation and separation, self-limitation and self-validation, parentification, and destructive idealising.

All of these concepts together contribute to a more comprehensive understanding of the existential entanglement of human lives. Due to the emphasis on the fundamental role of "justice" and "loyalty", it helps to shed light on the total human situation, framed by ethical confines.

Loyalty: The quest for an ethical approach to existential entanglements within human encounters

The fact that Nagy and Geraldine Spark used the concept of "invisible loyalty" for their joint publication, is already an indication that loyalty is a key concept in their design for an ethical approach to contextual therapy and humane encounters in the concrete settings of life. With humane encounters are meant relational interaction and dialogue determined by loyalty; humane encounters are qualified by loyal encounters.

With loyalty is not merely meant a noble attitude and personal virtue. It is a comprehensive concept, depicting many aspects of relational dialoguing. It is complex and consists of many layers of meaning according to the character of that specific relationship within concrete social settings. The paradigmatic background and social context determine how it is applied in theory formation. "It can have many meanings, ranging from individual psychological sense of loyalty to national and societal codes of civic allegiance" (Nagy & Spark IL:37). It is, therefore, important to translate the original juridical meaning of loyalty into terminology appropriate for the design of a relational theory within the dynamics of social ethics. Loyalty implies indeed more than merely a passion for loyalty (loyalty as an affect).

For the re-interpretation of loyalty, the meaning of the concept should be sought on the level of existential motivation and behavioural orientation. One should therefore probe into the multi-personal dynamics of systemic, interactional exchange. It is exactly on this level that many different driving forces come into play. There are, for example, a cluster of motivational factors operating on the level of individual impellent powers. To understand their role in the conative dimension of our being human, developmental theories in psychology are quite insightful.

CHAPTER 2

A second cluster of motivation refers to multi-personal driving forces. In this regard, theories in communication and systems models of interaction, are most helpful in order to understand the complexity of relational contexts.

Due to an arsenal of systems theories regarding communication in therapy, it becomes imperative to detect their value for a therapeutic approach. Within the kaleidoscope of many theories for family therapy, it becomes paramount for a multi-team and holistic approach to helping, healing and caring. A kind of synthesis could be most helpful for an integrative approach to helping and healing.

"One of the least constructive points of view in current writings about the family approach is the assumption of an either-or, mutually exclusive relationship between individual personality dynamics and multi-person relational or system dynamics. […] My own outlook has been dominated by a search for a creative synthesis of mutually complementary and antithetical factors in evaluation of the *total human situation*" (Nagy F:103-104; ital VR/MK). At stake, is the attempt to bring about an "integration and flexible expansion of our knowledge of *the human condition*" (Nagy F:101; ital VR/MK).

Part and parcel of an integral approach is the challenge how to establish constructive communication. Simultaneously, the phenomenon of transfer should be addressed, especially in cases where intersubjective conflict (destructive patterns of constant blaming) interpenetrates the dynamics of the family system (parent-child interaction). Healing is often delayed by unresolved conflict and exposure to unjustified guilt. Eventually, the burden of guilt becomes too much to bear. It can even contribute to attempts of suicide amongst adolescent youth.

Due to his clinical experience, Nagy concluded that any form of therapy should start with the subjective and existential reality of the person and the level of personal accountability. "As our point of view progresses from relatively impersonal formulations of psychic mechanisms to subjective experience and meaning of exchanges among people, we have to consider not only psychological reactions, but also the *ethical and existential entanglement of human lives*" (Nagy F:107; ital VR/MK).

Nagy's heuristic search (*dogged perseverance*) boils down to the following: It is about a clinical journey, starting from relative impersonal formulation of psychic mechanisms (urge for classification and accurate diagnosis), via subjective experience and the meaning of intersubjective reciprocity, to ethical and existential entanglements within concrete, human settings of life. One has to make assessments within "the total human situation", probing into the context of "the human condition". It is only when one is involved in the ethical and existential entanglements of life, that the interactional and psychological reality becomes recognised, illuminated and voiced in an appropriate manner. The challenge is then to discover, together with the concerned person, the inner preconditions that help human beings to live in meaningful patterns of coexistence. One such pattern within the human quest for belongingness, is the interactional dynamics of familial networking.

On recognising the familial reality of intimate belongingness

Familial interconnectedness constitutes a sense of belongingness that is irrevocable, despite exposure to destructive experiences such as enmity and the phenomenon of parental detachment. In one way or another, familial connectedness points to the desire for intimacy; the family system should guarantee security. The intimacy of familial interconnectedness is a given fact in life[8]. It brings about an existential feeling of security (*Heimat*) and could be viewed as an ontic form of trust; a nuclear sense of being-at-home. The latter constitutes a depth-structure of coherence; an invisible sense of irrevocable intimacy and space of belongingness (being a coherent group). And that is exactly what familial relationships are about. This sense of belongingness is stronger than even the affective dimension of hatred and jealousy. It transcends the cognitive idea of a close family and the liberating option of freedom of choice. It creates an archetype of trust (loyalty) and mutual reciprocity, incorporating even the outsider and stranger due to a pact of existential hospitality.

Familial dynamics: "A multi-personal loyalty fabric"

The cornerstone of familial dynamics is loyalty (Nagy & Krasner BGT:15). The concept "loyalty" constitutes a comprehensive framework for recognising the core or nuclear component of familial relationships in differentiation from other group dynamics. In this sense, familial relationships are

---

[8] See in this regard, the novel "*De harde kern*" by Frida Vogels 1992. The core of a nuclear closeness is about a basic sense of trust.

irrevocable, and, thus, cannot be contradicted or even denied. Together with James Framo, Nagy wrote an article with the title: *Hospital Organization and Family-Oriented Psychotherapy of Schizophrenia*. They made the very profound statement: "The notion of loyal support introduces the term, loyalty, into the literature of psychotherapy" (Nagy & Framo in Nagy F:71).

Loyalty describes the essence of family ties. Its basis is not merely feelings (the affective component), romantic associations of attachment, a sensual appeal or blunt attraction. It does not feed on power-impulses and intuitive dependency as in feudal systems. A family is a "multi-personal fabric" wherein more than one person discovers his/her humane tapestry of interconnectedness. It creates a space of intersubjective investment and graceful taking; a mutuality of giving and receiving. "We assume that in order to be a loyal member of a group, one has to comply with the internalized injunctions" (Nagy & Spark IL:37).

Familial loyalty is unique in the sense that it constitutes an ontic basis for existential coherence and sustainable trust.

Loyalty: The meta-dimension in inter-group identification

For Nagy, loyalty is a meta-psychological category. It is dynamic and not static. Its impact on individualisation is that the person receives his/her identification by means of the dynamics of group identification. The family as a unique mode of grouping constitutes a process of group-identification via other persons in the group. Simultaneously, group-identification always implies internalisation. And this internalisation with, and via the other, creates a whole chain of mutual internalisations and web of interrelatedness. In this web, loyalty functions as a coherence factor. "Loyalty as an *individual's* attitude, thus, encompasses identification with the group, genuine object relatedness with other members, trust, reliability, responsibility, dutiful commitment, faithfulness and staunch devotion" (Nagy & Spark IL:42).

The family system is complex. On the one hand, it safeguards continuity. On the other hand, it is constantly exposed to existential events like birth and death that point to discontinuity. Familial loyalty exists within the dialectical tension and contrast of continuity – discontinuity.

Despite possible paradox, loyalty as coherence factor, creates a space for vivid expectations. To be part of a group, implies immediately familial expectations. The expectations of members towards one another postulate requirements in the mode of imperatives and demands. The latter can be called rights. One's position in the group is not without obligations, and therefore requires that every group member should respect and acknowledge the right of the other. Unwritten codes of social regulation and social sanction immediately come into play. These codes are then established over long periods of time and become symbolically embedded in what one can call *the generational story* or *history of familial customs* – traditions or modes of interactive identification. These codes are essentially socially and culturally structured. They will be transferred in a very subtle manner from one generation to another. Most of times, the personal transfer and identification process happen in an indirect and subconscious way.

In conclusion: The aim of "loyalty" is to develop a satisfactory relation-theory that combines and unifies concepts of depth-psychology and developmental psychology within a holistic approach. Loyalty connects all of these theories with the dynamics of multi-personal and intersubjective systemic driving forces. Nagy, thus, understands "loyalty" as essentially a socio-dynamic and psycho-dynamic entity. The advantage of a dynamic understanding of loyalty, is that it contributes to an understanding of the basic constituents of familial interactions; factors that shape a family into a familial unit.

Loyalty sheds light on the irrevocable foundations of our being human within the confines of historic modes of belonging, and frameworks for meaningful existence in this world; "… loyalty is almost synonymous with the essential irrefutability of family ties" (Nagy & Krasner BGT:15). It creates fascinating opportunities for therapeutic self-insight, as well as insight into the dynamics of socialisation; that is, depth relationality as a structuring process in the becoming of families; families as contours for the establishment of human dignity; the family as educational environment for our becoming a humane human being. Thus, the notion of *"multi-personal loyalty fabric"*: A complex network of kinship affinity, unwritten codes, interaccountability, explicit human rights and obligations. Family links human beings to contextual realities in the process of becoming human. Within this network of commitments, loyalty contributes to the establishment of a kind of existential familial foundation; it provides the contours for an ethical approach to a contextual understanding of a psychotherapeutic anthropology.

Ethical entanglements: The interplay between "obligation" and "indebtedness"

"Loyalty" is a descriptive concept. At the same time, it entails more. Due to ethical entanglements, and the connection to the basic existential conditions of our being human within close relationships, loyalty articulates the primary, irrevocable and non-refutable connection for intersubjectivity. It contributes to the creation of a humane space for a meaningful sense of belongingness.

Loyalty as systemic dynamics displays a bipolar tension of "obligation" and "indebtedness". It brings about a concern for rights, debt, merit, reward and attachment. Human beings are then primarily constituted and determined by a complex, networking web of ethical entanglements. This complexity is on the one hand meaningful, but, on the other hand, often painful indeed. We become then involved in ethical intrigues and plots of scheming that eventually lead to severe forms of guilt. The loyalty system depends, thus, on a regulatory input of guilt (Nagy & Spark IL:38). "Naturally, various members have varying degrees of guilt thresholds, and a purely guilt-regulated system is too painful to maintain for long. Whereas the loyalty structuring is determined by the history of the group, the justice of *its* human order, and its myths, as well as each individual's extent of obligation and style of complying, is codetermined by the particular member's emotional set and by his/her *merit-position* in the multi-person system" (Nagy & Spark IL:38; ital VR/MK).

Nagy's postulation of "justice of its human order" is interesting indeed. It seems as if the justice can be derived from the order of the group. However, that is not the case. This mode of justice only refers to the specific code or text of the group as connected to the bipolar interplay between merit and obligation. The justice of the group, thus, reflects and represents the quality of our basic existential concern for human dignity in general.

Loyalty as exemplification of "preferential commitment to a relationship": The group dynamics of choice (different aspects)

Nagy's basic assumption is that loyalty represents a "preferential commitment to a relationship" (BGT:15). This commitment presupposes the making of choices because people always compare and make compromises. Comparison is part of reciprocity within group dynamics. In this regard, loyalty-conflict is intrinsically a feature of familial dynamics. Loyalty is not static and operates interactionally; it, thus, challenges individual assertiveness.

One aspect of the dynamics of choice is the notion of "*invisible loyalty*". "Invisible loyalty" is not in the first place a diagnostic or analytical tool for the hermeneutics of preferential commitments. Its function is to help therapy to become engaged with connecting actions in relationships (*rejunction*) and path the way for recovery of trust and loyalty.

The aspect of invisible loyalty

Loyalty as the ontic fabric of our being in this world is in essence "invisible". The flipside of loyalty is not the absence of loyalty. Loyalty as a feature of human existence within group dynamics and intersubjective communication, operates on a subtler level. Most of times, it is unarticulated and occur in an indirect way. This other, shadow side of loyalty, can be called an invisible display of loyalty. It features like a phantom and feeling of unrest (stirring of consciousness).

Within a veil of ignorance, Hamlet (in Shakespeare's play *Hamlet*) came back without knowing that his father was killed by his mother. The ghost/phantom of his murdered father stirred in Hamlet a sense of "invisible loyalty". It was manifested in his wavering behaviour and eventual decision to take revenge (Cox & Theilgaard 1994:64). Justice must be done so that guilt towards his dead father haunted Hamlet and started to direct history.

"Invisible loyalty" plays a decisive role in the inner conflict of Hamlet regarding the murder of his father, king of Denmark, by his brother and rival Claudius. The phantom reminds Hamlet of the tragedy until Hamlet called out loudly: "Let me not burst in ignorance …" The phantom exposes Hamlet's indecision regarding his invisible loyalty. Visible loyalty compels Hamlet to revenge the murder of his father; invisible loyalty articulates the quest for truth that evokes fear and anxiety. This haunting phantom, together with an acute sense of guilt, became driving forces in Hamlet" search for truth.

The burning question was how does one make a new start without the negation of guilt or just deleting the painful memory?

Hamlet's agony became a symbol of how painful responsibility eventually can become. To take up responsibility in order to guarantee the future of coming generations, can become a courageous expression of loyalty, even towards past generations[9].

The point is, when loyalty is neglected, it becomes a painful inner loss; the loss of an opportunity to act on behalf of the other and to deal with the indebted guilt. This failure enhances the awareness of relational guilt; it contributes to existential shame and the pain of indebted guilt – the lack of merit and loss of freedom. Along the lines of indebted guilt, loyalty starts to operate underground so that by means of indebtedness and shame, the loyal family member becomes even more obliged to the guilt that should be revenged. In this way, "invisible loyalty" can become a destructive obligation that eventually destroys trustworthiness.

In healing and helping the burning question becomes the problematic contention (dispute): To what extent is "invisible loyalty" a generational burden that limits own personal freedom?

The aspect of split loyalty – the abuse and exploitation of loyalty (exclusiveness and destructive after-effect)

Due to different modes and levels of obligation within intersubjective networking, loyalty can become exclusive. Nagy calls this phenomenon "split loyalty". Loyal obligation has a shadow side. Human beings can start to exploit the ethos of loyalty with eventual destructive after-effects.

This threat of exploitation is imminent in parent-child relationships. For example: The mother remarries somebody else, and deliberately tells her son how proud she is of him; he was her support and crutch through difficult times. However, he must now understand that his new stepfather needs more attention. On a deeper, invisible level, the son receives the message that his loyalty is so self-evident that she can now neglect his "merit" and exchange her loyalty to somebody else. This subtle presupposition eventually causes deep pain and sorrow to the child's loyalty which, in fact, was actually exploited by the mother's selfish needs. Exploitation can cause acute forms of jealousy. Eventually the latter can be transferred to other relationships as well.

---

9   For a more detailed explanation about Hamlet as exponent of invisible loyalty, see Aat van Rhijn 1996:21-25. Invisible loyalty can be seen as a mode of responsibility for past generations, but also for new coming generations. It becomes a mode of guarantee for the other; expression of intergenerational bonds.

"Jealousy is the most sensitive indicator of someone's hunger for trust and loyalty" (Nagy & Spark IL:132). Jealousy feeds the dialectics of trust and distrust and is quite typical of Nagy's dialectical reasoning.

Exploitation is a form of psychic wasteful damage. It can even be the cause of destructive triangulation; a mode of an "internalised triangle" that eventually influences other important relationships as well. Nagy uses the term "triangle" (triangulation) that is quite common in many other circles of systems theory. Triangulation means that in the systemic dynamics a new triad is created. Due to damage in the reciprocity between A and B, A turns to a third other (C) as compensation for the loss of trust experienced by A and B. In this way the loyalty of A is transferred to C, and a new pact is established (See Friedman 1985) with C as ally for A, or as mediator between A and B or as "lightning rod".

Nagy views "triangle" as a possible perversion of the triad mother-father-child; even of other triads in upcoming generations. Triangulation, however, is not always destructive and negative and does not necessarily implies pathology. "Not every triangulation, though, is inherently trust-demolishing or lasting in its destructive consequences" (Nagy & Krasner BGT:191).

In Nagy's dialectics of trust and distrust, the phenomenon of comparison plays an important role. The question is then how much one invests in the other and vice versa. The relational ledger constantly checks and controls imbalances. This ledger is based on quantitative calculations of merit and guilt. The factor of comparison in this process of book keeping, is about the question how much commitment one receives. This is much more fundamental in relational dynamics than the amount of commitment already experienced. The reason for this asymmetry, is that fairness in reciprocity is more important than a balanced symmetry.

One can therefore understand why the notion of "split loyalty" plays such a detrimental role in Nagy's theory. A very poignant example is the ministry of clergy. Their absolute loyalty is focused on God. But this loyalty is often maintained at the expense of intimate familial ties. A subtle form of religious exploitation takes place: The loyalty to God is abused and introduced as excuse for neglect of familial responsibilities. "In a strict sense then, God should never have to take the second place behind any loyalty to humans. However, the wife and the children tend to test the clergyman's comparative loyalties as a husband and father" (Nagy & Spark IL:132-133).

This is a perfect example of severe forms of "loyalty conflict" and its impact on familial dynamics. The other example was the already mentioned case of the mother who remarried. Acute forms of loyalty exploitation eventually lead to manifestations of split loyalties in children. The danger in "split loyalty" is that the child always receives the message "I am never good enough"; "I will never succeed to earn the trust of my mother/father"[10]. The further danger is that it contributes to confusion in later years and can even play a role in suicidal attempts.

"Split loyalty" endangers intergenerational trust. Due to "destructive entitlement", the motivation of children to obtain fair and constructive modes of justice, is impaired and could become obstructed. This personal obstruction contributes to distrust. Eventually the latter can curb further constructive development (adulthood). It could even damage the so called third factor in intergenerational relationships: The justice of the human order (Nagy & Krasner TGN:155). When the latter is violated due to a massive distrust in the relational reality, the eventual innocent third factor is grieved and deeply wounded. In fact, it even puts the unknown future about a humane society at risk.

The aspect of future commitments – the interests of coming generations

At stake, in loyalty is the concern for safeguarding a future for upcoming generations. Nagy's clinical experience helped him to understand that due to the ethical implications of dependence, the vertical (intergenerational loyalty) ties are probably stronger and more fundamental than the horizontal dimension (the connection to partners by means of choices and affiliation – like marriage relationships) (Nagy & Spark IL:105).

What became evident is that familial loyalty does not affect merely the existing children, but also a commitment to the next generation. Therefore, decisions in the now, determine the quality of the not yet. Thus, the reason why a choice for abortion can be rendered as a choice for the humane being of offspring. An absolute no to abortion under all conditions is therefore difficult to maintain when one takes into consideration an ethics that is focused on

---

10 See in this regard, the case study on split loyalty by Sigmund Freud. *The case of Dora* – an analysis of hysteria (Freud 1988:19-157).

the quality of life and the implications of choices in the present for the future (Nagy & Krasner TGN:427).

The reason why appropriate therapy in the present should reckon with future consequences, is captured in an article with the title: *Transgenerational Solidarity: The Expanding Context of Therapy and Prevention* (Nagy F:292-318). Transgenerational solidarity is fundamentally substantiated by an ethical concern for future generations, mostly one-sided. Future generations are so vulnerable "… due to its asymmetrical vulnerability to consequences, posterity commands an unconditional, inherent entitlement to consideration" (Nagy F:303). Nagy wanted to underline the fact that the most crucial generational consequences do not even constitute feed-*back*. "Even if they are part of circular transactions, they essentially feed forward" (Nagy F:297).

The aspect of felt loyalty (affinity) towards group identity, place and ideals

Original loyalty encompasses more than merely parents and family members. It can even incorporate a home, a city or cultural sub-group (Nagy & Spark IL:103). He calls the latter a kind of loyal emotion (felt loyalty). For him it is a psychological expression that wants to minimise guilt regarding not expressing original loyalty, fundamental familial and generational attachment. Attachment to land and other related issues are not automatically included in Nagy's understanding of the ethical dimension. But when it is about responsibility for relational justice, a comprehensive approach suffices. Even people from the second and third generation of migrants can still campaign for stately and political acknowledgement of its original national affinities. Loyalty to forefathers and parents has got a kind of backward value. Loyalty to past or future generations can even bring about differences and conflict between parents and their children. For example, the campaigns of Molukkens in the Netherlands, or extensions to historical buildings or holy places (church buildings).

As ethical category, loyalty is not about romantic affiliations. It does not represent emotional sentiments. It is a complex category that scrutinizes interrelational categories critically according to the interplay between justice and contextual healing. The previous outline underlines the fact and importance of relational interaction and its possible contribution to the well-being of a person, a group, a family, intersubjectivity and intergenerational dynamics. Relational justice constitutes a structural framework for interrelational modes of loyalty and trustworthiness. Relations are ethically founded; justice determines social coherence and public health.

Justice and social dynamics: The public framework for community and familial well-being (the invisible becomes visible)

In terms of the argument thus far, it becomes clear that loyalty is the core issue and driving force in the dynamics of intergenerational networking and communication. As motivational factor (conative factor), it operates as driving factor in human endeavours to enhance the quality of systemic and familial interaction. Loyalty is a kind of existential structure and component in the relational structuring of family processes, and the shaping of a humane space for identity formation. Loyalty as systemic driving force is structured by obligations, rights, guilt, merit, reward and trust. Together, these concepts describe the interplay between justice and ethical entanglements. The intention is to promote a systemic force that surpasses personal behaviour and disposition. As a result of this networking web, a systemic memory and data bank are established; a kind of "invisible ledger" containing verbalised stories, as well as unarticulated narratives of the family system. Loyalty operates within a normative framework. Thus, the need for a kind of assessment criterion, framework of reference, memorial script. Nagy call this framework a ledger: A kind of bookkeeping regarding the balance between merit and indebtedness of people interrelated.

Familial memory: "Invisible ledger" for "merited trust"

With "invisible ledger" is meant a kind of familial register with data regarding obligations, commitments to acts of indebtedness. The latter refers to a comprehensive understanding of time; to an integrative understanding of temporality; the interconnectedness of past, present and future events.

The hypothetical ledger functions as kind of bookkeeping of "merit-positions" reflecting the interplay between "merit-trust" and "reward". The bipolarity of merit and trust creates options within the relational obligations of the familial system. These options are even available to human beings, suffering from different forms of accusations due to the impact of a basic exposure to all kinds of *mis*trust.

This ledger (or "balance of fairness") provides opportunities for change and helping, even for further development and processes of identification. One is never excluded from different modes of care for the other; the giving of attention to the other, and the constant acknowledging of the other's human dignity and identity.

Sometimes, Nagy uses the term *"merited trust"* as alternative description for the "fourth dimension" of "relational ethics" (Nagy & Krasner BGT:59, 64-66). In the 1986 publication, "merited trust" is even called "earning constructive entitlement" (Nagy & Krasner BGT:65). All the concepts create together a family memory, in order to compile this imaginal script of a family ledger.

All narratives, written or not, visible or invisible, known or unknown (the family secrets), impact on the quality of loyalty-representations in the familial system, irrespective of the fact whether they were articulated or kept hidden. The narratives are sometimes dramatic or anecdotic in the storytelling-dynamics of the family. The disturbing impact, however, is that, despite their subtle or masked character, they can also represent judgement, even references to failure and damnation.

The whole of our existential being within the networking of familial interaction, is framed by this narrated and symbolic ledger. Even before birth or intended action, we are shaped by this invisible register. "The individual family member's slate, so to speak, is already loaded before he/she begins to act" (Nagy & Spark IL:53). An example used by Nagy in some of his workshops, is the process of name giving and choices for identifying the significance of the unborn baby. The eventual name becomes an association-tag, referring to meaning, significance and familial associations. Naming articulates relational contextuality. It should be viewed as an intergenerational ingredient of commitments and obligations that shape the quality of the human condition. Even if the child is not renamed, just toying with the idea of a name, brings about a whole network of associations. They are sometimes reflecting a subconscious dimension of family memories. In other cases, they are intended and articulate some form of familial connection or association.

The human quest for justice: The core issues of guilt and obligation within the networking dynamics of loyalty

Within intergenerational dynamics, family members have in common with one another: "guilt" and "obligation". These categories are existential features of our being a family. They are not in the first place about emotions (the affective dimension) referring to depth-psychological categories on the level of intrapsychic responses and intrasubjective turmoil. They should also not be restricted to, or neutralised by, "power game terminology", or paradigms emanating from abstract interactional and communication theories.

Guilt and obligation are in fact relational entities connected to the concrete existential human condition. They are determined by justice as driving force within the realm of social dynamics and intersubjective order. At stake, is the fundamental ethical imperative: Accountability for a more dignified, humane livelihood. This ethical imperative gives profile to the vivid existence of an "invisible ledger". It also shapes human life as a hospitable environment in continuous reciprocity with the other; the other as co-partner responsible for the intersubjective order of life. In terms of familial language, it means that intergenerational dynamics and intersubjective orders are structured by a triadic interplay: The relational dynamics of mother-father-child. The intersubjective order constitutes a prototype of this triadic existence, even when the child is with one parent, or with a caretaker, or under foster care. In every dual connection and relationship, there is always a third factor present – others with whom everyone in this dyad is interconnected due to entanglement with the primary triad. All the partners in the commitment are immediately engaged in the interplay "guilt-obligation". Within this dynamic interplay, even families of origin still have an influential impact. Eventually the whole network of intergenerational dynamics and interacting connections contribute to the personal development of every individual.

"In psychodynamic theory, guilt is assumed to result from infringements of taboos that the individual has internalized from his/her elders" (Nagy & Spark IL:55). The problem with psychodynamic theory is that most of times "guilt" and "obligation" are reduced to the level of intrapsychic emotions. However, for Nagy the concept of justice establishes the link with relational realities and an ethics of interactive exchange and reciprocity. In this sense, human beings inherit demands, commitments and connections from the familial system. Everyone in the system inherits obligations concerning the process of upbringing and identity formation.

Education is about an interdependent system of responsibilities and challenges: "... we benefit all of the past and we owe all to the future" (Thans 1991:30). With reference to Nagy's attempt to design an "operational anthropology" (the quest for a new nosology), the presupposition, namely that we all benefit from the past and we should all contribute together to the future, is of huge significance for the design and outline of an intergenerational theory for familial dynamics. Our whole being is intergenerational. Intergenerationality attains hereby an ontic and existential value. Intergenerationality is not about fate, but about structured being. Our being human is embedded in an inevitable generational "before" and "after" me. This ontic and existential givenness, attains furthermore a kind of objectivity; that is, being as shaped by temporality and characterised by responsibility. Our temporality (modes of being in terms of past, present and future) has got an ethical quality and is qualified by "indebtedness towards the past" and "merit towards the future". The terms "guilt" and "obligation" incorporate both "indebtedness", as well as "duty". Intergenerational inclusiveness is very comprehensive; it includes both the forefathers and descendants; together, we owe all to the future.

Gradually the ethical quality of our temporal existence gained more attention in Nagy and Kramer's thinking. "Contextual thinking stresses responsibility for the consequences of actions. The human order of being is seen in terms of transgenerational continuity. [...] Each human order requires that each person contributes to this solidarity. The justice of the human order requires that each human person contributes his/her share to this human order and receives his/her share in returns from it. Thus, an ethical ledger of rights and obligations exists between a person and a human order. *The context of the human order of justice and transgenerational solidarity is a silent partner to intergenerational relationships*" (Nagy & Krasner BGT:98; ital VR/MK).

It should be evident to the reader that this ethical quality of temporality, namely being obliged to the forbearers and being responsible for descendants, is an intrinsic condition within the existential fact of familial contexts. And the latter is always qualified by the ethical determinant of loyalty. The core intergenerational question is then: What is intrinsically right and fair for the maintenance of the humane quality of intersubjectivity?

To conclude: An intergenerational dynamic of temporality is essentially an ethical entity. It is based upon the diachronic venture of future, as well as present and past generations. In this diachronic structure, loyalty becomes a cohesive factor with justice as ethic norm for the establishment of interrelational fairness. Without this guarantee for an ethic of fairness, and a dialogical structure for the establishment of human dignity, our being human becomes a void struggle of nihilistic helplessness and hopelessness (Nagy & Spark IL:43). What is most needed is an ontic realm of meaningful relationships. The latter must be "motivated by mutually interlocking patterns of past and present concern and caring, on the one hand, and of possible exploitation, on the other. [...] The sum of all ontologically dependent mutual dyads within a family constitutes a main source of group loyalty" (Nagy & Spark IL:43). In order to differentiate between family relationships and casual group connections, it is paramount for therapy to at least understand the value of Martin Buber's theory reflections about what he called: The I-Thou dialogue.

The existential paradigm of I-Thou interactions is much more illuminating for contextual therapy than the paradigms of behavioural-interactionalism, or even the language of psychodynamic, individual psychology. Why? Because relational existentialism provides motivational layers for the kindling of hope; a hope that contributes to repairing hurt human justice (Nagy & Spark IL:53). Nagy believes therefore that the concept of "justice of the human order" is a common denominator for individual and societal dynamics (Nagy & Spark IL:54).

"The justice of human order" creates a multi-directional ethic and existential balance, as well as a consciousness of appropriate guilt. Justice is then an ontic form of human relationships (Martin Buber's notion of an intersubjective, interpersonal order of being) and the dynamics of close, familial relationships. Our human order is, thus, from a different order than merely the logic of cognitive reasoning. It is from an ontic order that founds loyalty, guilt and obligation as categories of existential human orientation within the dynamics of an I-Thou dialogue. Guilt and obligation are therefore not merely emotional impulses, but exponents of existential responsibilities.

Human connections cannot be defined by cybernetic thinking. It then becomes shallow and mechanistic without an ontic basis for ethics and a sense of justice. In existential justice, form and content come together. Justice is not about abstract idealism, but about the concrete fairness within the dynamics of human coexistence and intersubjectivity.

One must admit that human relations are not automatically fair. Most of times they tend to be abusive, unfair and unreasonable. They cause a lot of human suffering; suffering as exponents of revenge and retribution. But in the last instance, retribution can also become a form of justice.

Fairness and justice as existential structures for the maintenance of human dignity, contribute to an ethos of accountability and obligation. With reference to familial terminology, an ontic sense of fairness and justice sets the parameters for obligation to the parents: To repay the parents. "Binding obligation" is a contra-pole for the negligence of repayment of (adult) children to parents.

Justice and reciprocity: The realm of between

From a social perspective, justice is a cohesive factor in intersubjectivity. It operates within the reciprocity of contra-revenge. Within social dynamics, reciprocity is a normative principle. "The norm of reciprocity is a concrete and special mechanism involved in the maintenance of any stable system" (Gouldner cited by Nagy & Spark IL:56). The amount of justice for A versus B, is equivalent to the amount of guilt of B versus A. "… as family therapists we want to focus on a multi-person or systemic ledger of justice which resides in the interpersonal fabric of human order or the "realm of the between" (Nagy & Spark IL:56).

The reference to the "realm of the between" is a direct citation from Martin Buber (Buber 1965:277). Reciprocity implies the interplay between give and take (receive); achievement/performance and compensation. For every interpersonal achievement, there should be an interpersonal compensation. That should be the case for intergenerational, as well as family relationships. When justice dictates the quality of reciprocity, there will always be a "social bill" to be paid.

For example: For parents whom it is indeed difficult to receive compensation from their children ("non-receiving parents"), there will always be a ledger of guilt and obligation. Due to this ledger, the development of their children's personalities will be influenced by this ledger. The impact will be different in cases wherein parents cannot give ("non-giving parents"). In the case of "non-receiving parents", a permanent relationship of guilt will be established (in the receiving child). In the case of "non-giving parents", a relationship of the "bottomless pit" is established.; that is, the child is never compensated and rewarded. The child never receives anything. The unpaid bill becomes part and parcel of the ledger.

The revolving slate

In many cases, it is the coming generation that has to settle the inherited bill/account. The bill is always rotating. Eventually, this bill is settled mostly by somebody for whom this bill is not intended. "An innocent third person may be used [...] as a means for balancing the account" (Nagy & Spark IL:66). In intergenerational terminology, the "revolving slate" implies that the children inherit an account about something that was unsettled between the parents and their ancestors. The outstanding guilt of pre-generations becomes now the responsibility of possible "innocent children" (Nagy & Spark IL:65).

Therapy in this respect implies more than merely insight. At stake, is repayment and compensation; "… hope resides for repairing the hurt human justice" (Nagy & Spark IL:53)[11]. Within the dynamics of "rotating slate", justice attains the character of retribution. Justice and fairness are then connected via retribution to the encounter between subjects and past events. Justice has then a distributive aspect in the intergenerational ledger of intersubjective relationships (Nagy & Spark IL:67-73).

Relationships imply differentiation. A relation is about the articulation of difference; the difference between two or more entities. In fact, the difference creates connection and can, thus, be viewed as the instigator of the relational dynamics (Buber 1965:22). These differences establish in a living system/living organism (Bateson), the dynamic and vivid force of the system; that is, the principle of life.

In a systems approach to family therapy, these differences are described in terms of categories of power and dominance (see patriarchalism in extended families). Instead of merely referring to categories of power, differentiation in the human order is much more complex. At its root, it is the justice factor,

---

11 See in this regard, the event of settlement in the in "*Epitaph*" written by Sophie Freud Loewenstein (1981:3-10). Sophie wanted to repay the unsettled bill of her mother. She wanted to be emotionally available for her daughter, so that her daughter does not need to desperately claim it from her (Sophie) – "… the same kind of excessive closeness that injured us both". After settling the inherited bill, Sophie Freud wrote: "I have exorcized my mother's ghost. I no longer need to fear that it will take over my life" (Freud Loewenstein 1981).

as expressed in reciprocity, retribution and distribution, that accentuates difference. "Account and settlement", "guilt" and "obligation" are differential factors; they establish and constitute reciprocal processes of differentiation within different encounters with guilt and the guilty. All the derivatives of "guilt" and "obligation" ("care", "gratitude", "receiving", "merit", "gifts" and "compensation") are based on reciprocity – the binding factor in human interconnectedness.

What eventually is established within the reciprocity of human interconnectedness, should become concretised (making real). Realisation means to measure and to weigh. All the people involved in the dynamics of reciprocity should be measured and weighed in terms of guilt or innocence; they become judges to one another.

But how is this judging reciprocity founded and fairly justified? From which source is it derived?

This judgement and the right to judge should be derived from the third factor in the human order of justice: "Invisible loyalty" as an indication of the level of commitment to fairness.

A good example of this obligation and commitment, is the role of the Judge (fair director in Israel). The function of the Judge was to defend the case of the weak. The weak is not merely a physical defect. It refers primarily to people suffering from "guilt" and "obligation" due to commitments. The commitments create even more guilt and obligation. The burden becomes too much for them. Eventually a situation of unfairnesses develops – unbalanced fairness. Actually, "unfairness" is a variant of violent exploitation. Justice then means that the vulnerable should be protected and not furthermore be exposed to more violent exploitation.

The challenge to therapy is how to expose the injustice that contributed to the perversion of the justice of the human order (realm of injustice of the human order). It should be exposed to all people involved and connected; to the victims, the perpetrators, and to the therapist as well. One should really toy with the idea that in exposure and lucidity (to make "visible"), lurks the potential of healing and of becoming whole. Exposure implies a process by which all people involved, should be screened, making the invisible visible.

But where does one start with this process of revealing the invisible? Exposure and the process of making the unseen visible, of becoming aware of the unconscious factors, start with the other; that is, the differentiated other within the dynamics of reciprocity. The light that helps one to start to reflect, emanates from the other; dialogue is displayed in the interplay between differentiated others. In fact, dialogue starts when somebody starts to talk and verbalise in many different modes. The most profound way of verbalised articulation is what Nagy called: care (commitment to justice).

The interplay: Dialectics – dialogue (respondeo, ergo sum)

The basic thesis for formulating sound theory in helping and healing, could be the following:

(a) The *dialectic approach* of the researcher in psychology (a discourse between two or more people holding different points of view about a subject but wishing to establish the truth through reasoned arguments; solution by means of contradictions as basic point of departure), and:
(b) The *dialogical approach* of the therapist, (articulation/communication and verbalising by means of conversation as basic point of departure). The two are in fact complementary (Trüb 1971:42). The interplay between dialectics and dialoguing are two complementary perspectives in the reciprocity of humane encounters, and *the-one-for-the-other* intergenerational dynamics.

Already on the first pages of Nagy's publication: *Invisible Loyalties* (1973), the notion of dialectics surfaces. He refers to "paradoxical laws" that function like familial dialectics. These laws are shaped by the principle of loyalty and represented in familial dynamics, a framework of interconnected modes of intergenerational loyalty. "The martyr who doesn't let other family members 'work off' their guilt is a far more powerful controlling force than the loud, demanding 'bully'" (Nagy & Spark IL:xii). This is the reason why the significance of human relationships cannot be derived directly from visible behaviour by means of sheer observation. It is disclosed within the complexity of dialectical interaction. In many cases, it is the hurt person or victim, the exploited factor, that (in making an appeal on the other), displays the meaning of significant encounters. "The manifestly rebellious or delinquent child may actually be the most loyal member of a family" (Nagy & Spark IL:xii).

The question at stake is: How can you observe and understand entities that are not directly visible and comprehensible?

"It has long been recognized (Boszormenyi-Nagy 1965a) that the dialectical model of thesis, antithesis, synthesis is eminently suitable for the understanding of relational dynamics" (Nagy & Krasner BGT:33). In an early article (1966), later published in *Foundations of Contextual Therapy* (F:54-78), Nagy referred to his theory as "dialectical relational". "In a Hegelian sense, we use dialectic as a challenge to the one-dimensional limitations of the definitions of phenomenon. In this sense, it can be predicted that life's basic unpredictability will introduce challenges to any equilibrium. The qualitatively new event will upset the whole principle of equilibrium instead of simply tilting its balance from one homeostatic phase to the next" (Nagy & Spark IL:19). Thus, the following proposition: The understanding of the structure of our relational world, demands a dialectical mode of thinking; "… dialectical *rather than absolute or monothetical way of thinking*" (Nagy & Spark IL:18; ital VR/MK).

There is a difference between the autonomous necessity of Hegel's immanent regularity (mechanistic dialectics) and Nagy's much more paradoxical interpretation of dialectics as embedded in a dynamic mode of either-or (Kierkegaard). A paradoxical approach to dialectics opens up options for ethical decision-making and the unpredictable realm of faith. In a new approach to dialectics, opposites are not anymore absolutes (Van Tillo 1989:6). Dialectics is not about a static predetermined historical process (Hegel). It differs from a mechanistic interpretation and positivistic prediction that develop automatically in terms of a fixed structure of thesis-antithesis-synthesis. Dialectics is about powerful competing forces of confirming, and simultaneously, about negating. Thus, the notion of change and development (Van Tillo 1989:6) as significant expressions of the dynamics of social realities.

In this regard, Nagy's presupposition is: "… prevalence of movement over stagnation" (Nagy & Spark IL:19). Change as a category in itself, isolated from relational dynamics, easily falls prey to static thinking, and does not suffice for theory formation and the design for a contextual approach to therapy. Dialectics should be relativised in terms of a relational dialectics and the dynamics of systems theories. In this respect, Nagy was influenced by Helm Stierlin (see Stierlin's publication *Conflict and Reconciliation*. New York 1969). He used the term "dialectics" as indication of the non-mechanistic dynamics that occurs in personal interaction. The mutual interrelational dynamic is between driving force and resistance, developmental forces and counterforces. Within intersubjectivity, there is an ongoing dynamic field of tension; that is, between connectedness – freedom; "committed to" – "autonomy". One can even dare to say: between perpetrator and victim. It is therefore extremely difficult to arrive at a final conclusion or static condition wherein one of the anti-poles is disconnected. Dialectics is about a vital process of interconnectedness. "The dialectical resolution is never a bland, grey compromise between black and white, it is living with live opposites" (Nagy & Spark IL:19).

The point in Nagy's argumentation is that dialectics is not neutral. Therefore, the necessity to introduce the principle of ethics and its connection to "invisible loyalty". This is exactly where Nagy influenced Stierlin, namely, to reckon with the ethical dimension in psychotherapy. Despite the fact that Stierlin acknowledged the strengths of an ethical emphasis, he eventually applied a more mechanistic interpretation of dialectics. Stierlin's approach was too static for the more open process of dialogue that Nagy had in mind. Therefore, Nagy turned to "the I-Thou model" of Martin Buber.

The dynamics of individualisation and separation: An ethical assessment

In a dialectical theory of relationships, it is important to understand that "autonomy" is attained by means of "heteronomy". In Nagy's approach of systems theory, as directed by the paradigm of reciprocity, autonomy comes into play when one's legacy is received as a transgenerational mandate. The appeal for self-realisation comes to us by means of an order, formulated and created by the intergenerational ledger.

The obligation to grow and develop into maturity, is a result of the dynamics of parenthood. The challenge to grow into adulthood could, thus, be viewed as a kind of "repayment" from the side of the developing child. This "developmental repayment" is part of a "revolving slate". To repay the parent, becomes a vital component within the dynamics of an intergenerational triad. The "repayment" is at the same time a reward to the forefathers, as well as to the coming generations. Eventually, the reward is an investment in the future; that is, to safeguard human welfare. In fact, it contributes to the establishment of a future humane society.

The essence of the legacy is the following mandate: to care for the future. In order to perform this mandate, one has to use in the now what already has been achieved and established. The challenge in the mandate is to enhance the advantages of the past. At the same time, its aim is to prevent the repetition of mistakes made in the past (Nagy & Krasner TGN:156; BGT:129-133).

A further implication: The triadic dynamics has got an impact on anthropology. When anthropology is merged with a dialectical approach, the whole process of individualisation is changed. "While the traditional individual point of view thought in terms of monothetical or absolute concepts: instinct, power, control, love, hatred, intelligence, communication, etc., the dialectical approach defines the individual as partner to a dialogue, that is, in a dynamic exchange with his/her counterpart: the other or non-self" (Nagy & Spark IL:19). The individuation of a person must, thus, be viewed in terms of a process of reciprocity and the finding of a "dynamic balance" with symbiotic forces that resist processes of individuation. Therefore, every human being struggles to find his/her own direction within the realm of antithetical paradoxes. "As one self becomes an antithesis to another, a relational dialectic requires implicit and explicit accounting of credits and debits" (Nagy & Krasner BGT:76). Individuation is then connected not only to the centripetal forces (a concern for the needs of the human I in many psychological theories for human development), but also to centrifugal forces and attitudes.

As already mentioned, dialectics is for Nagy not about a monistic paradigm. In a monistic paradigm, both the I and the person of the other, are absorbed within a totality. The comprehensive whole, defines both, and encircles them within a closed system.[12] Dialectics is not about a comprehensive understanding of the I-dynamics so that my conceptualisation absorbs and encapsulates the dynamics of the other. For Nagy, dialectics is about *pluralism*. Even when Nagy refers to polarisation between the selves, it is much more about the psychic and social dynamics of poles within the bipolar tensions of our being human, than about a monistic absorption.

"Genuine autonomy" or "autonomous maturation" display both a sensitivity for the concern of the other, for the individuation of the co-partner, especially in cases of the vulnerable (elderly people) and wounded other (oppressed people) (Nagy & Krasner BGT:77). For Nagy, the complexity

---

12 See Peperzak 1995 in a remark on a text of Levinas 1995:220.

of the dynamics between internal and external components, and how to be related to the other within reciprocity, were always a challenge in therapeutic endeavours. "My reason for such close consideration of certain modes of the relational process originates from the recognition of certain often-overlooked dialectic aspects of social motivation" (Nagy F:96).

Individuation presupposes the option for "relational self-delineation" and of "boundary-formation". This option implies an understanding of relational commitment and its impact on individuation. In 1967, Nagy identified six relational modes that have an impact on processes of individuation and the eventual challenge of separation. It will be described in a sequence from minor forms (modes) of self-delineation to more dynamic forms (modes) of boundary-foundation as connected with relational commitment.

1. The intrasubjective mode of delineation.
2. The mode of internal dialogue with focus on the subject. Both 1 and 2 describe a dyadic structure. The point is: In both of them the determinant factor is still the I of the subject.
3. The mode of intersubjective fusion or merger. It describes an interim mode of delineation which is at the beginning non-dialectic but can lead eventually to pseudo-modes of dialectics (pseudo-dialectics).
4. The mode of becoming an object to, and for the other. The implication is that one becomes isolated from all meaningful ties with people. Despite the tendency of an incomplete phase in the dyadic development, one is still being encapsulated.
5. The mode of being subject within reciprocity. This mode implies that the other becomes an object. One therefore, negates temporarily the predicament of the other, in order to set boundaries for the dynamics of the me-focus. One then ascribes object roles to others. The danger in this other-objectification (in order to discover and maintain oneself) is the phenomenon of scapegoating. The identification of a scapegoat implies that the other, as scapegoat, is now robbed of the opportunity to set him/herself off from the one who is scapegoating, and from establishing his/her own "self-delineation". Scapegoating moulds the other into brute objectivity.
6. The mode of *dialogue*. This last mode is qualitatively different from mode 4 and 5. Dialogue is more comprehensive and cannot be reckoned as the calculated sum total of both 4 and 5. Dialogue in

reciprocity implies that the other is fully acknowledged by me as a unique subject, and even rendered the opportunity to maintain his/her being a subject. Nagy further describes dialogue as in principle a symmetric relationship, established by the subject within the process of self-delineation. This establishment occurs within the reciprocal dynamics wherein the other is also acknowledged as subject. At the same time, the human I (subject), acknowledges the necessity of self-delineation (self-demarcation) as existential option for the other. The act of paying respect to the other, creates an opportunity for the self-delineation of the other. In this reciprocal dynamic act of mutual self-demarcation, resides the qualitative value and unique character of dialogue. It contributes to differentiation from the other modes of self-delineation[13]. "The simultaneous examination of both participants' undesirable subject and object roles may result in the uncovering of specific obstacles to the genuine dialogue" (Nagy F:95). In an in-depth dialogue, it is not about the individual person as an interacting entity. It is essentially about the basic existential conditions for being an individual human being. In this regard, Nagy cites the philosopher Fritz Heinemann: *Respondeo ergo sum* (I am *respond*-able and responsible therefore I am) (in Nagy F:89-97).

One can conclude and say that for Nagy individuality means: "Being a partner in dialogue". Dialogue is basically founded by a "mutuality of commitment" (Nagy & Krasner BGT:415). Commitment refers to both connection and indebtedness. We owe one another trust. In a dynamic exchange with one's counterpart, the other, or non-self, our humanity and self-delineation is established. To be established as subject, presupposes also "trust" and "trustworthiness". Identity is in fact a basic ontic structure and therefore surpasses all the counselling skills of the psychotherapeutic expert. The irreplaceable other, within the mutuality of reciprocity, constitutes a unique self-understanding that contributes to change, healing and hope. Co-subjects constitute one another. In this respect, the researchers want to pose the critical question: To what extent is the unique otherness of the other maintained in separation of the first subject? Or is the other eventually only an extension of the needs

---

13 According to later developments, Nagy incorporates the other modes of self-delineation (intra-psycho-dynamic modes) as vital components of dialogue.

and expectations of the first subject? Can one still speak of a dialogue? Is the other completely and absolutely a unique other, or only a relative and extended other?[14] Within the parent-child interaction, how should one understand the interplay between symmetry and asymmetry?

For Nagy, dialectics is not a neutral entity. Gradually it attains in Nagy's thinking an ethical connotation. An ethic of dialogue and dialectic reciprocity presupposes a basic form of mutual trust, as well as an existential mode of trustworthiness and loyalty. "Ideally, what is being learned and developed in this earliest phase in the relationship between parents and children is a capacity for mutual trust and loyal commitments based on the law of reciprocity and fairness" (Nagy IL:248; Friedman 1992a).

In therapy the paramount question is: How can the basic trust be restored in cases where trustworthiness and loyalty have been violated? Furthermore, this question implies that the therapist has to enter the vulnerable space of human beings (realm of the between) as determined by the quality of dialogue and the level of spontaneity between co-partners. More than therapeutic skills are needed. At stake, is the quality of the dialogue. And dialogue is in Martin Buber's understanding, a meta-psychological event. Even "self-delineation" and "self-validation" is within the interplay and dialectics between self and the other, not an intrapsychic event, but the happenstance of a reciprocal encounter.

Two aspects (phases) of the dialogue are: self-delineation and self-validation. "Self" does not point to an ego-detachment. The "self" is differentiated in the dialectics between self and the other. Self-delineation or self-demarcation refers to the capacity of demarcating my own autonomous self in order to articulate own needs and rights regarding receiving and giving. In this sense, the relational process contributes to self-differentiation.

An advantage in this event of dialogical encounter, is the fact that "self-delineation" is about the enriching capacity of giving and receiving. "Self-delineation" is therefore a major source for healing, offered by the relational process (Nagy & Krasner BGT:421).

A further advantage is that "self-validation" is about the capacity to safeguard relational integrity and human credibility. Integrity and credibility

---

14 This question needs to be answered in the exposition of Levinas' thinking on the meaning of our being human.

reckon with the self-delineation of the other; it is about an existential openness to receive what the other can give in order to invest meaning and enhance significant existence. The power of mutual empowerment is not about the destructive impact of power abuse. Based on justice and loyalty, empowerment is about the advantage of investing in the mutuality of dialogue. In this way, people can "earn" relational credits. Merit is gained while the abuse of power is being reduced.

The intrinsic, relational dynamics within a dialectical context, determines the quality of important dimensions in the therapist-client encounter. The challenge in therapy, is to always approach the client from the perspective of the other (visible/invisible others). Therapy must constantly reckon with all the others related to the client. This perspective is quite relevant for:

- The field of visible and invisible behaviour; unarticulated expectations and needs.
- Temporal dependency, growth in assertiveness and maturity.
- The realm of strength and empowerment within apparent weakness.
- In all these therapeutic situations, the following assumption is applicable: The subjective experience of one's personal identity is meaningful only in a relational, intrinsically dialectical context (Nagy F:79).

This assumption is based on Nagy's **dialectical relational theory**: *It is a theory wherein giving is a mode and form of receiving and receiving is a mode and form of giving; activity is a mode and form of passivity, and passivity is a mode and form of activity. This whole process promotes a kind of dialectics. The only condition is (and this is decisive in order to surpass the threat of dialectics as an autonomous, exclusive process) that the process is not dictated by the totality of a predestined, mechanical outcome (a closed, predictable system in terms of cause-and-effect). A closed, predictable system implies that one can predict from the character of what one has given, the character of what has been received. Thus, the reason why authentic dialogue should always describe an open process that transcends the autonomy of a predestined result. The point is: In the open space of human encounters, and the dynamics of relational reciprocity, nothing happens automatically. In human encounters lurks the surprise of unpredictability. Unpredictability is one of the main characters of authentic dialogue.*

This theory should be applied to hermeneutics of familial interaction. Every stage in the development of a child, is characterised by this dialectic of dependency and striving towards maturity/adulthood (autonomy and independence; responsible freedom; informed decision-making; trustworthy interaction). To hold and to be set free, are ingredients of the educational dynamics and parental, intergenerational responsibility. Stagnation in this dialectical process, can eventually contribute to regression instead of progression. Stagnation can cause emotional obstacles that curb processes of growing into maturity.

In early works, Nagy referred to "pseudo-mutuality" (Wynne in Nagy F:14, 21, 30-31, Nagy & Krasner BGT:54). This is about a counterautonomous super-ego. Murray Bowen describes this phenomenon as "undifferentiated (family) ego-mass" (in Giat Roberto 1992:11).

One can, thus, understand why Nagy refers to "collusive postponement of mourning". The normal process of detachment (mourning as detachment from parental guidance and authority) can become stuck. Eventually, the task to differentiate within reciprocal dynamics, becomes postponed so that the child surrenders his/her autonomy (collusive postponement of mourning and the danger of disloyalty) (Nagy F:35, 49). In such a case, loss of autonomy points more into the direction of the ethical dimension in relationships (relational obstacle), than psychopathology (internal dysfunction). It touches the duality of loyalty – disloyalty.

Decisive for personal growth is the following challenge: How to delve into the foundational ledger of loyalty. The challenge is then how to remove the obstacle in order to promote viable reciprocity (Nagy & Krasner BGT:32). Healing resides in the establishment of authentic reciprocity wherein the rights and needs of the different persons involved, are acknowledged with the expectation that a kind of "need-complementarity" (Nagy F:14) will bring about a "silent, complacent balance" and "dialectical stability". The balance is always in flux, and sensitive for changes within the interplay: individuation – loyalty. Fundamental in this balance, is the notion of "care". With care is then meant: sensitivity to maintain justice; to create an opportunity for the other to take care of his/her "self-delineation, and to receive with grace what the other offers to give.

The innate tendency to care for the other, refers to all parties involved in the reciprocal dynamics – parents, children and caregivers (Nagy & Krasner

BGT:78). Care promotes "constructive entitlement" with the aim to prevent unjustified abuse. For example: The danger in "*parentification*" is that people with authority do not acknowledge the contribution of the children to justice loyalty. This is specifically the case with the pathology of scapegoating and one-sided objectification of the other.

Another form of abuse is the phenomenon of "*destructive idealisation*" (Nagy & Krasner BGT:163). When the demands exceed the capacity of the child, the latter becomes a victim of destructive idealisation. The criteria and rules do not take into consideration the developmental stage. The pressure on "performance loyalty" becomes an unbearable burden with the message: I must be perfect. Due to the danger of "split loyalty", the pressure becomes a stressor, and the sound dynamics between self-limitation and self-validation becomes hampered.

In education, the opposite should be true. In normal parenting, there exists a balanced interplay between "giving" and "receiving"; between validation and repayment. When the ontic need for acknowledgement, validation, and loving care is ignored, the destructive reaction of peevish revenge becomes a subtle mode of reciprocity sabotage.

Loyalty based on longing for receiving justice, and the danger of "reciprocity sabotage" (relational short-circuiting), are imminent in all forms of relational networking, very specifically in inter-group interaction and communication. See for example, the border between "we" and "them" in inter-group dynamics. "We may resent them, but we need them" (Nagy & Spark IL:21). The identity of the "in-group" is therefore indissolubly connected to the border/limitation (differentiation) of the other – the so-called outsider or "out-group". "Even movements which search for universal human goals can flourish only as long as they see themselves in opposition to ignorant, reluctant, or antagonistic outsiders" (Nagy IL:21). In the same way, the rejected other is always present in the act of rejection.

"Reciprocity sabotage" and "relational short-circuiting" bring about stagnation. An example of this is the threat of "intrusive in-laws". They should in fact reinforce family solidarity and shared meaning. However, they can become perceived as the greatest obstacles in the familial quest for peace and "absolute unity". That is especially the case when subject-roles in familial interaction become fixed. The eventual outcome is "*pseudo-dialectics*"; the antithetical dialogue has become a "polarised fusion" (Nagy IL:24).

A sound mode of relational dialectics in theory formation, is for Nagy about the continuous interplay between individuation and systemic interactional networking. "The dialectic of social life revolves around a constant ebb and flow of conflict and resolution of give-and-take, loyalty and disloyalty, love and hatred, etc." (Nagy L:61). The interrelational reality of life is multi-dimensional. Within this multi-dimensional networking, the "ledger of justice" brings about stability, because it deals with the other's need for justice and fairness. "As one self becomes an antithesis to another, a relational dialectic requires implicit and explicit accounting of credits and debits" (Nagy & Krasner BGT:76). In this accounting of credits and debits, there is no external judge present to safeguard fairness. Not even the family therapist can guarantee fairness and justice. The implication is that the quality of the relationship is dependent on the possibility of dialogue between the separated persons, parties or groups. The dialectic dynamics attains in the dialogue a humane face. Dialogue is about a face-to-face reciprocal encounter, and the establishment of justice. It does not mean that all people involved, start to talk about justice and verbalise justice as normative direction. The fundamental question is whether the dialoguing partners represent in word, act and intention, an existential and ontic mode of *"being just"* and *"doing just"* – the enfleshment and exemplification of justice as a mode of being in this world (the how of humane being in human encounters).

Possible consequences for therapy

The core question at stake is: What is the basic task of therapy?

The basic challenge in therapy is to guide a human being how to cope with the "basic nature" of him/herself, and of the other in caring encounters, despite conflicting aspirations that determine the intersubjective structure of systemic reciprocity (Nagy BGT:200). The first step is to try to understand the relational structure of our existential reality, and to realise that underneath the spoken word, lurks a minefield of unspoken and unarticulated human experiences. Under the visible subsists the dynamic of the invisible. Subjectivity is encircled by a multitude of dimensions so that a unilateral approach to therapy will be totally inappropriate. Therefore, most needed is a multi-dimensional approach to the therapeutic hermeneutics of human encounters. A reductive approach will not suffice. On the contrary, therapy urgently needs a more comprehensive understanding of our relational reality and complexity of dialectical dialoguing. In this regard, the oversimplification of traditional psychotherapy will be totally inappropriate.

The problem with traditional theories in psychotherapy is that they overemphasise the technical and instrumental dimension of counselling. The emphasis on counselling skills and communication techniques, does not reckon adequately enough with the fundamental and personal presuppositions of the therapist. It often happens that the questions about the eventual goal, outcome and impact of the counselling process, are not properly discussed and defined (Nagy DB:117). In most cases, therapists do not deal with four very basic dimensions of relational ontology and epistemology, namely: (a) biological and socioeconomic facts and information; (b) intra-psychic processes (needs); (c) the systemic dynamics of transactions, and (d) the impact of relational ethics on the relational context and human individuation (Nagy F:191).

The point in Nagy's argument is that the fundamental principle of relational ethics, and its connection to obliged consideration and merited trust, are overseen. For Nagy, the dimension of relational ethics is the key to healing. Thus, the emphasis on a more synthetic approach in prevention strategies. Prevention is not merely focused on the triggers of the past, but also on the implication for future generations. At stake, in the complexity of human encounters, is the ethical principle of *"fair multi-laterality"*. Such a multi-approach guarantees a trustworthy and fair "democratic" "inter-group", as well as "inter-national" community incentives. Thus, the reason why Nagy always came back to the most fundamental concept for appropriate counselling and familial healing: *transgenerational solidarity*.

The space of counselling, humane relating, therapeutic human encounters and intergenerational change must not be reduced to a mono-approach. The concerns of all people need to be taken into consideration. Even the temporal dimension of time is important. The coming, future generation must be incalculated in the therapeutic dialogue. The future is an indispensable component of personal autonomy and the dynamics of individualisation within the realm of interactive intergenerational dialogue and the framework of ethical assessments. "Our psychological need to be generous may help us choose the option of self-validation by way of earning entitlement" (Nagy BGT:77).

The further implication of multi-dimensionality in dialectical relationality and systemic intergenerational dynamics (the systemic ledger), is the challenge how to deal therapeutically with the inclination and need to be in one way or another dependent (the need for support) of the other ("good" or "bad"). The further challenge is how to deal with projective identification (with "good" or "bad" objects). Due to the principle of heteronomy in the developmental process of intersubjectivity, relational dialoguing and ethical justice, therapy should deal with the multi-dimensionality of dialectic interaction. Relational healing is about guiding human beings into autonomy within the dialectic dynamics of systemic and reciprocal networking.

Individual autonomy is understood as a dialectical process: I am in a process of becoming via the co-presence of the other (Thou) (Martin Buber). Individual autonomy, assertiveness, responsibility and co-caring (Nagy BGT:200) are not about the achievements of merely an individual (individuation), but about dialectical interaction. It is established by means of the interrelational dynamics in systemic reciprocity: The whole is more than the sum total of the parts (particularity of every individual).

Therapy implies more than diagnostics within close relationships. Psychotherapeutic diagnostics and classification reduce healing to the confines of personal achievements and characteristics. Psychotherapy should rather be embedded in an a priori of systemic reciprocity. "The therapist's offer of simultaneous concern for the balance of fairness in relationships is thus a priori and not dependent on diagnostic criteria, the family's awareness of shared problems, or the particularities of feelings and hidden motivations in family members" (Nagy F:163; Buber 1965:31). The therapeutic endeavour is not to trace down all the details of the genealogical tree, but to extend involvement to "multi-directed partiality" and prevent, thus, relational stagnation.

It is not possible for individuals to create their own relational spectrum and control. The latter approach (independent self-control) is more or less the model of the traditional, linear, non-dialectic point of departure. Nagy even goes so far as to call the "age of narcism" a deformed mode of colonial or dogmatic imperialism wherein one society dominates the culture of the other. When "adult freedom" becomes a cover for minimizing (playing down) the asymmetric character of the responsibility of the parent for consequences of the upbringing in the life of the child, then this is blunt narcism according to Nagy and eventually harmful for descendants. Authentic adulthood and parental freedom "… results from a balance between individual spontaneity and accountable caring about the reality of consequences to others, especially to defenceless posterity" (Nagy F:xvii). In terms of Buber I become through my relation to the Thou; as I become, I say Thou (Buber 1965:15, translated by RG Smith).

"I and Thou" is not about the stagnation and fixation of a dualistic polarity (see Hack 1993:26). The endeavour is not to create a synthesis by uprooting the dialectics. The challenge is rather to maintain the dialectics within a systemic reciprocity and creation of a just human order. The latter functions as a kind of "intergenerational eschatology". This order is in terms of the researchers" understanding not synchronically the same as the evident reality, but indeed simultaneously present (diachronically). Due to relational entanglements, "justice of the human order" is about a kind of oppositional criticism of social entanglements and contextual chaos. The "justice of human order" displays an ethical opposition with unruly, even rebellious characteristics (Levinas: "*Le Moi et la Totalité*").

Within the paradigm of a "just human order", one can even speak of a "worldly" or "secular" morality. The latter does not imply that life is encapsulated in the here and now of happenstances; life is not isolated from a transcendent dimension, nor is the present like a flat screen. Networking is about several horizontal layers and open systems, especially an openness to the "invisible other"; the third person or factor that is most of times excluded due to our selfish modes of love. Justice liberates humans from discriminatory exclusiveness and oppressive injustice. In this respect, dialogue constitutes an open space of negotiation that transcends the narrow confines of romantic and idealistic expressions of societal intimacy. The regulations of the ledger, the law (*torah*) of a justice order, surpass neighbourly love (Levinas MG:118-119; Nagy *Interview* 1995). What is most needed, is that all forms of fixed syntheses should be converted into patience (Levinas HAM:32). For this transformation, more than dialectics is needed. It is by means of a person-to-person dialogue that justice is gradually established, so that ethics contributes to "repairing hurt human justice". The latter is what Nagy's legacy is about.

CHAPTER 2

In retrospect: Short concluding remarks on healing and repairing the hurt human justice

One can conclude and say that chapter IV in *"Invisible Loyalties"* (1973), contains the core elements of Nagy and Spark's theory about the ethical dimension of the intergenerational and systemic dynamics. The first pages can even be rendered as their credo for the design and outline of an invisible family ledger of justice within a relational context. It provides the motivational layer in which "… hope resides for repairing the hurt human justice" (Nagy & Spark IL:53).

The following twelve postulates capture the gist of Nagy's basic propositions for relational repairing and healing.

- *Postulate one: Therapy needs a paradigm shift from probing into past causal factors for distorted human behaviour, to the motivational layers for healing and hope.* "However, we have felt that it is more important to explore the motivational layer in which hope resides for repairing the hurt human justice" (Nagy & Spark IL:53).
- *Postulate two: The interplay between the family ledger, relational contextuality and systemic justice constitutes a framework for detecting the ethical quality of the interactional and dialoguing dynamics.* "The invisible family ledger of justice is a relational context, it is the dynamically most significant component of the individual's world, although it is not external to him/her. The essence of this realm is related to *the ethics of relationships and it cannot be mastered by intelligence or shrewdness alone*" (Nagy & Spark IL:53-54).
- *Postulate three: Systemic homeostasis and the structure of reciprocal obligations are determined by entanglements in the invisible realm of relational dynamics.* "Thus, though motivationally we must consider other factors in loyalty – ties of blood, love, ambivalence, common interest, external threats, and so forth – we have been interested in the structure of reciprocal obligations itself. We postulate that deeper, long-range motivations have their own familial, systemic homeostasis […]. The family therapist can be greatly helped in his/her work by the knowledge of the deeper relational determinants of visible behaviour" (Nagy & Spark IL:54). Deeper than visible personal behaviour, there are layers of unarticulated relational networking with ethical implications that shape human identity and processes of individuation.

- *Postulate four: The justice of the human order opts as coherence factor and common denominator for establishing fairness in interpersonal-familial dynamics.* "We believe that the concept of justice of the human order is a common denominator for individual, familial, and social dynamics. [...] Justice can be regarded as a web of invisible fibres for running through the length and width of history of family relationships, holding the system in social equilibrium throughout phases of physical togetherness and separation. Perhaps nothing is as significant in determining relationship between parent and child as the degree of fairness of expected filial gratitude" (Nagy & Spark IL:54).
- *Postulate five: The notion of distorted judgement of social justice points to obstacles in relational healing.* "Individuals who have not learned a sense of justice within their family relationships are likely to have distorted judgement of justice" (Nagy & Spark L:54).
- *Postulate six: Justice functions as a priori in hermeneutics of humane human relationships.* Justice functions as a presupposition, a kind of meta-framework for the understanding and conceptualisation of human relationships within the basic human quest for dignity and rights. Justice features as a kind of Kantian postulate for a meta-ethics, and comprehensive human awareness of trust as an ontological order for the ought of humane being[15] – a kind of just, a priori of being in itself (Buber).
- *Postulate seven: For appropriate language (in order to articulate the invisible layers of authentic human being) an eclectic approach is paramount in theory formation for the different disciplines in the field of healing and helping. In this regard, juridical terminology is most helpful.* The justice of human order concerns every human being; every human being contributes to fairness in this systemic dynamic of life. The key to disclosing the deepest motivational layers of family dynamics (close relationships), is *the language of justice*. To articulate this deeper language, Nagy made use of an eclectic approach probing into the body of knowledge: Psychodynamic and systems theories;

---

15 It is indeed a question whether the order for the essence of being can be in itself, ontologically speaking, ethical. The question is whether ethics is more about a qualitative category indicating "the ought" of humane forms of being?

cultural-anthropological concepts; the continental philosophy, specifically the anthropology of Martin Buber; the judicial science and history of law.

- *Postulate eight: Dialectical relational theory (learning to read the visible and invisible dimensions of interpersonal behaviour backwards and forwards) is decisive for the articulation of hidden/invisible agendas in a hermeneutical approach.* According to Nagy, it is the dialectical relational theory that helps therapists to read the invisible dimension of human behaviour. It functions as a kind of "mirror writing". It even helps to understand the invisible side of interpersonal behaviour. The visible and invisible dimension in human interaction is not merely about an intrapersonal hermeneutic but also about an interpersonal hermeneutic. Who we are in ourselves, is predetermined by who we are in relation to the other. The human mind is structured relationally; the internal dynamics is embedded in a multi-person-system.

- *Postulate nine: "Loyalty" as meta-psychological and meta-systemic category, establishes and promotes clusters of interconnected commitments.* The concept "loyalty" as meta-psychological and meta-systemic category makes it possible to connect the two clusters (the psychodynamic cluster and systemic cluster) with one another. Loyalty as a lived category, exhibited and demonstrated by people living in a "loyalty-bound", creates a mode of living for every human being separately. The reason? Because every human being is born within generational connections. "Guilt" and "obligation" are the indicators of "loyalty-commitment". "Guilt" and "loyalty" are in the first instance determined by the interpersonal dynamics. Out of this dynamic, emanates the intra-personal dynamics. "Guilt" and "loyalty" also shape the whole of our actions, decision-making and behaviour due to the dynamics of interconnectedness (sense of belongingness). They are relational categories and assess all human behaviour within the dynamics of reciprocal commitment to one another. In order to perform a normative function, systemic networking is directed by a code that is supposed to be just, and hopefully, not directed by mischief and injustice.

- *Postulate ten: Stagnation and the threat of becoming a "closed system" harm relational openness and reciprocal dialoguing.* A loyalty system can (due to "guilt", "obligation", "indebtedness" and the correlates of expectations and demands) become (and eventually remain) a closed system. In this sense, a loyalty system can become a source for total, relational stagnation, and brute injustice: material and/or emotional exploitation, victimisation and "scapegoating". The mechanism of "revolving slate" eventually sets in. The principle of "*summum ius summa injuria*" (The highest law the highest injury). It is the intention of Nagy, that the introduction of the concept of "justice of the human order" functions as a normative critique on different modes of our being human and expressions of behaviour. It should help to prevent the system of becoming closed, and in cases of stagnation, its task is to make the system functional and open again. "… we have reviewed some of the reasons for our turning to justice as a suitable conceptual framework for the examination of crucial, guilt-laden obligations and loyalty-binds. A discussion of justice may seem extraneous to a dynamical clinical theory of relationships. Yet, like 'basic trust', justice characterizes the emotional climate of a relationship system" (Nagy & Spark IL:97). Furthermore: "The concept of equity presumes the individual to be in a constant action dialogue, responsibly dealing with the important others around him/her. It stresses the ubiquitous but implicitly quantitative subjective scale which all of us are constantly – if in-consciously – using to determine where we stand in our family's multigenerational obligation hierarchy" (Nagy & Spark IL:96).

- *Postulate eleven: The therapeutic function of loyalty in the establishment of intergenerational "trust" and "trustworthiness" is about: the establishment of obligations in the family pact.* The concept of "justice" makes it possible for the therapist to be engaged in family conflict, especially in educational dynamics concerning the autonomy of the developing child. The challenge is then to convert "loyalty" into "trust" and "trustworthiness". Loyalty is not per se ethical. Justice, however, presupposes dialogue. This dialogue does not take place in an empty space. It is connected to a basic form of loyalty towards a kind of intergenerational pact, constituted by binding laws. Autonomy is therefore, as a relational category, embedded in the dynamics of ethical concerns. It is also dialectically connected to loyalty-obligations stemming from the family of origin. At the same time, individual freedom transcends the limitations of familial loyalty. It is also engaged in relations outside the family of origin. "Trust" and "trustworthiness" are therefore both intra- and interrelationally structured; both are determined by past loyalties, but also open for future generations as well.

- *Postulate twelve: The differentiation between different orders is important in order to repair relational injustice.* For Buber, it was important to differentiate between the ethical order of being (an ontic order of justice), and other orders such as the order of society and the confines of a cultural order (Buber 1962:223). According to the researchers, this is also applicable to the familial order. The intention is not to isolate the "justice of the human order" from other orders. Within all the other orders, there is indeed a longing for justice. There subsists indeed an existential longing to do justice to others. It is about the need that justice should be done to both the sender and the receiver. This longing for justice is often unarticulated and lurks in the subconscious of the human mind, waiting for somebody to be voiced and to be responded to appropriately. Of paramount importance is, that due to the "justice of the human order", relationships should be restored and repaired. "We believe that the major avenue toward interrupting the multigenerational chain of injustices is to repair relationships, not to magnify or deny injury done to particular members" (Nagy & Spark IL:95).

The "justice of the human order" inevitably implies in contextual therapy, restoration, reparation and meaningful, significant, re-orientation. It also implies in professional therapy, the exploration of new avenues to escape from closed circuits, and from the encapsulation of causal thinking (the necessity of cause and effect), as well as from linear reasoning (the outcome is already given in the beginning and becomes unfolded – visible – in predictable events in time).

Nagy in a nutshell: Hope within relational repairing and caring encounters

Chapter II was helpful in order to understand processes of conceptualisation and basic argumentation. It is therefore important to attend to the basic components that contributed to the moulding of Nagy's theory, and his presuppositions regarding contextual therapy and relational anthropology. As already pointed out, one needs to understand how notions like "justice of the human order", "the realm of the between" and "dialogue" shaped his therapeutic skills and professional approach to the practice of care, helping, reparation and healing.

The following perspectives capture the essence of Nagy's thinking:

1. Dialectics helped Nagy to break through polar limitations and the threat of stagnation which lurk in many psychoanalytical approaches and theories by means of the reciprocity in a relational approach. Most of times, the theories became one-sided with merely an intra-focus. Dialectics helped to discover that the human order is determined by many layers of reciprocal interactions. For example, the notion of loyalty is structured by the interplay between "visible loyalty" and "invisible loyalty". Loyalty describes a relational structure wherein dialogue plays a fundamental role. Its role is to establish fairness in caregiving. Especially, in the between of intergenerational dynamics; the intersubjective, educational realm between parents and children; the intimacy of close relationships, spouses and members of the extended family. The dynamics of relationships are not instigated by the bipolar tensions in themselves, but by the ethical dimension of relational reciprocity. The driving force in the dynamics of systems resides in the principle of justice. Justice is the motivational factor; it determines the character and content of social dynamics.

2. In his quest for an "operational anthropology", Nagy applies the categories of Martin Buber, namely "justice" and "the order of being". In terms of Nagy's reformulation: "The justice of the human order" and "the realm of the between" (Buber: "*Zwischen*") (relational dynamics) should be ethically based. The dynamics of intersubjectivity cannot be reduced to merely bipolar reciprocity. It represents an independent realm of interconnectedness (sense of belongingness); a kind of a priori that precedes the bipolar tension. Relationality constitutes being; it is primordial. Intersubjectivity is the ultimate mode of objectivity within the reciprocity of relational dynamics. Within the parameters of "the order of being", and within "the realm of the between", the key concept is without any doubt the credo of "justice". When familial

relationships (their form and content) are not informed by an ethos of justice, they can cause huge damage to all people involved in this system.

3. The hermeneutical horizon that helps one to understand the mode of the other's daily orientation in life, as well as one's own actions, is framed by justice as enfleshed and exhibited in dialectical systems of loyalty. It does not matter that the script of our life, even familial pacts of lawful obligations – the ledger – are indeed complex, and often the cause of confusion and conflict. What counts is that the hermeneutical horizon for meaningful interactions is still determined by the principle of "justice". Without this hermeneutical framework of reference, it would become virtually impossible to differentiate between what is fair and what is unfair in different contexts. For therapists, as well as for pastors, "justice" is the framework for all modes of hermeneutics within the humane space of intersubjective encounters.

4. The process of therapy is for Nagy about "re-balancing". It is about an attempt to restore balance and trustworthy equilibriums. The metaphor of "balance" refers to a dynamic equilibrium in loyal family systems and intergenerational dynamics: The equilibrium between guilt and obligation, disadvantages and advantages; merit and reward.

5. Nagy coins terminology borrowed from civil law. It helps to understand the dialectics of "guilt" and "obligation" within a familial context. Even care is determined by the obligation to repay what has been received. In giving and receiving, "crediting" plays a role. Especially, when trust is established without the condition to earn trustworthiness. In receiving a credit, one has immediately the obligation to act accordingly and not to disappoint. Therapeutic terminology can indeed be defined by intrapsychic categories (Fairbairn), or theories stemming from systemic/interactional thinking (Bateson). However, these categories do not necessarily imply an ethical dimension. This is the reason why Nagy imported categories from the juridical sphere of life and the practice of bookkeeping. These categories help to understand what is at stake in familial systems as shaped by justice and loyalty. Thus, the need for an ethical framework in the hermeneutical attempt to understand therapeutic interventions in relational and intergenerational dynamics. Also,

for the understanding of psychodynamics and interactional driving forces, judicial categories contribute to an ethical assessment of intersubjective interaction.

6. The reparation of the relational reality of human beings, and "caring attention" to the dynamics of interconnectedness, are predominant, because in the human order of being, obstacles should immediately be addressed. It does not matter whether helping interventions are partially, they need to be repaired. Because this order is determined by the notion of justice, and the fact that the being order of human relationships is always in flux and ethically based, the quest for one or other form of reparation and healing becomes evident. Thus, the reason why Nagy introduced terminology such as "guilt", "obligation", "merit", "merited trust", "acknowledgement", "accountability", "responsibility", and "entitlement" to indicate the vulnerable state of the relational reality of our being human. All of these categories point in the direction of relational reparation. The relational dynamics of our being human is always in need for authentic care and attention. This is indeed the case in intergenerational dynamics. Thus, the reason why the quest for justice and fairness in the healing of intergenerational conflict and violence, is in need for a kind of lawful framework of reference (the ledger). The latter helps to guarantee and foster a humane approach in the enhancement of the quality of life for all human beings. The introduction of a metaphor, rendered from the practice of bookkeeping (*ledger*), serves as motivational layer for action. It also serves as a form of hope for repairing the hurt of human justice – the violence of injustice. The hurt and wounded dignity of our being human must be repaired. The process of care is an ongoing endeavour, because as long as there will be human encounters, and relational interaction, the final balance is outstanding and the ledger still an open book.

In this regard, it is necessary to note that balance and reparation can appear in many different modes. One very unique mode is silence in human encounters. To keep quiet, can be an attempt to cover injustice. On the other hand, it can be a serious mode of "saving the other" and "speaking" the truth.

In therapy and caregiving, patience is healthful. It is about the art of silence: waiting for the other. But silence can also be harmful.

CHAPTER 2

The art of re-balancing: The healing power of "loyal silence" within the spiritual dynamics: Justice – mercy (ḥēsēd)

Silence (to keep quiet and to say nothing) is a human response with many layers of meaning. That is indeed the case when silence is connected to the interplay between loyalty and disloyalty. Not to say anything, can indeed be a meaningful way of talking and verbalising a very complex situation. Due to very subtle nuances, the speaker can convey a message without being bounded to the eventual outcome.

The many faces of a spirituality of silence

An example of the deceptive character of silence, is the case of the false prophets in the Bible. They don't act according to their mission and religious identity. They said what the people wanted to hear, but by doing this, their silence about God's will violated the revealed truth.

Furthermore, silence can be an indication of guilt due to anxiety and fear that the group could take revenge.

On the other hand, silence can sometimes be the most appropriate mode of talking. This mode of keeping quiet can be sanctifying, articulating the truth in such a way that it can be called the royal privilege of holy silence.

Within human encounters, one can deliberately decide not to speak and to draw a line in verbal communication. The reason could be not to hurt the other, or to render respect, or even to save the other.

In the publication *L'Exil de la Parole* (*The Exile of the Word*), the author, André Neher (1992), refers to the phenomenon of silence in Auschwitz, as well as to the case of David and Jonathan. Silence became a holy deed of keeping quiet in order to save the other.

In the book of Samuel, the author refers to King Saul and the fact that the Spirit of the Lord had departed from him. An evil spirit tormented Saul. Saul's attendants knew about his torment but kept quiet. Instead, they suggest that Saul gets someone who can play the harp so that he can be soothed. David, the son of Jesse of Bethlehem, was called to play the harp. David came to Saul and entered his service. Saul liked him very much, so David remained in the king's service. "Whenever the spirit from God came upon Saul, David would take his harp and play. Then relief would come to Saul; he would feel better, and the evil spirit would leave him" (1 Sam 16:23, NIV).

Chapter 17 is about the challenging encounter between David and Goliath. David was armoured only with stones and a sling. The huge figure of Goliath approached the boy David with sword, spear and javelin. However, David triumphed over the Philistine with a sling and a stone. Without a sword in his hand, he struck down Goliath and killed him. Saul was tremendously impressed and asked Abner, commander of the army, whose son David is. Abner responded and said: "As surely as you live, o king, I don't know".

In his novel, Neher interprets the response of Abner as hypocrisy: He pretended not to know. Even though all people who surrounded David should have known who David is, they said nothing, while David in a very profound way declared: "I am the son of your servant Jesse of Bethlehem" (1 Sam 17:58). Although Saul and his whole family were very vulnerable at that time, David did not give Saul away. The narrative continues as follows: "After David had finished talking with Saul, Jonathan became one in spirit with David, and he loved him as himself" (1 Sam 18:1, NIV).

According to Neher, the silence of David overwhelmed the spirit of Jonathan. Very deliberately David finished talking to Saul. That was literally what David did. We can hear David limiting his speech and then he kept silent. Jonathan, in this act of respect for his father, recognised the spirit of a true brother. Hereafter, brotherly love connected Jonathan to David until his death. According to the researchers, the friendship and love between David and Jonathan started from Jonathan's side due to Jonathan's loyalty to his father. The impact of this silence from David's side, is that loyalty became the bonding factor between the two[16].

With reference to the fact that silence is a many layered concept, the silence of David is viewed by Neher as an indication that silence can become a vital expression of an existential mode of ethics. The silence implies more than merely uttering a "word". In fact, it verbalises more than a word can express ("*au delà de la parole*"; beyond a word), or even a cause. When silence expresses an unspoken truth that is linked to, for example, justice, silence is not about a conspiracy, but becomes an expression of love that surpasses the boundaries of a pact. This kind of silence expresses trust and symbolises the cause of trustworthiness.

---

16 For the meaning of the word "*na'ar*" in I Samuel 17: 55, 58, see the article of KA Deurloo 1967 and KAD Smelik 1977:154, 189.

It is quite remarkable, that Nagy's contention that loyalty forms the cornerstone of relationships in the human order of justice, finds an analogy in the Hebrew concept of "ḥēsēd" (merciful grace). Between David and Jonathan, a covenant was established with obligations from both sides. One needs to understand that a covenant is not merely about a pact or formal contract. Both parties are now in a reciprocal way connected to one another. This connection attains the status of a bond with legal implications. The latter is then determined by the interplay between justice and mercy (ḥēsēd)[17].

Applied to loyalty within familial dynamics and intergenerational interaction, loyalty and fairness imply that people (adults as well as children) experience trust and safety – they will never forsake or betray one another. Thus, we can say that the criterion for the ethical quality of loyalty (a core issue in Nagy's theory) corresponds in general with what the Bible means with ḥēsēd.

---

17 Nelson Glueck translates ḥēsēd in I Samuel 20:8 with "brotherly love" (Glueck 1961:12).

CHAPTER 3

The ethical dynamics of contextual encounters: On entering the unpredictable space of humane reciprocity

In terms of the research question and basic research problem, namely the quest for a contextual approach to the dynamics of intergenerational intersubjectivity, it became crystal clear that therapy is embedded in dynamic contexts that transcend the limitations of psychotherapeutic theories with their narrow focus on intra-processes of psychic individuation. The networking dynamics of social interaction encompasses not merely the characteristics of the separate personal entities; it represents and constitutes something "more": an interacting web of coherent "wholeness". The whole of human encounters constitutes a web of reciprocal relationships that are directed by the interplay between loyalty and disloyalty, fairness and injustice, responsibility and ignorance, trust and distrust. At stake, is the quest for indicators that can guarantee the humane quality of this networking web of human encounters.

Human encounters are embedded in and framed by what Nagy calls "a just human order". Relationships should be directed by an ethos of trustworthiness. Immediately one realises that this order is not a neutral space dictated by brute power play, or the fatal determinism of linear, causal thinking. It should be a moral order founded by an ontology of being; it should deal with the human quest for dignity and meaning (significance).

Therefore, the challenging question: What are the indicators for meaningful encounters, trustworthy relationships and hopeful living?

In order to "save" the "web of dynamic interrelational networking" from becoming stuck (stagnation), processes within this "whole" should be steered by dialectics, as well as by dialogical encounters that establish human bonds with "covenantal characteristics"; that is, characteristics like merit, obligation, accountability and trust. Together, they reflect a kind of mercy that contributes to healing and reparation.

The intriguing question to be researched is: If it is indeed the case that psychotherapy implies more than merely the intrapsychic capacity of individuals in their attempt to overcome obstacles in their personal life and complicating relationships; if it is indeed true that our existential reality and social dynamics are intrinsically determined by a meta-realm that constitutes a moral order for our being human, what then is the link between "the justice of the human order" and the "ontological structure of humane being"? In other words, what is the link between dialogical ontic structures in human encounters and moral orders of overarching ethical paradigms that direct human behaviour towards the establishment of continuous, trustworthy and humane encounters?

The reciprocal system of humane interaction and trustworthy encounters within intergenerational transactions, constitutes a web of social structures that can be called "context". It is this context that Nagy wants to incorporate in what he calls: "*Contextual therapy*". The argument is that context is not a neutral entity and should be framed by an ethical dimension.

What now is the relationship between this context and the ontic reality of being (the ontological dimension of life)? Or, are they so intertwined that, systemically speaking, differentiation is virtually impossible?

The further goal and aim of the research project, is to explore the character of the relationship between "context" and "ethics" in Nagy's theory for intergenerational family psychotherapy. In one way or another, an ontology of relationships and ethics are linked. Thus, the further research question in this chapter: How appropriate is Nagy's appeal on Martin Buber's relational ontology? Can one accommodate Levinas' critique on Buber in Nagy's application of Buber's dialogical approach to his therapeutic model for care?

As argued, context is in the first place for Nagy a construction to assist the therapist in diagnostic assessment and healing interventions (reparation). A contextual approach could also be most helpful in the social dynamics of family interaction. The assumption is that it could play a decisive role in the opening up of existential reciprocity. Specifically, when the encounter becomes stuck. It could reinstall meaningful connections in reciprocal human encounters. The latter can indeed be very unpredictable. It is in this regard, that Buber's notion of "encounter" could become relevant. The fact that the human I can be connected to a human Thou in meaningful encounters, can be viewed as a gift of "grace". One cannot achieve and constitute this mode of gracious encounter by means of own psychic capacity. It is established in the very act and event of an encounter: I find and discover the Thou. Precisely, because this "Thou" is *there*, always *present* within all modes of dialogical encounters. Presence is established by the very fact that the other (Thou) is there. Being there, is part and parcel of the existential event of a dialogical encounter (Buber 1965:15-16).

Gabriël Marcel refers to the term "encounter" (*Begegnung*) in Buber's thinking: "… in the presence of human beings, there is created among them, let us not say even a field of forces, but a creative milieu, in which each finds possibilities of renewal. The term 'meeting', *Begegnung*, is here far more adequate than that of 'relation'" (Marcel in Schilpp & Friedman 1963:45).

In the previous outline, the question surfaced: Is Buber's understanding of "order of being" the same as Nagy's contamination of "the justice of the human order"? Is the human order of justice identical with the ontological order of being? Or is this human order of justice, an order *sui generis*; that is, from a total, different sphere – a kind of meta-order (metaphysical entity)? Is this order in fact an ethical order a priori, in other words, is it preceding the order of being? Is it indeed the case that the "order of justice" does not belong to the "order of being", but in fact judge the quality of being?[1]

For the research project these previous questions are of vital importance. The reason? For the understanding of Nagy's therapeutic model, "the dimension of relational ethics" has a fundamental impact on systematic reflection in theory formation. It shapes the therapeutic outcome of helping interventions.

One has to wrestle with the question whether there is place in Nagy's theory formation for an ethics that does not reside in the autonomy of the subject, but in the reciprocity of dialogical, reliable, trustworthy, fair human

---

1   See in this regard, Levinas (DL:41): "Ce que soutient le langage théologique, mesurant tout le merveilleux d'une telle liberté, en disant que Dieu seul juge." This quotation means more or less: Theological language is supported by the fact that, despite the marvel, privilege of freedom in the articulation of God, God is in the last instance the judge who will assess how valid and appropriate it is.

encounters? When Nagy's understanding of "ethics" and his notion of an "ethical dimension", are merely founded by an autonomous subject, the real danger lurks that ethics could merely become a personal view and subjective opinion. Even if it is about a kind of meta-view, it is still subjected to the historic arbitrariness of intrasubjective inclusiveness. Also, if personal opinions are excellent and indeed appropriate within the relativism of postmodernity and the milieu of historical contextualism, it will soon be extinguished and become irrelevant within global pluralism with its cacophony of confusing social voices and multiplied electronic options.

Against this background, the core question is: What is true and just in intersubjectivity? What are the foundations for a humane society? Instead of subjective moralism, what is the basis for the establishment of authentic humanity and humane coexistence? (Meulink-Korf 1990:143).

These questions put us before an enormous challenge. Ethics and morality are complex issues in processes of globalisation. When morality pretends to have universal consequences, it immediately revives scepticism and resistance. In this regard, the cruelty of Auschwitz and the racism of apartheid cause immediately harsh criticism. Even Levinas wrestled with the question whether morality and ethics eventually change human beings into puppets and fools. Many violent actions like riots and war took place under the disguise of so called sound moral campaigns (See further Levinas TI:ix).

One cannot avoid the critical question whether ethics, the ethical dimension, and relational ethics in Nagy's thinking, are not merely the product of disguised misconceptions and false deceptions. Contemporary scepticism in postmodernity, and processes of global relativism, pose very seriously the question regarding the legal basis for alleged ethical and moral exponents of authority. Without any compromise, sheer scepticism in contemporary society is based on a critical rationality (Goud 1992a:16). However, there are also serious attempts to search for normative principles that infer the human mind and direct human actions (Goud 1992a:16). The search for sound normative indicators cannot be denied. Although it seems that human goodness has been replaced by evil, the aesthetical dimension of life still prevails in one way or another[2].

---

2   See the poetry by Lucebert over beauty, and the quote by De Boer. See also the possible link with Levinas in his critique on Western thinking (De Boer 1976:122).

The interplay between "context/contextual" and human well-being (therapy)

The attempt to link the term "context" to "therapy" is difficult, even complex. Everything is nowadays contextual. It becomes "fashionable" to refer to "contextual" in order to claim: My approach is quite relevant.

In her attempt to translate Nagy's theory into Dutch, this complexity is captured by Ammy Heusden (in Schlüter 1990:9). She pointed out that the term "contextual therapy" is problematic because it is a many layered concept with many different nuances. Without any doubt, the term needs thorough attention.

With reference to Nagy's publication *Invisible Loyalties* (1973), his approach is primarily "dialectical" and "intergenerational". This characterisation is confirmed by Albert Neeleman (1995:108) and others in their research on the disciplinary contribution of Nagy within the broader paradigmatic framework of systems therapy.

However, Nagy himself called his approach "contextual". This term sets for Nagy the confines for theory formation in therapy. In the publication *Between Give and Take* (1986), the subtitle gives a clearer indication of the direction of his argumentation: "*A Clinical Guide to Contextual Therapy*". This tendency is confirmed in the 1987 publication: "*Foundations of Contextual Therapy*" (see also *Interview* 1995).

In the traditional approach to family therapy, the focus was on pathology, that is, the problematic aspects and causes for dysfunctional behaviour, specifically for psychotic behaviour. Terms like "sickening behaviour" and "game-rules", contributed to the blaming of family members for improper communication and the impact thereof on the "identified patient". A pathological approach to dysfunctional behaviour goes hand in glove with a very strict approach to "disciplinary classifications" and intrapsychic diagnosis. For example, it is not only the patient that becomes labelled. The classification strategy even affects the family. The latter also becomes diagnosed as "schizophrenic", "dysfunctional", "symbiotic" or "rigid". The impact of these "disciplinary labels", is that they don't necessarily contribute to healing. On the contrary, they increase the impact of the problem by alleviating guilt and piling a lot of blame on family members. By doing this, classification runs the danger to even contribute to complification, rather than to head for human well-being. The family system becomes entangled in the attempt to cope with the demands of the so called "identified patient". The further problem is that professionals eventually leave the impression that the "guilt" and "blame" for problematic behaviour should be put fully on the shoulders of one of the family members. This approach reinforces the pathology and pathogenic components rather than contributing to alleviating the burden.

With this background in mind, one should understand why Nagy opted for a quite different approach. His model homes in on a quite different angle. Thus, Nagy's fundamental critique: A pathological approach to helping and healing eventually falls prey to sheer moralism. It victimises rather than cares. The focus on abuse and pathology leaves the impression that therapy is a kind of "technical intervention"; the manual dictates the therapeutic strategy, and not vice versa, the concrete setting of the relational dynamics determining the therapeutic intervention.

Nagy's approach is based on the interplay between ethics and reciprocal dynamics. With a "contextual approach", or "contextual therapy", Nagy has in mind the redefining of context in terms of ethics – "… an ethical redefinition of the relational context" (Nagy F:196). From the outside it seems as if "relational context" is merely about networking as such. This could leave the impression of superficiality. However, this will be an optic illusion. For Nagy, a "relational networking context" refers to an existential web of human interaction and the quest for authentic being. It is about the dynamics of an ontic orientation within the existential realm of life. *Existential orientation* refers to the daily happenstances of life within concrete facticity. To be situated, points to both the embodied (somatic) and social factors that constitute the character of our being human. It encompasses the reality of psychic processes, the affective dimension of life, and the interactional reality (known as redundancy[3] – the plenitude and positive plus/extra factor as by-product of different modes of being within mutual interconnectedness and multiple interactional interpretations).

Nagy's ethical redefinition is quite a radical correction with reference to existing viewpoints on the systemic dimension of relational and familial networking. For Bateson, context refers to the basic framework for

---

3 *Redundancy* is quite a technical term. It refers inter alia to the duplication of critical components or functions of a system with the intention of increasing reliability of the system (it refers to an extra and overflow); furthermore, redundant communication refers to having multiple back-up communication modalities which become imperative in prevention care.

meaning-giving; a kind of foundational structure for the interplay between meaning-giving and meaning-finding. Communication is, thus, not possible without a situational context that signifies our being human in this world. Communication is about some organic dynamics. Every pole in the communication system creates his/her own context in terms of stimuli emanating from other organic components. The stimuli need to be decoded in terms of the code system, as connected to the character of that very specific organism (Bateson 1980:15-16). This unique organic dynamic is called by some of Bateson's scholars, "*autopoiesis*"[4] (Maturana & Varela 1980).

What one needs to understand, is Nagy's concern for an objective anthropological foundational structure (basis for meaningful existential orientation) that is both relational and ethical, is focused on the establishment of interactive trustworthiness. In this respect, the difference between a cognitive-technical conceptualised style of doing family therapy, and a therapeutic intervention that focuses on ethical resources, is quite remarkable; they differ hugely from one another. At stake, in ethical resources are different modes of trusting that promote individuation, family interaction and community building.

The endeavour of an ethical redefinition is not about an attempt by the therapist to redefine the "relational context". The redefinition is a process wherein all significant members, belonging to somebody's relational reality (the other/others), are involved as persons or individuals within the mutual dynamics of relationships. According to the intersubjective order of being, all people involved are subjects of the ethical redefinition of the relational context. "Contextual therapy aims at the goal of *eliciting* trust resources of close relationships" (Nagy F:191). What the therapist should do, is to evoke "trust resources" in order to establish trustworthiness. For this new approach, a radical mindset is imperative: "Reversal has to start in the therapist's own mind" (Nagy IL:374).

The terms "contextual" and "contextual therapy" should, thus, be understood as a *process of redefinition of relationships* and not as a diagnostic endeavour.

---

4   With reference to living organisms, *autopoiesis* refers to a system capable of reproducing and maintaining itself. *Autopoiesis* is about the dynamics of a closed circuit. "We are such stuff as dreams are made of" (quote by Bateson from Shakespeare, *The Tempest* (Bateson 1980:15-16).

Context represents an ultimate framework of meaning, a kind of horizon that renders significance to separate objects or text-components. This significant horizon instils a sense of meaning to the functioning of each of the separate elements. A significant horizon is, therefore, a networking whole that can be called a context due to its interrelational dynamics and connection to the notion of justice. Horizon as context, thus, compiles an ethical web of meaningful interactions that inflict in the mindset of the contextual therapist an ethos of fairness. Contextuality, thus, transforms paradigms, that is, patterns of thinking. As already pointed out: "Reversal has to start in the therapist's own mind" (Nagy IL:374). Therapeutic engagements should, thus, direct human behaviour according to this paradigmatic change. Therefore, the imperative for the conversion of therapeutic mindsets.

The term "context" consists of four aspects at least. (It is not always easy to identify them in Nagy's theory formation. They are so intertwined and interconnected that separate identification is quite difficult).

1. The interplay: Context – text within social settings and familial dynamics

In order to understand what is going on in the patient/client, a thorough scrutiny of his/her social context is paramount. The patient is then the "text", and the family the "context". The context functions as a kind of spotlight that illuminates the sectional text – the patient. Dysfunctional or psychotic behaviour, even the reference to the so-called "schizophrenic salad", attains meaning from the context. Context is then viewed as a significant framework due to social interaction and familial networking.

2. Justice as an ontic feature of human orientation in concrete situations

Context gives an ontic profile to the dynamics of being. Being then viewed as an existential endeavour within reciprocal relationships. This dynamic is unique, because in all these interactions, it is about the ethos of justice. Everyone is engaged in this existential endeavour. The realm of the between, determines in both the patient and the relational context, the character of the human encounter – the between of I and Thou (Buber). Intersubjectivity is, thus, a being entity. It even entails more: It touches the essence and ontic truth of being; "the truth of personal uniqueness" (Nagy IL:54).

The relational reality is a kind of "common denominator"; it profiles the unique personal orientation in life (ethos); it functions as a kind of differentiation-factor and delineates identity. The relationship with the significant other, as well as the relational dynamics between significant others, are simultaneously constituted as a vivid interplay between "context" and "text".

3. Context as a dialogical "feed-back-/feed-forward-system" within the surprise of giving and receiving

Context is never a closed "feed-back-system". It is not a complete book with a final chapter. The driving force in this contextual system is the acting out of justice. The system is, therefore, open for surprises due to the unpredictability of relational dynamics. In significant mutuality and co-existence, dialogue is always imminent and contributes to the surprise of unexpected events and unforeseen outcomes. Dialogue contributes to openness. "Context is shaped by the openness of people's realities, and by the malleability of people's fate" (Nagy & Krasner BGT:9). Within stagnation and relational obstacles, there is always the option for renewal and the establishment of new relationships. Human beings are not crippled by fate nor encapsulated by past events. Life is not rigidly determined, circular or homeostatic (Nagy & Krasner BGT:9).

"Openness" does not mean that people merely give new meaning to one another. The danger then lurks that the signifier dominates the process of signifying and receiving. "Openness" is predominantly about an ethical dynamic; it interrupts the momentum of being; it exposes courageous vulnerability; reveals existential truths, and profiles empathy and even vulnerability for the fate of the other (see also Levinas HAH:12). Openness is even about a patient's passivity, a mode of wait until …; until the "significance" of the "significant other" starts to appear.

4. Context represents a kind of future anticipation and ontological predisposition

For Nagy, the concept "context" refers to future as well. The dynamic interconnectedness between human beings, does not hold human beings captives of the past. Context includes past, present and future. "… context implies consequences that flow from person to person, from generation to generation, and from one system to its successive system" (Nagy & Krasner BGT:8).

Besides influences of Carl Rogers's client centered therapy ("person-to-person"), and Edwin Friedman's systems family approach ("generation-to-generation") Nagy and Krasner added another dimension to "context", namely the fact that invisibility is a vital ingredient of "context". Context includes coming generations and unborn children; "… context is an ontological realm. It *consists of pre-ethical reality, that is, the fact of personal accountability for relational consequences*" (Nagy & Krasner BGT:10; ital VR/MK).

The hunch is that Nagy uses the term "pre-ethical" to indicate that there is a kind of ontic appeal to our being human. One should respond with a kind of responsibility that does not stem from external normative frameworks. It is about a predisposition (*habitus*) to instantly respond according to the fact that we are created beings. As living organisms there is an ontic urge to respond appropriately. Other than any other created entity, our being human is structured ontologically to act in such a significant way that, other human beings and coming generations will benefit from our being human. The appeal is in terms of a phenomenology not designed by us; it rather envelops from the facticity of being itself. The order of being implies a personal accountability that encompasses "transgenerational solidarity". "The context of the human order of justice and transgenerational solidarity is a silent partner to intergenerational relationships" (Nagy & Krasner BGT:98).

In conclusion

One can capture the following basic assumptions regarding the meaning of "context":
- The notion "context" in Nagy's approach is many layered and always in flux with many variations. It is open to multiple interpretations. It varies from a hermeneutical horizon that interprets phenomena in terms of observational appearances, to something that is not-yet.
- Context instigates change and conversion: "The reversal has to start in the therapist's own mind" (Nagy & Krasner BGT:374).
- Context is about the dynamic reciprocity of "I-Thou": "The family-therapist must be able to conceive of a social group whose members all relate to one another, according to Buber's I-Thou dialogue" (Nagy & Spark IL:43).
- Context is intergenerationally structured: "… consequences that flow from […] generation to generation" (Nagy & Krasner BGT:8).

- Every human being, in his/her unique personal identity, should be rendered as subject, irrespective of the question whether one is the victim, perpetrator or insignificant other.
- The meaning of a human being can be changed from a meaning rendered by others, to a meaning that is intrinsically significant for that human being in her/himself, even without knowing it or contributing to it.
- As context, the "justice of the human order" is an open concept due to the fact that the "ledger" is not closed yet.
- Context as a "pre-ethical" entity (Nagy & Krasner BGT:10), features as personal accountability for relational consequences and coming future generations still to be born. Contemporary generations are accountable. Context is even "the account" to be inherited by the coming generation (Nagy & Krasner BGT:8).
- Context is a methodological term that portrays the framework of reference for therapeutic actions, and the justification of helping interventions. This framework of reference articulates close relationships wherein people are interdependent from one another and committed to one another; it creates an ethical situation.
- The process of redefining human connections is an ethical process due to the fact that everybody is a subject and stays a subject. The intersubjective order constitutes everybody as subject. Thus, the reason why ethics redefines the context, and not vice versa.

The networking framework of heteronomous relationality and the ethics of intersubjective obligations

At this stage the reader should understand that two features of Nagy's approach characterize his theoretical approach:

(a) "Contextual therapy" is coined due to Nagy's basic assumption that intersubjectivity is founded in an ontic and dialogical structure which displays the fact that coexistence within the interhuman dynamics is intrinsically determined by the ethical dimension of life. Thus, the reason why contextual therapy is engaged in therapeutic leverages, namely in mobilizing trust (Nagy F:191). "Contextual therapy" is shaped by the interplay between relational ethics and merit (*merited trust*).

(b) *Intersubjectivity* is viewed as a kind of a priori; it constitutes an ontic predisposition and mode of being (Nagy F:4-7). Our being human is basically structured by "being-in-relationship". Being situated in relationality, is not the by-product of personal autonomy or the outcome of free choice. I don't choose my mother, father, brother or sister; it is a given fact within the dynamics of relationality. Relationships are heteronomous.

Intersubjectivity does not rob human beings from their unique, independent identity. Important is to reckon with the fact that the heteronomous character of the relation precedes the autonomy of the person. Being unique (individuation, subjectivity), should be interpreted from the perspective of heteronomous intersubjectivity. "The system itself (the parenting others in their trustworthiness) begins to place structured ethical demands and expectations on the child long before this sort of obligation has a chance of becoming conscious" (Nagy & Spark IL:45). Already in the process of name-giving, intersubjectivity is presupposed. Name-giving confirms our being a subject within the dynamics of intersubjectivity. "Furthermore, as long as the child lives, he/she will never be really free of the existential indebtedness to his/her parents and family" (Nagy & Spark IL:45). The family loyalty system is the "multi-person-fabric". Every human contributes to the quality of this system; the quality of this system invests in the formation of our being human. "The invisible ledger of justice is a relational context, it is the dynamically most significant component of the individual's world, although it is not external to him/her" (Nagy & Spark IL:53-54).

This ledger contributes to the essence of our being human; it constitutes an anthropology of life. It functions as a kind of invisible, existential bookkeeping system about shortcomings and abilities, merit and guilt within the dynamics of familial interaction. Familial relationships create memories wherein the developing child receives his/her unique identity; it is about the most intimate and meaningful component of our being human in this world.

With world is meant a pre-reflexive, pre-scientific mode of orientation and experience; a world-wide web and horizon of meaningful frameworks. In this world-wide web, the constitutional factor is "justice". "Justice" is even the form and content of relationships in our world of becoming human. The invisible ledger of justice enfolds within the dialogical interplay between "external horizon" and "internal framework"; it is a vital component in self-development.

Every component of our human self is defined by the conditions of our existential environment (Nijk 1978:208). Independent self-assertiveness is in this approach, a myth and existential lie. One can, thus, conclude that intersubjectivity is the pre-condition for our becoming our-*self*. *Self*-awareness, responsibility and re-*spond*-ability are all exponents of intersubjective dynamics; of the interplay of "external world" and "individual's world" (Nagy & Spark IL:54); of the dialogical dialectics between attachment and detachment; differentiation and a sense of belongingness; separation and trustworthy intimacy. This dynamic "between" (the realm of the "between") constitutes our ontic relationality. It is within this realm that the metaphors of the ledger and the process of bookkeeping envelop the account of our ethical existence, as well as the dynamics of an intrinsic ethics (see for example Nagy & Spark IL:81-82).

The ethical system does not function as a fixed precondition and kind of moral fatalism dominated by religious dogmatism or denominational affiliations. "The criteria [...] for judgement could never be predicted from religious, cultural, or superego morality of any particular type" (Nagy F:309). Intrinsic does not mean "immanent". It signifies a mutual sensitivity and reciprocal sense of (co-)responsibility. Responsibility is hereby shaped by the triadic structure of relationships. "The dilemma here is the presence of a third party, often imaginary, who is supposed to hear and decide the issue between you and me" (Nagy & Krasner BGT:224)[5].

Despite the large amount of injustice between people, Nagy maintains that justice is still more primordial than injustice. Thus, the reason why the therapist is eliciting the trust resources of close relationships (Nagy F:191). Relational resources possess the character of "trust" and "reliability" (Nagy & Krasner BGT:141-143). Without the postulate that justice is primordial to injustice, "eliciting of trust-resources" would have been a hybridised, even in vain, endeavour – a kind of hypocritical therapeutic "as-if".

One such "resource for trust", is what we (the researchers) propose to call "the giving child".

---

5   See the commandment in Leviticus 19:18b: "Love your neighbour as yourself."

CHAPTER 3

Children as reliable resources of care and reinforcement (the giving child)

As said, intersubjectivity constitutes a preconditioned space for becoming one-*self*, for the development of identity, processes of individuation, and authentic self-awareness. These processes correlate with the presupposition of "personal accountability", "responsibility" and "commitment". Loyalty presupposes a fundamental commitment that precedes even the freedom of decision-making (including children). It is because of these premises and a reckoning with the fact that they are imperative for self-development, that the notion and right of the "giving child" becomes evident. Even under conflicting marriage tension, children can, even despite tension between the spouses, still make valuable contributions. Thus, the proposition of the "*giving child*"; the conviction that even children can give help, support and care. According to Nagy and Krasner (BGT:356), children could become the most reliable resources available to reinforce family stability. Children are enormously giving and caring entities. In fact, Nagy is even prepared to speak in this regard of the "right" of a child to give and to be acknowledged. One should give credit to children's capacity for giving and caring.

The following question immediately surfaces: But is the child not so dependent on the goodwill of the parent, that by giving, children can become exploited and eventually partake in the game of mutual manipulation (being collusive)? In such a case, freedom and the making of choices, become gameplay.[6] Albeit, Nagy's response will be that even in giving and receiving within the mutuality of freedom and dependency, the receiving child can still contribute to giving, despite the risk of becoming overwhelmed by parental authority.

It is inevitable that children contribute to the quality of familial interaction as well. The educational space is in fact exposed to retributive dynamics. "Our assumption is that learning amounts to giving to rather than receiving from the teacher" (Nagy & Spark IL:31). Thus, the importance of acknowledgement and the awareness why merit plays such a paramount role in the ethical redefinition of the relational context and the dialectics of comfort and compassion.

---

6   See the mimetic theory of René Girard 1961.

It is indeed the case that merit can become manipulated and exposed to abuse of authority – the so-called threat of *"parentification"*. Due to respect for the parents or fear of becoming punished, there is always the imminent danger that the child could eventually surrender his/her autonomy (Nagy F:21). In the light of this lurking danger, it is paramount to reckon with the child as an autonomous subject. The child is also a unique subject endowed with the capacity to renounce external autonomy without the danger of becoming a victim. To maintain the right of a child as subject, it is for Nagy important how to designate a family within the framework of a multi-person systems approach, rather than merely prefacing traditional individual diagnostic terms or phrases (Nagy & Spark IL:10).

Surrendering autonomy is often not voluntary. It could even become self-destructive. However, it can still be rendered as a contribution due to the presupposition that it is in essence a contribution to intersubjectivity founded on the ethical principle of justice – the just human relational order. In the last instance, there is the option to appeal to the mutuality of fairness towards one another. The closed system should therefore be redefined in terms of loyalty in order to safeguard fairness and openness. In this sense, family loyalty can be viewed as the pathway for founding an ethical framework.

Nagy's view has implications for the ethos of the therapist. Psychotherapeutic interventions should, thus, be ethically based. It is the task of the therapist to help both the parent and the child. "How could you (the child) and I, the therapist, work as a team to help your family?" The principle is not either – or, but together we can! "Therapeutic acknowledgement is essentially didactic in nature" (Nagy & Krasner BGT:413). In such a didactic environment, it is important to learn how to differentiate between personal contributions to fairness within different layers of the relational dynamics. This differentiation is immediately connected to validation and acknowledgement.

The systems therapist Murray Bowen, calls families who cannot distinguish and differentiate, an "undifferentiated ego mass" (Bowen in Nagy & Framo 1965:219-223). The family pathology is then about a kind of familial fusion and inability to differentiate and understand the value of ethical cognition, recognition and acknowledgement. Differentiation is based on an ethics of intersubjectivity. In the question "How could you and I work as team to help your family?", subjectivity as differentiation and responsibility is instigated and promoted (Nagy F:115). Within such an approach, and with this question in mind, the therapist enters the vulnerable space of the other (the child). In the language of Levinas, this vulnerability is primarily an "ethical vulnerability".

In the quest for clear differentiation within the space of familial interaction and the demand for an ethos of trustworthiness, the focus is on the exposure of human frailty; that is, the emphasis is on the weakest component, namely the vulnerable child. For example, the new-born baby is embedded in a kind of weakness that can be called corporeal helplessness. In his/her corporeal helplessness, the infant is totally dependent on the other for nutrition, warmth and care. This need makes an appeal on the other and can be viewed as a contribution to the quest for care. "Even very young children can contribute to family life [...] and can do so without understanding the adult world and its specific problems. Thoughtful utilization of a child's care requires adults to recognise an offspring's contributions rather than belittle them" (Nagy & Krasner BGT:356-357). In cases where parents cannot correspond to this reality of vulnerability appropriately, but still have to meet the demands of parenting, their inability can be projected to the vulnerable child, by blaming the child for not coping with demands. The child becomes the object of blaming, namely an "identified patient" – the child as cause of guilt for not coping. "Perhaps the most excessively destructive parentification is perpetrated by unfairly blaming the victim" (Nagy & Krasner BGT:329).

The argument is that the quest for care does not originate from a shortage or kind of "existential deficit", or even from a desperate need for attention, but from the urge to "do good" to the adult/parent with whom the child is existentially connected or "committed" to. This kind of commitment seems to be quite strange. One can argue as follows: But parenting is automatically about caring and doing good. However, that is not the case. Appropriate parenting and trustworthiness correlate with the demand that the parent should also acknowledge the contribution of the child to fair treatment and loyal parenting. "A major relational resource [...] frequently goes unrecognised: The young child's offering of loyal devotion and trust to the adult world" (Nagy F:303). Fairness is reciprocal, namely for the children, but also through the children. One should realise, without any doubt, children "count" and are intrinsically part of the moral order. It is a moral issue how one goes about with the problem of "more" and "less", "strong" and "weak".

Paradigm switch in psychotherapy: From psychic terminology to legal terminology (judicial language)

It became evident that Nagy has got a special affinity for legal terminology. For example: "Justice", "entitlement", "trustworthiness", "fairness", "ledger", as well as concepts like "exoneration". Most of times we make use of terminology stemming from psychotherapeutic endeavours, or from the sphere of politics and power. Nagy, however, derives terminology from law and the legal context.

For many professional psychotherapists, it will be very strange to use words like "justice" and "trustworthiness". It sounds like sheer moralism. If one is not willing to change, it will be difficult to associate with Nagy's terminology (Van Heusden in Schlüter 1990:9). It could indeed be that, by making use of terminology that stems from a total, different discipline, new light is shed on stereotyped and "zombie categories".

Pitfall of moralism

The advantage of legal terminology is that it helps Nagy to articulate the importance of justice in therapeutic endeavours. This paradigm switch to legal terminology is not easy because it is difficult to grasp that justice in contextual therapy is about a secret code and systemic ledger; justice as part of systemic homeostasis. The system needs justice; justice becomes an organic entity; it functions like a guardian to prevent the pitfall of moralism and unjust manipulation (Meulink-Korf & Van Rhijn 1990).

In a contextual approach, justice takes on the role of a "lawful caretaker" in order to make sure that the interaction between therapist and client is fair. It is not about judicature by the therapist, but to make sure that justice will be done to each person involved in the familial dynamics, as well as in social interconnectedness. In this sense, justice as a legal term, describes the character of ethics in intergenerational dynamics. Fundamentally it is about a perspective and ingredient of being. Ethics, therefore, is not about a meta- or superstructure, also not about sub-atomic depth (underneath); it is an expression of the ontological character of fairness as a being quality.

Nagy's focal point was subjectivity within dialogical intersubjectivity. The advantage of a dialogical point of departure is that it describes subjectivity within the multiple dynamics of two selves, interacting mutually with one another. This interaction between selves should be studied from a multiple subjective vantage point. This is exactly what he had in mind when he started to wrestle with the question how to structure caregiving and helping so that the subjectivity and individuality of the two selves stays intact and not become objectified from an "above-position" (a helicopter view). At stake, is to understand the interactional dynamics from the "dialogical between" from the perspectives of the interacting subjects. Intersubjectivity is in essence a multiple endeavour (Nagy F:241-242).

The pitfall that Nagy wanted to avoid is to approach human intersubjectivity from the abstract viewpoint of theoretical objectification. The observer is then like a therapist from the planet Mars, landing on the tip of the Empire State Building, looking down to the hustle and bustle of city life and the rummaging of people on the streets. However, it becomes totally inappropriate to make suggestions from this vantage point to what should happen on the streets in order to avoid traffic jams, but, in the meantime, one cannot spot the desperate attempts of somebody looking for a taxi. "No understanding of the transactional pattern is complete without regard for coexisting multi-personal criteria" (Nagy & Krasner BGT:30). The notion "multi-personal criteria" does not imply that the therapist develops multiple subjective perspectives, but that he/she is able to reckon with the unique subjectivity of every family member involved in the familial conflict area, and simultaneously with the dynamics of multiple coexistence. This multiple-approach puts the challenge before the contextual therapist to adopt a kind of versatile bias ("multidirected partiality").

It is difficult to develop such a versatile bias within the paradigmatic contours of most psychological models. Psychology alone does not suffice. Not even if psychology is complemented with viewpoints borrowed from family systems theory. What is most needed in psychotherapy and a contextual approach, is the meta-psychological categories stemming from Martin Buber's dialogical philosophy (Nagy F:72).

The interplay: Buber (dialogical encounter) – Nagy (therapeutic context)

"… I did not rest on the broad upland of a system that includes a series of statements about the absolute, but on the narrow rocky ridge between the gulfs where there is no sureness of expressible knowledge but the certainty of meeting what remains undisclosed" (Buber in Friedman 1976:3).

Without any doubt, one can say that the dialogical philosophy of Martin Buber plays a fundamental role in Nagy's relational model for contextual therapy. On many different occasions, Nagy referred to Martin Buber.[7] Although direct citations are few and very fragmented, he often made use of Buber's terminology. For example, "the I-Thou dialogue", "the just order of being", "the realm of the between". Albeit, one can say Martin Buber's paradigm of thinking about the dynamics of the dialogical, human encounter is definitely a kind of theoretical framework of reference for his theory formation regarding the relational dynamics of contextuality.

On the one hand, Nagy's theory on subjectivity can be linked to the individual, client-oriented therapy. On the other hand, systems therapy plays a paramount role in his understanding of intergenerational dynamics and dialogical dialectics. It was Martin Buber who inspired him to link an individual approach to a relational approach. "Buber's concept of the dialogue came closest to a requisite framework which can describe two or more individuals in a personally engaged relationship" (Nagy F:241; VR/MK 1995). This explains why it was sometimes difficult for the classic individual focused psychotherapists to accept Nagy's paradigm switch with its emphasis on the a priori of dialogical relationships (I – Thou dialogue). In many systems theory representatives it seems as if the personal dimension was reduced to the transpersonal, anonymous interplay between systemic dynamics and autonomous interactional forces. One can even toy with the idea that the message of Nagy to abstract systems theory therapists like Haley (Nagy F:273), could be: Go and read Buber to find out what relationships between people are about.

In an interview with Margaret Markham in 1981, Nagy said: "Interesting to note, the key to the door of depth relational phenomena and to contextual extension of system-based thinking in classical family-therapy came from Martin Buber, and only to a lesser extent from relationally based ego theory" (Nagy F:241).

According to Nagy, therapy is about the dynamics between two of more selves. The condition is that the one "self" will not negate the other "self", and vice versa. Rather, the one should promote the other, without underplaying

---

7 On Buber, see Hans Kohn 1979; also, Paul Arthur Schilpp & Maurice Friedman 1967. Also M Friedman, *Martin Buber: The Life of Dialogue*, 1976. Nagy referred mainly to the following texts of Buber: *I and Thou, Guilt and guiltfeelings* (Buber 1965a), and also *Heilung aus der Begegnung*, this last text in Hans Trüb (1971:9-13).

one's own unique individuation. The inter-relational dynamic between the two selves is in fact involved in the reciprocity of "dialogical dialectic". This dialectic is not about a flat relationality wherein one renders the other not as a conversational partner, but rather about the "*thou-antithesis*" over against the "*I-thesis*".[8]

Instead of an autonomous dialectic, Nagy's emphasis is on familial reciprocity between subject-selves, balanced by justice and fairness. "A capacity for *responding* and being open to the other's responses is the core of the genuine dialogue" (Nagy F:72). At stake, is what Nagy calls "interpersonal responsiveness" and "subjective self-assertiveness". "It is a means of developing and maintaining selfhood through meeting the other, as well as having one's own needs met" (Nagy F:72). For Nagy dialogue is a means to social development, growth and maturity, because dialogue entails processes of constructive self-maintenance.

For Maurice Friedman (1992a:93), the most difficult aspect in dialogue is to take responsibility for one's own behaviour and decisions, as well as the challenge to appeal to the other's responsibility. Another aspect of dialogical dynamics is mutuality: The mutual implications of responsibility for the reciprocal quality of the human encounter. To maintain this viewpoint in theory formation, as well as in clinical work, is the most exigent aspect in applying the dialogical paradigm to healing interventions.

The "I-Thou" reciprocity: Interpreting intersubjectivity as the origin of authentic human being

The texts of Buber played a notable role in Nagy's paradigmatic reinterpretation of psychotherapy and its very narrow focus on the intrapsychic processes of the human person. In this regard, Martin Buber's enigmatic publication, "*I-Thou*" (*Ich und Du*), made a huge impact on Nagy's application of systems theory. Especially, the application to the "familial between" within intergenerational interaction. In *Ich und Du*, one finds the cornerstone of Buber's theoretical reflection and dialogical philosophy.

---

8   In this respect, there is a difference between Nagy's dialogical dialectics and Stierlin with his emphasis on a Hegelian dialectic of thesis and antithesis and reconciliation as synthetic ideal.

Despite mutual differences, together with Martin Buber, Franz Rosenzweig, Eugen Rosenstock-Huessy, and Ernst Simon, they formed a new pact regarding the interpretation of existential, life problems. They called their thinking and methodology, a new thinking and a paradigmatic renewal. The new paradigm was to view intersubjectivity as the beginning and origin of authentic human existence. The "truth" about human orientation resides within human encounters and the happenstances of daily living. The "I", within the reciprocity of "I-Thou", is from a different order than the "I" in relationship with "It" (*Ich-Es*). The two I's differ from one another.

In the introduction to "I-Thou", Buber distinguishes between two basic modes of being: The one mode is about the "word pair" (merely like a doublet): "I-Thou". The other basic concept is about the doublet: I-It. This "It" is not merely material (not only concerning things). It encompasses the possibility of "he", "she".

The implication is that the human "I" is indeed a doublet, but in the different connections, the I attains different meanings (I-differentiation).

The primary concept and word pair "I-Thou", can only be articulated when it is spoken and expressed with "the whole of being"[9]. Integration into the whole of being can never be established by the "I" in itself, by itself. Nor can integration be established without the contribution of the "I" (me-function). "I" am in becoming, through and by my relation to the Thou. As I become and am established, I say (pronounce) "Thou" (Buber 1965:15)[10].

The foundational word-construction "I-It", indicates a subject-object relationship. This "It" includes everything that can become an object, as well as content for rational reflection and conceptualisation. The "It" is object for the thinking (*cognitive dimension*), feeling (*affective dimension*) and motivating (*conative dimension*) of the human I. This reciprocal dynamic differs from

---

9   The capital "I", "Thou" and "It" is used in the English translation in order to indicate that with the German "*Ich*", "*Du*" and "*Es*" are meant some very unique relational dynamics that implies more than merely a *general pronoun* – a word that can function as a noun phrase used by itself, and referring either to the participants in the discourse (eg, *you*), or to someone or something mentioned elsewhere in the discourse; eg, *she, it, this*. For example, within the German, "I" is implied as a dialogical and reciprocal interaction and systemic dynamics.

10 This is a paraphrased translation by DJ Louw. Translation of the German quotations will not be put into inverted commas ("…") because a direct translation from German into English will become so technical and philosophical, that it will be difficult for the reader, without knowledge of German, to capture the significance of the specific philosophical articulation.

Freud's understanding of *it*, and his connection to urge and drift. It is about the authentic reality of objects.

"I" and "Thou" represent a subject-subject relationship and reciprocal dynamics: pure presence as a "*presencing* being there". Objects exist due to the factuality of their "already" – they already had been (Buber 1965:16). "I-Thou" is pure actuality – a kind of dynamic now (actuality as *presencing*). "Thou" is also not merely an awareness in the human mind, or merely the by-product of experience and observation. In fact, one can experience actually nothing from "Thou", because then "Thou" becomes objectified. One cannot speak "about Thou"; one can only encounter "Thou" and discover "Thou" by means of a continuous mutual encounter with "Thou". The vivid, existential encounter implies reciprocal continuity of dialoguing and mutual addressing.

The becoming of "I" (the developmental and growing person) is intrinsically interconnected with the "Thou"; addressed by me, and to whom my words are making an appeal to respond and to establish a reciprocal interaction; that is, a reciprocal interaction that constitutes the "Thou" as a "Thou" for me.

Buber did not directly write on "the dignity of our being human"; on being a humane human being that can be described in terms of objectified characteristics of being, something one can possess or achieve. Human dignity is much more a foundational, ontic structure of our human orientation in the dynamics of life. Thus, the reason why the concept of "encounter" as a living mode of coexistence, took such an important place in the German text[11]. It became gradually an indication of the dialogical ground structure of being, and the fact that dialogue displays some intersubjective dynamics. Intersubjectivity is about the unpredictable and surprising dynamics of happenstances in life. A "humane between" is always about the creative event of establishing human beings by means of reciprocal dialogue and intersubjective relationality.

The attractive dimension in Buber's model is that reciprocity does not imply the pathology of being totally dependent on the other. The fact of "I am", is autonomous. This is the reason why two people who are totally not even spiritually related to one another, even belonging to two totally different family traditions and cultures, can relate. In a reciprocal dialogue, the two can

---

11 Later Buber started to also use concepts like "the dialogical principle".

start acknowledging one another, constituting and identifying one another, even establishing the dignity of the other within the here and now of the encounter. This establishing of dignity and identity can take place even within conflicting situations, in combat and fighting with one another. Even when they are opponents to one another, without a common ground, they are still two dignified subjects within the ethos of reciprocal co-humanity (see Buber in Levinas NP:52; also in Schilpp & Friedman 1963:723).

It is not only the notion of dialogue that had an impact on Nagy's thinking, but also Buber's notion of guilt. Buber's publication on guilt and guilt feelings (SuSg 1962) helped him to start working with the reality of guilt and guilt feelings in therapy regarding problematic relational issues (Nagy F:107). The interesting fact is that Buber, in an introduction for the publication of Hans Trüb (*Heilung aus der Begegnung* – The healing impact of encounter) made the challenging remark: References in psychoanalytical literature are too general and vague. The ontic dimension and experience of guilt have not been addressed appropriately (Buber in Trüb 1971:11). Guilt does not reside merely in the intrapsychic processes of the human person but is fundamentally seated in the ontological ground structure of being. In fact, the human being exists within the realm of ontic guilt. Not to acknowledge guilt and to suppress it, surpass the confines of psychoanalytical observation.

Guilt is for Buber essentially "*existential guilt*". Buber connects existential guilt to the notion of the "human order of being" (Buber SuSg). Guilt is an exponent of the order-of-being, and, thus collective. Due to collective guilt, all human beings contribute to harming and damaging of our common world. Retribution and healing, thus, implies that every guilty person starts to do introspection by identifying yourself with your "self". When I harm the human order, I am the only person that can repair it. Our being human is at stake in the way we acknowledge personal guilt.

Nagy gave an own unique connotation to guilt and guilt feelings in the sense that he linked them to the notion of loyalty and the justice of the social order (civil societal justice and public of loyalty). In this regard, Nagy differs from Buber. For Buber, guilt is personal. It is established and caused by damages to the reciprocity of the dialogical interaction and the ground structure of being. With Nagy, guilt is the outcome of damage to the dimension of loyalty and violation of the principle of fairness inherent to relational and intergenerational dynamics. Guilt operates within the meta-realm of a metaphoric ledger and is connected to merit and responsibility. Irresponsible behaviour harms the validity of the ledger and causes distrust. Healing and reparation of the hurt human order of justice, is essentially an ingredient of therapy and care to the family system. When guilt contributes to stagnation of the dialogue and schismatic disruptions in relationships, healing can only be established by dialogue within a vivid humane encounter. Nagy call this process *rejunction*; *reparation of connections*.

Dialoguing: In search of a common ground for the a priori of relationships

A year later, after his visit to the United States of America in 1957, and his lectures at the Washington School of Psychiatry, an essay of Buber had been published under the title: *What is Common to All?* (included in the publication Buber 1962b; see also Friedman in Buber 1965a). This very unique essay is about Buber's attempt to probe into the common ground and principle for our being human. He linked his thinking to Heraclitus (pre-Socratic Greek philosophy) whom he estimated as the edifice of Western thought (Buber 1965a:79). Heraclitus postulated that the logos is the most common factor (*xunos*) in the constitution of the cosmos (Kirk & Raven 1982:188). The whole cosmos enveloped (gushed forth) and came to pass from this logical principle; all entities came into being according to this *logos* (reason, account). Thus, everything is in flux and subjected to change; everything flows (*panta rhei*). The human spirit or reason partakes in this *logos*.

Buber re-interpreted this logos principle as "the word". The common world order is constituted by a word event, so that even language, communication and all encounters are about the act of "wording". As we speak to one another, we contribute through dialoguing to a common world. The word is in principle the word of an ontic dialogue between "I and Thou".

The ontic dialogue gradually attains the character of a transcendent event as well. Heraclitus' meta-principle of logos played a role in Buber's reference to a kind of *"eternal Thou"* that can be linked to the notion of a world order that contributed to the concept of a common cosmos. The Eternal, only begotten "Thou", is in fact identified with the whole, most comprehensive exponent of the world order. The whole of the cosmic order emanates from this Person as most authentic representation of common *logos* (Buber 1962b:64-65). This common *logos* is a kind of sovereign unifying factor, and beyond logos there is no other mode of transcendence. Logos and cosmos are completed in this pact and contribute to the fact that human beings exist as "a we" in the presence of a divine factor (God). This is more or less the language of faith with its roots in the faith tradition of old Israel.

Although Nagy found Buber's concepts of "common order", "logos" and "dialogue" indeed appealing, he skipped the notion of "Transcendence". Another difference between Nagy and Buber is his introduction of justice as an ethical principle inherent to the character of the common world order. One can, thus, conclude and say that, despite correspondence, there are essential differences between the two. His position can be summed up by the following remark: "I didn't get it from Buber; but Buber gave wording to it" (Nagy & Spark IL; VR/MK 1995). His attempt to link dialogue to "loyalty" and "justice" developed before his contact with Buber. References to Buber are much more indirect, namely through Maurice Friedman's introduction of Buber to psychotherapists. Nagy's interest was much more in Buber's emphasis on dialogue than in Buber, the interpreter of the Bible.

To conclude: Nagy's affinity for Buber is to be traced back to Buber's emphasis on the a priori of relationships. This a priori with its link to justice is intimately related to the factor of guilt and guilt feelings in our human existence. Guilt and guilt feelings are not merely about external, moralistic projections or intrapsychic feelings. It is even not evoked by a kind of judging caretaker; the guilt is about an ontic conscience and existential condition; in fact, it is a being quality. It is to this ontic factuality that Nagy connects his notion of intergenerationality and responsibility, as well as the consequences thereof for "relational ethics". "In this sense loyalty pertains to what Buber called "the order of the human world" (Nagy & Spark IL:37).

Nagy's appeal on Buber: Basic questions about the status of a "human order of being" and the interplay with "a common order of justice"

It is quite understandable that researchers in theory formation will refer to other professionals in the field. It is evident that Nagy used Buber's thinking to support some of his most basic hypotheses. The question now is whether the appeal on Buber's concepts reflect Buber's intention and paradigmatic frame of reference. It could even be that, due to paradigmatic differences, some of the concepts are not appropriate for the argumentation and theory formation of Nagy. One should therefore indeed question whether the dialogical situation "according to Buber", and Buber's concept of "an order of being", correlate with Nagy's application of the notion of justice to the meta-realm of "a common order of justice".

The following questions need to be posed in order to assess Nagy's application of Buber's dialogical model to his ethical understanding of inter-relational networking (intersubjectivity).

Question one

Buber made a sharp distinction between the "I" within the "I-Thou" dynamic, and the "I" within the "I-It" dynamic. The "It" can also refer to other pronouns as well (Buber 1965:7). The "I-Thou" relationship is immediate and without any mediation. The relationship is established by "the word-event" wherein this voice is making an appeal and is received by means of an act of listening, even in moments of silence.

The question is whether a dialogue is possible without referring to or representing an "*it*": Some-*thing* is always evident and at stake. When somebody speaks, is the act of verbalising not disconnected from the intention and input of the dialogue? Can the *it* be from a lower order as the "*thou*" or even the "I"? If the it is from a lower order than the "thou", even the "thou" could be degraded and reduced to the level of an illusion by the "I," and, thus, become non-essential (De Jong 1971)?

Question two

Nagy wrote: "The family therapist must be able to conceive of a social group whose members all relate to Buber's I-Thou dialogue" (Nagy & Spark IL:43). The problem, however, Buber's "I-Thou" is unmediated and dual. The question now: How does one deal with a social group compiled by diversity and multiple forms of communication, following a zig zag pattern and without being dual? Buber's I-Thou dialogue, consisting of a very definite dual structure of reciprocity, does not make space for a triadic pattern. The fact is, that relationships in social groups are never merely dual, but indeed triadic. Nagy himself indicated that group interaction is about multiple subjective vantage points.

Loyalty is described by Nagy and Krasner as non-dual. "At a minimum, loyalty is a triadic, relational configuration: the preferring one, the preferred one and the one who is not preferred. [...] Loyalty and loyalty conflict are, therefore, difficult to separate" (Nagy & Krasner BGT:418). If the relational context is not predominantly determined by loyalty conflicts, it is paramount that all sides of the interconnected systemic components (*connectedness through consequences*) will be in-calculated and reckoned with (Nagy & Krasner BGT:89). All that are affected should be enclosed: "*Inclusive fair multilaterality*". The therapist should, thus, operate from a "*multi-directed partiality*". The basic argument is: "… no dyadic ledger can be involved in fair give-and-take without consideration given to all those who might be affected through consequences" (Nagy & Krasner BGT:88).

According to Buber, and his understanding of the I-Thou relationships, the dynamics in time and space is not structured by any kind of cohesion. Necessarily, after the ending of the relational event, the Thou should emerge in the form of an "It". For Nagy, however, a family is desperately in need of cohesion in time and space. The cohesion is established in time, because members are companions within temporal conjunctions. Members share space with one another, encounters are about concrete settings. Furthermore, what exactly is the shape and form of "It" after the ending of the relational encounter and interactive event?

Question three

Is dialogue merely interrelational without a cause or subject, especially in family interaction? The relationships in Nagy's theory are mediated relationships. The people in Nagy's contextual therapy, are interrelated because they do have something in common. According to Nagy, the dialogue is fundamentally about the maintenance of justice. Nagy postulated "justice" as a common ground for dealing with the ethical dimension of intergenerational interaction. Justice is the paradigmatic framework for the understanding of "the dimension of relational ethics". Facts, feelings and interactions are interpreted within a hermeneutic of juridical fairness: One needs to act in a trustworthy and right way. Justice needs to be done within all circumstances. The following "sub-terms" support Nagy's ethical approach to relational interaction: "Accountability", "reliability", "acknowledgement", "entitlement", "merit", "due", "recompensation", "loyalty", "legacy" and "exoneration".

Question four

It is clear that Nagy's emphasis is not so much on authenticity, but on a *"genuine dialogue"*, informed and directed by justice. Can his ethical model be merged with the ontic model of Buber? More fundamental than "genuineness", is the quest for justice and the ethical responsibility to acknowledge one another.

It is indeed the case, that in close relationships the dialogue can become stuck (stagnation). The reason: Damage (hurt) in the quality of the interaction due to injustice, improper perceptions and fixed images of the other. The skewed image becomes a fixed perception that determines the dynamic of *self*-understanding. These images become destructive filters, determining true observation and trustworthy experiences.

What is the reason that images become destructive? According to Nagy and Krasner: The images block the authenticity of relationships. It damages the trustworthiness of relationships.

On condition that one takes into consideration that relationships are fundamentally determined by ethics, and that the factor of justice is not becoming ignored or minimalised, Buber's quest for genuineness, could be accommodated in contextual therapy. How? Because self-acknowledgement and family dynamics are also about processes of "self-delineation" and "self-validation". For the latter, authenticity and genuineness is important in order to deal with Nagy's emphasis on accountability and therapy. Authenticity is imperative in order to attain intergenerational balance, merit and fairness.

Question five

With reference to Buber's emphasis on reciprocity and mutuality of cross-identification in the between of "I-Thou", what is the position and status of the subject before the reciprocal dialogue; that is, the status of the subject at the beginning of the interaction; the subject as instigator of reciprocal acknowledgement? Subjects establish and cause intersubjectivity; everybody is subject in the process. What is the disposition of this subject, irrespective of reciprocity? Who am I, and what is the ontic quality when I pronounce the "Thou"? This question is unanswered in Buber's dialogical reciprocity.

Question six

The basic hunch of the researchers is that Buber's "between" (the realm and space of the between) differs from Nagy's interactional between. Nagy's model is determined by ethics, and in fact, regulated by a lawful ledger. Such a regulating factor is not possible in Buber's reciprocal model. The dynamics in the "I-Thou" event is momentary and only accessible for those involved in the duality of the encounter.

"An order of being" is not per se also "a just human order". The "being order" and the "justice order" are not identical. And this dissonance is the main objection to Nagy's appeal on Buber's ontic model for reciprocity.

It is the same with a universal declaration of human rights. The human rights do not exist in terms of an ontic reality. What exists is merely a declaration or statement that needs affirmation and consent. One has indeed a human "right"; that is, the right to claim a humane space in the realm of being. This right corresponds with an obligation to adhere to a basic form of free expression without the danger to become manipulated or degraded to the status of an object; the danger namely: The purpose justifies the means, but in the meantime the subjectivity of the I is totally violated (Levinas 1994:266). This is the reason why one should differentiate between an "order of being" (an ontic status) and a "justice order" (a regulation with obligations). To make an appeal on Buber's being model, and still to maintain the notion of legal obligations, becomes virtually impossible.

Question seven

Is the realm of the "between" a neutral space or indeed regulated by ethical concerns and an interconnectedness that is guided by different modes of loyalty and commitments?

For Nagy, the "realm of the between" is portrayed by legal terminology. In the publication *Invisible Loyalties* (1973), the notion of "loyalty" is a vital ingredient of "the between-space". In *Between Give and Take* (1986), "the realm of the between" is approached from the perspective of connectedness itself. Loyalty and interconnectedness are not neutral entities. Interconnectedness is a differentiated concept and attains ethical substance within the dynamics of guilt-and-obligation. At stake, is the quest for care. Connectedness attains meaning and provides meaning due to the qualification of justice. The question regarding the status of the I, is determined by this qualification of justice. The status of the I, is qualified by Nagy's basic choice for the motivational layer for hope and reparation of hurt human justice; "… we have felt that it is more important to explore the motivational layer in which hope resides for repairing the hurt human justice" (Nagy & Spark IL:53).

The realm of the between can be portrayed as the dynamics of legal regulations while intersubjectivity is qualified by justice. And the latter, is only possible due to the fact that subjects exist with the ability to promote justice, to repair injustice, and to instil hope for fair treatment. The fact is, subjects owe one another justice. This indebtedness is the prerogative of the subject. Within this status of indebtedness and rendering one another justice, the subject is differentiated and profiled as an "I" – the separation of individuation. This differentiated and unique position of the person in the non-duality of intersubjectivity should, thus, be researched further.

Levinas and Buber: The discourse about dialoguing within the ground structure of subject-responsibility

The outline on Martin Buber's "I-Thou" approach, made one thing clear: To enter the field and landscape of reciprocal human encounters, and to step into the dialogical space of "a dynamic between" wherein the other appears as a constitutive partner for the quality and meaning of our being human, even for our identity as a unique entity (differentiation, individuation, self-acknowledgment), are to immigrate into a new and foreign territory without knowing beforehand that the landscape is rough and tough. This is more or less the warning of Levinas (TO:159). When one enters the landscape of an intimate society ("*une société intime*") and encounter one's fellow human being (neighbour as co-partner in coexistence), one discovers "a third" ("*un tiers*") (a third factor outside the close space of intimacy). This "third factor" is immediately also a fellow human being (my neighbour). Then the challenging question about righteousness and justice surfaces as a primordial and ontic imperative (Levinas EN:30-38).

Already in one of his early essays, Emmanuel Levinas (*Le Moi et la Totalité* 1954)[12] wrote that the notion of a very close and intimate society beholds a

---

12 Cited as EN Paris 1991; Dutch translation: Baarn 1994 (To), or even in Baarn 1978 (4) (MG).

kind of existential secret, a clandestine atmosphere that lurks in many modes of dualities. Suddenly there is the mystical appearance of a third factor. This is the reason why the relationship between I and you should not become so exclusive and absolute that there is no space for "the third". It could happen that the I is so embraced by the you, that they become like two spouses in a romantic encounter, detached from the outer world. Since the appearance of "the third" disturbs this romantic exclusiveness and poses the question of justice; "the third" challenges and demands critical reflection.

It is against this background that one needs to read Levinas' critiques on Buber. Despite Levinas' critical stance, he had a huge admiration for Buber's work. Levinas clearly stated that everybody who has the courage to enter Buber's territory, owes Buber some respect even if you get lost in his "I-Thou" dialogical landscape. One needs therefore to acknowledge Buber's contribution to the interplay between dialectics and dialoguing.

In 1963, with the commemoration of Buber's birthday (85 years), a *"Festschrift"* (a collection of essays to honour Buber), was published by Kohlhammer (Stuttgart 1963, English edition; Schlipp & Friedman 1967). In the English edition, there is a contribution by Levinas under the title: "*Martin Buber and the Theory of Knowledge* (Levinas in Schilpp & Friedman 1967:133-150). The essay deals with the question about theories for knowledge (epistemology). He argues that a theory on knowledge should be rendered as theory of the processes of knowing by and through the cognitive dimension of the human mind. It is the reflecting subject that probes into the realm of truth with the endeavour to understand and grasp what truth is about.

In this article, Levinas points out that truth in Buber's approach is not merely a rational or cognitive content; it is not an object of the knowing mind within the knowing subject. Thus, the reason why language and words cannot capture the essence of truth. Truth is always subjective. According to Levinas, Buber's intention is not to pose that everybody has his/her own truth. Buber's approach differs totally from idealistic subjectivism and positivistic rationalism, namely that the essence of being is determined by the cognitive dimension of the human mind: *I think therefore I am* (*cogito ergo sum*). On the contrary, truth is more subjective than all modes of subjectivity. It is extremely important that this ultimate exponent of subjectivity should totally be distinguished from the idealistic and postivistic interpretation of the subject (subjectivism). An ultimate mode of subjectivity provides a very unique entrance to the realm of objectivity; it opens up a kind of ultra-objectivity that is even more objective than the objectivity provided by the object-subject split of rationalism. It renders entrance to a dimension and realm of life that a subject can never fully comprehend, namely the entrance to that which is absolutely and wholly different (Levinas NP:31).

For Levinas, Buber is an exponent of contemporary philosophy. It is the new paradigm of existential encounters and relational dynamics that brings about a total brake with causal thinking and the explanatory model of metaphysical speculation. The certitude and firmness (ontic dimension) of the human I, is now displayed by the interactional and reciprocal dynamics of relationships within contextual human encounters. Within these encounters, the "I" looses (gives away) its prefixed substantiality; it is released from being encapsulated by itself. The "I" in Buber's dialogical model is not a separateness: The "I" in and on itself[13]. With Buber, the relationship precedes the "I"; in the beginning is the relationship.

According to Levinas' interpretation of Buber, the dynamics of dialogical relationships are about the following paradigm shift: From the traditional philosophical subject-object split with the dualistic separation of truth (meta-realm) and being, to relational thinking within the concrete setting of existential relationships; it is from the ontological realm, with the corresponding question: How can a limited and finite human being reach and embrace the eternal, infinite and authentic truth?, to the realm of relational ethics; it is about the shift from causal thinking to the contextuality of social dynamics. Truth (existential, personal truth) is embedded in the social interaction of a reciprocal between: Person-to-person exchange. The dynamics of "I-Thou" constitutes authentic being. Truth is not anymore about verification (classic mode of positivistic rationalism), but about existential hermeneutics. The realm of the between is predominantly accessible for the two interacting entities involved. Truth is not about the content of the analytical and rational human mind, because truth will then be reduced and objectified to the realm of "I-It". The dynamics of truth is rather established within the actuality of an "I-Thou" dynamic. This subjective dimension

---

13 "*Le moi humain n'est pas un sujet qui constitue, il est l'articulation de la rencontre*"; the human ego [thus Buber] is not a subject that is constituted in and by itself (on its own); it is being articulated in and by the encounter (Levinas NP:37, in a rather disapproving interpretation of Buber's work).

should strongly be differentiated from the impersonal realm of "I-It". The relationship precedes the "I"; the starting point and origin is the relationship (Levinas NP:37).

This paradigm shift from a mechanistic and rationalistic objectification, to the existential dynamics of relationships, is indeed a dramatic progress and advantage. The emphasis is now on existential realities and intersubjectivity. However, to reduce the unpredictable dynamics of relational interaction to the confines of a reciprocal "I-Thou between", is not unproblematic. The paradigm shift of Buber implies for Levinas that truth becomes an exclusive relational matter within the reciprocity and actuality of an "I" and "thou" encounter. Levinas' critique on such an exclusive inter-space, boils down to the following:

(a) Truth is now reduced to a formal event between two dual poles. This formalisation should be linked to the fact that the encounter is in fact volatile and without real content. The "I-Thou" relation is merely a happenstance without real cause and direction. The core of Levinas' critical argument is that "truth" remains merely an ontic status of being – authentic being (Levinas NP:42). This reduction implies that Buber's ethics is formal and shallow despite the ethical elements attached to the "I-Thou" encounter. A further critical aspect is the fact that Buber connects "I-Thou" with transcendence. Being becomes determined and comprehended by the "Eternal Thou". The central question prevails: Can transcendence, without a connection to content (dogmatic theses and doctrine) still be qualitative enough to function as a meta-realm that is open to the dynamics of relationships? (Levinas NP:43). In other words, can there, without the dimension of "height" (vertical perspective) and "depth" (foundational perspective) in the "I-Thou" relationship, still be place and space for a dynamic and open interpretation of transcendence?

(b) The further problem is that every encounter is merely momentarily, unique and a separate event. It happens suddenly and abrupt like a spark and "bolt from the blue" within a moment, without continuity and sustainable history. For Buber, only the world of "It" possesses in space and time, order and coherence. The realm of the "Thou" has in space and time no order or coherence (Buber 1965:37). The implication is that the "I-Thou" dynamics is ahistorical and surpasses the concrete realm of word and language. The impact, however, is that truth becomes inexplicable[14].

(c) The spear point of Levinas' critique on Buber, is his emphasis on the reciprocal character of the "I-Thou" relationship. For Levinas, the question boils down to the following: Is it possible to explain the otherness of the other without importing merely a paradoxical plateau-difference between the "I" and "Thou"? Reciprocity is reduced to an exclusive intimate I-Thou interaction, without multi-partiality: I am in becoming, exclusively in, and via, the relationship with "Thou", and vice versa – it does not even matter whether from right to left, or from left to right. The impression is left that an outside factor operates like an external spectator, watching the reciprocal encounter from above (objective, analytical viewpoint). The happenstance is exclusively only approachable for the two involved (two insiders). The further implication is that the "I" (me experience) of the "I" (constitutive I) that is in becoming within the "I-Thou" event, also becomes an outsider and spectator that can oversee the happenstances within the event of encounter. Buber, thus, attains a double position: One becomes an "I" in the reciprocity with "you", but one is at the same time, also an "I" that can oversee the event between the "I" and the "Thou".

The problem in a nutshell: The philosophical "I" of Buber synchronises the two, into an encapsulated reciprocity.

The intriguing question should, thus, be posed: Is the reciprocal relationship that one can read either from right to left, and vice versa, as well as the fact that the two concepts, as well as the applied terminology, are virtually more or less the same, still be called an ethical relationship? Despite the fact that Buber describes the "I-Thou" relationship in ethical terminology, Levinas still questions its validity.

For Levinas, the appropriate ethical relationship is one wherein the other

---

14 See Levinas (NP:43): "*Peut-être cette façon de voir tientelle aussi au libéralisme relgieux de Buber, à sa religiosité opposée à la religion, plaçant [...] le contact au-dessus de son contenu, la presence pure et inqualifiable e Dieu au-dessus de tout dogme et de toute règle*". In a more paraphrased translation, it means that the reason for the description of the ahistorical position of "I-Thou", is Buber's more liberal stance over against traditional religiosity, namely his opposition to a mode of religion that places contact above its content with the implication that the presence of God becomes inexplicable, even above dogma and any doctrinal formulation.

stands at the same time higher than the "I", but also lower than the "I", being less important. This is essentially the core and paradoxical difference between the two levels of existence. The otherness of the Other, exists in the fact that the other is much more exposed (poorer), much more deprived than the me of the I. This is not about attributes or relative characteristics of an accidental other. "Higher", "poorer", and the fact of "being much more deprived", are for Levinas descriptive categories to explain the otherness of the other. "Higher", "poorer" and "much more deprived", portray the otherness of the other.

The ethical relationship between "me" and "you", is not constituted by the authenticity of being, or the ontic validity of the between, because then the ethical relationship is primarily an ontic relationship of being and not in principle an ethical one. The ethical relationship can only start, and take exclusively root in "me", within my existential situation, earthliness, materiality, because the otherness of the Other, possesses a dimension of "height": "You" differentiated from merely "thou" ("*Vous*" and not "*Tu*"). The otherness of the other invites me into a vivid discussion.

The reason for Levinas' critique on Buber, is that he (Levinas) wants to align the I, from the start, as being responsible. This position should be maintained from the beginning. The responsibility is not a consequence of the relationship. There is not firstly the relationship and thereafter responsibility. The ethical relationship is the irrevocable responsibility of the one over against the other; it is a relationship wherein the terminology is not mutually exchangeable; it is not reciprocal and not simultaneous. Responsibility is a position of oneself; a position sui generis. This position is more or less an investiture.

What is meant by a position of self-hood that is at the same time an investiture?

Levinas indicates with the notion of investiture, the venture of becoming; the becoming of the subject, (the subjectivity of our being human). The latter does not start with the subject in itself, but from the other with whom I share his/her destiny. I don't start within a nominative case, but in the accusative: The me-voice (*Me voiçi, Here I am*) is the starting point. The Other challenges me to start thinking about myself, and evokes my-*self*, in taking responsibility for my-self. A human being is in fact on his/her own. That I am a being in and for my-self, is established within a process of subjectification (on becoming an I). Subjectification does not occur merely due to the boomerang effect of the pronoun "you". And this is the problem with Buber's position: He underestimates the irrevocable character of being a subject in and for my-*self* (autonomous subjectivity) (Levinas DTA:62).

In fact, it is impossible for the human being to forget his/her subjectivity. Our being a subject, is not an imperative a posteriori or a moral aftermath. On becoming a subject is an avatar, a metamorphosis. The "I", before the (I-Thou) encounter, is within the happenstance, or thereafter, never again the same. Thus, the importance of a total new philosophical paradigm when one wants to detect the truth of intersubjectivity. One needs a total new paradigm switch, namely to a dialogical mode of thinking. In this model the impetus is in the first place not the concern for the relationship. Primarily at stake, is the longing to safeguard the independence of the "I" within the structure of interconnectedness.

Summary of critical aspects

Buber did not take the separation and individuation of the I (differentiation) from the total whole seriously enough. An ethical relationship presupposes the irrevocable responsibility of the I. It can only be established in and by myself.

The I-Thou relationship, as an ethical relationship, is an access of the me, into the space of the other, in his/her bare simplicity, nakedness, poorness and hunger. It is not about an esoteric or spiritual friendship. One needs to ask oneself, whether the clothing of the other and the feeding of hungry people are not by far the most concrete access to the other (Levinas NP:48). Ethics is not merely formal; it is also material. It touches the material, as well as the bodily needs of a human being. If not, the all comprehensive "Thou" is becoming an esoteric phantom. Buber seems to be rather more a word-artist than dealing with the hardcore realities of daily living in his theory of relationships (Levinas NP:48).

The I that comes into being by, and through, the "Thou", should inevitably receive personal knowledge about him/herself; should necessarily have to reflect about the cosmos and reality. In other words, it seems quite incomprehensible that Buber accepted so easily the hypothesis that in the ground word (I-It), the "It" can be substituted by "she" or "he, without changing the meaning of this ground word. Philosophising, and to reflect on the character of truth, are perhaps exactly a most needed breach with undifferentiated participation in the totality of the whole. When you ignore this separatedness, then you run into danger to forget your subjective avatar[15] – a kind of metamorphosis and painful transformation.

In an article about Buber (1968: *La Pensée de Martin Buber et le Judaisme Contemporain*), Levinas (HS:15-33) made anew some positive remarks on Buber's contribution. However, he also criticised him, and accused him of applying a total German paradigm within the tradition of religious liberalism of the nineteenth century. He approaches the Hebrew text, without taking into consideration the Rabbinic tradition of Talmudic literature that deals with the text in the history and creative Jewish tradition (Levinas HS:26).

One should understand the paradigmatic background of Levinas' criticism. It is about the intriguing question: What are all the conditions for one's ability, the capacity of the subject, to act in a just and trustworthy manner within the confers of intersubjectivity. Justice needs to be done under all circumstances. In order to promote this perspective, Levinas digs deep into the philosophical and Hebrew tradition of the Bible. In a nutshell, his attempt is to maintain and promote the independent status of the subject.

In the volume *Noms Propres* (Levinas 1963), Buber's response to Levinas' critique is incorporated. For Buber, the critical remarks hurt him, and were indeed painful. He wrote that Levinas made a huge mistake in his interpretation. The "I-Thou" relationship is not volatile; it is not about a spiritual friendship as Levinas thought. The relationship attains its grandeur and spiritual power, when two human persons (who are not like-minded, belonging to different, even to totally opposing spiritual families) despite these discrepancies, and even in fierce controversies, orient themselves (the one over against the other) in such a way that the one acknowledges, intends, identifies, permits the other as this person in the here and now. It is exactly in this kind of encounter, that one discovers true human companionship and true communality (Levinas NP:52).

Immediately, Levinas responded in a letter (incorporated in *Noms Propres* 1976). He made the profound statement: To say "Thou", is about *giving*; it is established through and with my whole body. To converse and to talk, are instantly about embodiment. The latter implies more than physical organs (physiology and biology); it is about corporeal existence and a unique entity. Furthermore, my personal embodiment/corporeal existence is a pre-condition

---

15 See Nijhoff 1964:215-223; D Kroon 1981.

and about a possibility, prior to the appeal on my responsibility for the well-being of the other – the other in his/her inhumane predicament (hunger, poverty, nakedness). Exactly, because one *is* one's body, one can become a brother/sister for the other. Brotherhood/sisterhood is through and by the brother/sister, and not due to freedom of choice. The word as responsible answer is my concern, my responsibility. The Other as Other is always the poor and vulnerable, but at the same time my superior. The relationship is, thus, always asymmetric.

According to Levinas, the starting point is not the eventual reciprocity that could even under certain conditions be about justice, but my existential embodiment as enfleshment of sheer acts of responsibility.

One should always keep in mind, that Levinas' approach is about a phenomenological description of intersubjective responsibility, built upon an analysis of living in this world. The "I" lives out its embodied existence according to modalities that feature as concrete presentations of responsibility and proof of the fact that the "I" respond indeed. It consumes the fruits of the world. It enjoys and suffers from natural elements. It constructs shelters and dwellings. It carries on the social and economic transactions of its daily life. Yet life entails "more", and this more portrays the "*meta*-realm[16] of subjectivity". Levinas does not use this term so much, but the implication is that no event is as effectively disruptive for a conscious holding sway in its world than the encounter with another person.

Encountering the humane but vulnerable space of the other, can be called spiritual indeed. In this encounter (even if it later becomes competitive or instrumental), the "I" experiences firstly itself as being called (predestined), and liable to account for itself. It responds. The response of the "I", is

---

[16] "*Meta*" refers to the fact that life, even human encounters, human experiences entails more than what can be observed by the human senses. *Meta* as an indication of "the more" in life, implies that there are determining factors and dimensions in relational interaction that are not immediately and directly "visible" for the human eye; they are in this sense "invisible". Invisibility is not about a "beyond" as principles for causative and rationalistic explanations regarding the essence of being as in for example traditional ontology, or as in the case of Platonic metaphysics. It is an indication of the fact that the realm of transcendence does play a role in the significance of our being human (transcending direct experiences of observation). With reference to the role of norms, values, philosophical ideas, belief systems, religious thinking in life events, this *meta*-realm plays a decisive role in the human quest for meaning and human dignity. It is even possible to use the concept of "spirituality" as an indication of the "more", *meta*-realm, in life (explanation by translator).

as response, a reaction to a more or less nebulous command: With all your heart! – "affective self-positing".

There is no direct indication that the other gave a *de facto* command. The command, or summons, is part of the intrinsic relationality. With the response (re-*spond*-ability), comes the beginning of language as dialogue. For Levinas, the origin of authenticity is always about a response; an act of responding to and for the other; one is summoned to respond. Dialogue arises ultimately through that response. Herein resides the root of intersubjectivity; intersubjectivity as lived immediacy. In other words, responsibility is the affective, immediate experience of "transcendence" and "fraternity" – indicators of what one can call: the *meta*-realm of engagement with the other. This engagement takes place within the vulnerable space of the other; encounter as a "spiritual" category; as a face-to-face meeting with visage (the other as subject: Being-there and available). In the face of the other, the "I" discovers its own vocation. The expression of the face is interrogative and imperative. This imperative says, "do not kill me". It also implores the "I", who eludes this "saying" only with difficulty. Nevertheless, the command and supplication occur, because human faces (the visage) impact on us as affective moments, or, what Levinas calls "interruptions".

In order to explain what one can call the "spiritual character" (interruptive character) of encountering moments, Levinas turned to *The Midrash text*. The *meta*-realm of the text (*bekol me'odéka*, Deut 6:5), helped him to explain how the command, namely being called and summoned to enact in a responsible mode, reframes the meaning of subjectivity. The point he wants to illustrate, is that being carries on as continuous presence within the sequence of many encounters with the other. The face-to-face encounter inflects itself toward the possibility of responsibility and hospitality (the *meta*-realm of subjective responsibility).

The meta-realm of subjectivity: "Mammon" (bekol me'odéka)[17] *as an embodied soulful investment in life*

Levinas' remark on the Hebrew text of Deuteronomy 6:5 entails more than merely being a concern for a correct philological translation of the ground

---

17 The following outline is a somewhat changed version of an article written by Van Rhijn 1995.

text. At stake, is the meaning of the word *me'od*. Taking as a substantive, it is actually a hapax. It is only here in Deuteronomy 6:5 that it appears. The text is quoted in 2 Kings 23:25: "Neither before nor after Josiah was there a king like him who turned to the LORD as he did—with all his heart and with all his soul and with all his strength (*me'od*), in accordance with all the Law of Moses." In other places where *me'od* is used, the word functions as adverb. It can then be translated with strong, very much, great.

In ancient Aramaic translations of the *tanakh*[18] (*Targum Onkelos*), *Bekol me'odéka* is translated with: *bekol niksak*. The Aramaic word *nekes* refers traditionally to a herd of cattle. Later it was used for "possession", wealth, account or treasure of the king. One can accept that in the first century, it was used for financial purposes like financial reserves, financial abilities, or financial transactions. *Me'od* had been used within material contexts; things like possessions could be described in terms of material value like money.

A century later, *The Mishna* used *bekol mamonèka* for *bekol me'odéka* (Berachot 9:5). Within this context it was translated as: With all your mammon; that is, with all your money. Rasji, in his commentary on the Mishna version (circa 1100), took this Mishna explanation over. He argued that there were many people who loved their money more than their life/soul (*nēfĕsh*).

One can accept that this argument is not about sheer moralism, or merely irony. It is more about a factual declaration: For many people, it is indeed the case that they devote their life/soul/vitality to the spending of their money, or to make financial gain. In fact, it is not so strange that people spend their life/soul/vitality to make money, or to make financial investments. In fact, it is not so strange to think about moneymaking of financial investments as modes of being a subject, especially, in our global rat race for material gain and financial achievements.

When one translates this commandment in the Shema within the tradition of the rabbis, and its hermeneutical context, it is quite understandable

---

18 *Tanakh*- the Jewish scriptures which consist of three divisions--the Torah and the Prophets and the Writings. *Tanakh* is an acronym of the first Hebrew letter of each of the Masoretic Text's three traditional subdivisions: Torah ("Teaching", also known as the Five Books of Moses), Nevi'im ("Prophets") and Ketuvim ("Writings")—hence TaNaKh. It is related to the Targum Onkelos. Targum Onkelos (or Onqelos), סולקנוא םוגרת, is the official eastern (Babylonian) targum (Aramaic translation) to the Torah. According to Jewish tradition, the content of Targum Onkelos was originally conveyed by God to Moses at Mount Sinai. However, it was later forgotten by the masses, and recorded by Onkelos.

why Levinas preferred to translate *bekol me'odéka* in financial and material terminology, namely as money making/money spending/powerful wealth[19].

It is quite remarkable that in many modern translations of the Bible, *bekol me'odéka* is translated with equivalents of power. Even the Septuagint translates it with *ischus*. Other translations are: "Power", "force", "might" and "strength". Buber and Rosenzweig considered financial capacity/wealth/material assets or gain. Eventually, they rejected this material framework, and decided on "power". It becomes clear that the preference is for energetic and emotional categories. In our postmodern context, it points in the direction of zest for life; the powerful input of the free, democratic subject as operational agent for magnificent achievements.

Albeit, whether it is with my "mammon" or my "body", "I" am obliged and under the imperative of the law (Levinas) to treat the other (*Autrui*) as my "master" and "lord". Thus, the reason why I should act in all inter-human relationships with justice and dignity. If not, I am guilty and could be fined. The meaning of "money"/ "mammon" is therefore primarily to be determined by its functioning within the realm of intersubjectivity; that is, mammon as meta-category (righteousness), promoting the dignity of the other. The intersubjectivity precedes my being a subject. Intersubjectivity could be for better (good) or for worse (bad). "Good", for humans, come to pass often in the mode of triviality. Nevertheless, the good enhances the significant and humane meaning of the other (human well-being). In this sense, responsibility and generosity become visible in human affairs.

Albeit, intersubjectivity is not vague, empty or neutral. For sure, it is not "spiritual" in the sense of transcendental metaphysics. "For me", mammon indicated that "I" do not exist on and for my own benefit. From the start, "I" am connected to the order of intersubjectivity. This order of intersubjectivity refers to a non-reciprocal, asymmetric mode of coexistence with the other. With my "mammon/possessions", I can inflict evil or good (see in this regard the parable of the unjust steward/treasurer in Luke 16:1-9). The inter-subjective order wherein I am connected to the other, can only flourish

---

19 See in this regard, the memoirs of a German, Jewish mother and business woman *Glikl Hamel* (1645-1724) (Amsterdam 1987). She understood *bekol me'odéka* as reference to all one's possessions, and this implies: with all your money. Thus, the reason why one should not save your money for your children. You are in fact responsible for yourself, your own neighbour, and should, thus, spend your money with responsibility in service to God.

within the indicative of a justice order. This is the reason why mammon should become under the commandment of the "poor other", an investment in the humane quality of life.

With my "mammon" and "body" I am re-*spond*-able and responsible. Responsibility is not anymore about personal competence, or the exercising of power/ego-strength. Ability/capacity and power are about stewardship: Stewardship and servitude put the "I" on the "throne" of subjectivity. Even "mammon/money" connects me to the other, and that is part and parcel of the powerful command to love God!

According to the researchers, to translate *bekol me'odéka* with "power", is not to reckon with the paradigmatic background of the Talmud. One should not "spiritualise" the text and ignore the direct, and very powerful material meaning of religious and faithful actions like "eating" and exercising love. One should love God also with one's money (*"Ah! Le matérialisme juif!"*. When paraphrased: "Viva the profound realism of Jewish materiality"; Levinas HS:33).

These critical questions resonate with Nagy's attempts to link ethics with a relational model: The subject as container, and representative of the ethical imperative, but, then in such a way, that the human I, the subject, is not the autonomous and final decision-maker about what is good and what is bad (injustice).

In the next chapter, the quest for ethics and the link between justice and intersubjectivity, will be addressed. It is therefore paramount to give more attention to Levinas. Thereafter, it will be possible to return to Nagy in order to detect thoroughly what is the status of the subject in Nagy's thinking. It will then be possible to critically compare Nagy's view with Levinas' philosophical stance.

CHAPTER 4

"The silent partner" and the founding of subjectivity (the subject) within the theoretic discourse between Nagy and Levinas

The topic of this chapter should be read in conjunction with the central phrase in Nagy's theoretical oevre: The context of a human order of justice and its connection to the notion of transgenerational interaction. As an ethical category, transgenerationality describes a kind of solidarity. Thus, the concept of transgenerationality as "silent partner" to intergenerational relationships (Nagy and Krasner BGT:98). This "silent partner" should play a fundamental role in the grounding and status of subjectivity.

In the dynamics of dialogue, silence is not the starting point and therefore first. First is the initiative to start speaking. Therefore, silence as mode of speech is prior. As an act, silence functions as a kind of genesis.

With "silent partner" (Nagy & Krasner TGN:122) is not meant an abstract concept. It should be understood personally. The "silent partner" is actively contributing to the whole endeavour of trustworthy interconnectedness (intersubjectivity); the other as a kind of "hidden ally" in significant human encoubters. The other as partner invests in the undertaking of interconnectedness and responding encounters according to merit. Eventually the "silent partner" even partakes in possible losses and eventual bankruptcy.

The preference for "silent partner" serves as an example of Nagy's heuristic search for a formula, that can serve as source for subjectivity and indicator of authentic origin. "Silent partner" also corresponds with Levinas' expression: "The voice of silence" (Levinas HAM:32; TO:80; 1991:71). This voice articulates truth that is manifested in humbleness. In the background of his mind, was I Kings 19. Elijah sat under a broom bush in the desert. He sat down under it and prayed that he might die. Then the profound revelation in verses 12-13: "Go out and stand on the mountain in the presence of the LORD, for the LORD is about to pass by."

"Then a great and powerful wind tore the mountains apart and shattered the rocks before the LORD, but the LORD was not in the wind. After the wind there was an earthquake, but the LORD was not in the earthquake (12). After the earthquake came a fire, but the LORD was not in the fire. And after the fire came a gentle whisper (13). When Elijah heard it, he pulled his cloak over his face and went out and stood at the mouth of the cave" (NIV).

The voice of the other, operates in terms of a gentle whisper that sounds in fact as a kind of silent speech. It stirs a sound conscientiousness and therefore needs an ethical framework that founds subjectivity.

The status of the subject: Grounded in ethics

Levinas' critique on Buber is about the notion of reciprocity within the "I-Thou relationship". Problematic is the fact that the relationship is assessed from a kind of "above"; *meta*-perspective above the relationship. This above, takes on the character of a synchronising perspective. The implication is that the subject becomes neglected. Within the ontological status of the "between", the relating poles tend to disappear. Even the subject loses his/her independent status and eventually evaporates.

The "I-Thou-relationship" is ethically speaking void. And the reason for this is that Buber does not refer to a coherence factor. In fact, within space and time, there is no indication of any kind of order linked to the "I-Thou" dynamics. The relationship has no duration and clear profile; it is like a mirage disappearing in the air.

It is now important to pose the question whether Nagy's notion of an ethical dimension addresses and could eventually overcome the shortcomings in Buber's model.

In the light of these critical remarks, another question surfaces: Is the encounter per se about human well-being? Can one still maintain: "Healing through meeting" (*Heilung aus der Begegnung*), despite the shortcomings in the "I-Thou encounter"?

The "ethical dimension" requires a definition of the subject wherein the surfacing of ethics is about an original event, and therefore not the result, or by-product of factors defined and formulated by psychology or social psychology. To ground ethics in the "I-Thou", or even the "between" of Buber, is not to be maintained. The reason: Because from the start there is no ethical subject. The subject-poles just evaporate in the relationship. Without an ethical subject, prior to the relationship, the whole ethical construction of a just human order in Nagy's approach, will be destroyed.

The decisive question: Is there any reference in Nagy's model to a subject that represents ethics as proposed by Levinas? Ethics then as a category sui generis, and a kind of commandment that cannot be reduced to something else (irreducible). Therefore, the responsibility of the "I" for the other, does not start at first with the reciprocity.

The implicit critique of Levinas on the dialogical model, is about the fact that the "I-Thou relationship" is anchored outside the society, and, thus, attains a clandestine character. The point is: A subject always exists within the society, and the other is always *in* the society. The consequence is that there is always a third factor, the other, that falls outside the exclusivity of the "I-Thou relationship". The problem with Buber's "I-Thou" is that it is only accessible for the two interacting poles, while the third other is ignored and in fact absent. "I-Thou" is never clandestine. The third factor, the other, is always involved. Especially, when encounters are essentially about "split loyalty" (Nagy).

With reference to the further exposition, it is paramount to turn to the meaning and content of the concept "subject" in Levinas' thinking.

We now turn to the second phase of the research project: What is meant by "subject" in Nagy's theory formation? What is meant by subjectivity? Does Nagy succeed to maintain the independent status of the relating poles in the encounter, or are they dissolved by the event of encounter?

Furthermore: What is the intention and purpose of Nagy's appeal on Buber? The question is valid, because Nagy's anthropology is built on the thesis that the ethical dimension is intrinsically connected to an order of justice. And it is because of this founded ethical basis, that Buber's model cannot fully carry Nagy's contextual therapy. It only covers Nagy's argument partially. In this respect, Levinas' critique on Buber opens space for Nagy's notion of a "genuine dialogue", supported not by an external authority, but by justice.

The attractiveness of Buber for Nagy resides in the fact that Buber wants to maintain the irreducible character of the relational reality, as well as the unicity of the human person. For Nagy, help and caregiving, are not strictly individual. On the other hand, Nagy refused the temptation to reduce the personal realm to the totality of functions within a trans-personal and neutral system.

"In our view, transactional patterning remains a formal and shallow therapeutic framework if it fails to allow for the *simultaneous coexistence of several individuals' rights and motives*. In point of fact, every relating person responds from the reality of his or her separate and distinct biological life. There is a discrete existential realm in which people are born by themselves, live for themselves and, perforce, die by themselves. […] What useful assumptions might be made about relationships that can transcend both the psychological reductionism and an absolute "psychic determinism" and the sheer chaotic power confrontation that Sartre[1] seems to imply?" (Nagy & Krasner BGT:32).

The previous reference to Jean-Paul Sartre, indicates that Nagy does not view coexistence as absurd and exposed to total nihilistic negation. Coexistence it not about sheer chaotic power confrontation. Coexistence is for Nagy about living together with people whose existence is intransitive. Every human being is born as a unique entity, one lives and dies on one's own. Nobody can substitute the individual person, and nobody can be born, or will die as substitute for the very being of that person. I cannot even delegate my life and dying to somebody else.

Conceptualisation should maintain both: The fact that life is intransitive, as well as the reality of coexistence. Living together in interconnectedness with other people, should simultaneously preserve the discrete existential realm of every person in his/her differentiation from the other.

---

[1] Nagy refers to Jean-Paul Sartre's *L'être et le Néant*. This is one of the very few places that Nagy refers to the existential phenomenology of French existentialism.

The emphasis on the importance of a specific personalised order, is the reason why Nagy on this point turns to Martin Buber's dialogical paradigm of the "I-Thou-dynamics". "Martin Buber's grasp of the relationship which he termed 'I and Thou' pointed to a paradigm for healing that comes from connectedness itself" (Nagy & Krasner BGT:33). Because "… the self and his or her relating partner create a personalized human order in the realm that exists between an 'I' and a 'Thou'" (Nagy & Krasner BGT:33).

The quest for the option of a coexistence that maintains separation and differentiation of persons without exposing them to "sheer chaotic power confrontation", implies furthermore the question whether it is possible to design an ethics that is anchored in the subject. But then one must reckon with the inability of human beings to maintain their humanity, and the constant failure of human beings to escape the danger of neglecting their humane identity (Levinas 1972:11).

The weak point in Buber's argument is that for him the ethical dimension starts with intersubjectivity and is also founded by intersubjectivity. However, our being human is intransitive and determined by the discrete existential realm of individual separation and differentiation. Power is part of the interaction in human relationships. But then, ethics cannot be founded by intersubjectivity. The attempt to anchor ethics in intersubjectivity will not be able to deal appropriately with Sartre's notion of "sheer chaotic power confrontation".

What needs to be overcome is both the psychological reductionism of psychic determinism, as well as this chaotic power confrontation. For Nagy it is imperative not to follow Buber to the end. The paradigmatic challenge for Nagy is to switch from a theoretic-objectifying discourse, to an ethical discourse. The ethical discourse should be differentiated from the theoretical-objectifying discourse, because the latter inevitably leads to totalitarian power play in epistemological processes of subjective knowing. The danger, however, is that the ethical discourse can easily fall prey to ideology. Eventually it will be virtually impossible to maintain its ethical integrity (De Boer 1991:133).

It was already underlined that cohesion in the realm of the between is not neutral and should be qualified by "justice". Justice remains a systemic force when the appeal for righteousness would not come to the hearing subject from an external, transcendental realm (exteriority). It is displayed in personal encounters face to face. The hunch of the researchers is that this force is indeed extraordinary; it is personal, but not dialogical in the sense of Martin Buber.

Emmanuel Levinas – biographical sketch[2]

Emmanuel Levinas was born in 1906 in the city of Kaunas (in Russian: Kovno), Lithuania, a province in the Russian empire of the tsar. He came from a middle-class Jewish family. From the three boys in the family, he was the eldest and brought up in the Jewish culture and tradition. He spoke Russian and was exposed to Russian literature from quite a young age. Without any doubt, he was influenced by Russian authors like Pushkin, Tolstoy and Dostoyevsky. In this respect, Dostoyevsky's *Brothers Karamazov* made a huge impression on his thinking (see Lescourret 1994:43).

In the understanding of Levinas' philosophy, one should reckon with his Jewish upbringing and background. In the tradition of the so-called Mitnagdim (a former Jewish denomination of opponents of the mysticism and lack of Talmud-study in Chassidism), he developed a sound critical, even scrupulous approach to Jewish texts[3]. Throughout his lifespan, he maintained a critical solidarity with the state Israel, and can be called a Jew in diaspora (Levinas 1968; see also his lectures on the Talmud 1990).

Between World War I and World War II, he was gradually exposed to antisemitism. When the German army invaded the Baltic States (in WW I), his mother fled with the children. Later, his father joined them to settle in Kharkov in the Ukraine. They returned to Lithuania in 1920 and Levinas embarked on an academic career.

It was difficult to become accepted at a university in Germany. Eventually he ended up in the prestigious French university of Strasbourg. He studied philosophy and became involved in what one can call a "spiritual career" (Lescourret 1994:54). He became attached to, for example, Maurice Blanchot

---

2 For detail information on biographical data, see Lescourret 1994. See also *Het menselijk gelaat*, Baarn 1978. The researchers also used data from interviews with Levinas: *Entre nous, essais sur le penser-à-l'autre*, Paris 1991:121-139, 237-243, 253-264. Furthermore, see the memoirs of Elie Wiesel 1994; R Cohen 1994:115-121.

3 Levinas never broke with his Jewish background. There was a time when he became slightly disoriented with Jewish discipline. However, since 1957 he joined the colloquiums of French speaking Jews. He even extensively lectured on the Talmud (*Lectures Talmudiques*) (Levinas 1968).

who later gave his first novel the name of a brother of Emmanuel (see Blanchot 1942) and was quite fascinated by the French life style.

During 1927-1928 he lived in Freiburg-am-Breisgau and started to study the phenomenology of Edmund Husserl and Heidegger's existential philosophy. A new paradigm of thinking illuminated his mind and inspired him to complete his studies with a doctorate on Husserl's phenomenology: *La Théorie de L'intuition Dans la Phénoménologie de Husserl* (*The Theory of Intuition in Husserl's Phenomenology*).

After his marriage with Raïssa Lévi[4], they settled in Paris[5] as an administrator at the school of the *Alliance Israélite Universelle*; an institute devoted to the education of teachers for francophone North Africa. Here he worked for nearly thirty-three years. He became befriended with the philosophers Leon Brunschvicg and Jean Wahl. He attended their lectures, and gradually developed the basic pillars for his philosophical methodology. Eventually, his academic studies contributed to a paradigm shift away from dialectical totalitarism and mechanical causality (Lescourret 1994:85) to a phenomenology of intersubjective responsibility. He became interested in topics like evasion, exodus, passivity and patience. These topics appear in both his philosophical reflections and Jewish essays, as well as in other publications (Lescourret 1994:356).

The previous remark is important. It gives an indication of the fact that Levinas' engagement with the fate and suffering of the Jewish people does not start due to what happened to them during World War II. One should not reduce Levinas' sensitivity for the other to the mere fact that he himself was a victim of war. Levinas' search for a more humane future should not even be explained by the fact that he came from a Jewish background. He was in search of a concrete expression of philosophy, based on a valid methodology, without ignoring the roots of his being human (see introduction by Peperzak, Levinas 1978:12).

After World War II, he became director of the institute: *Alliance Israélite Universelle*. The war indeed had consequences for his philosophical reflection. When pope Pius XI died in March 1939, he wrote a tribute which was

---

4   They had three children. The middle child, a girl, died after a few months. Her name: Andrée Eliane (Lescourret 1994:128). See also Levinas 1947:348.
5   Later, in 1936 he became a French citizen and was proud of his affiliation with the language and culture.

published by the journal of the *Alliance Israélite Universelle* (*Paix et droit*). In this tribute, he clearly revealed his deepest concern about the link between national socialism and brute naturalism.

In 1940 he was captured by the Germans. He became prisoner of war and sent to the concentration camp at Maagdenburg. Despite the awful conditions, Levinas read books from the prison library and started with a study, published in 1947 under the title: *De l'existence à l'existant* (1986) (*From Existence to the Existents*)[6]. He wrestled with the pain of suffering, the threat of loneliness and the human quest for hope regarding a more humane future. Eventually, he became aware of the fact that his parents and two brothers were killed by the Nazis. Other members of his family in Lithuania also suffered and died. With this painful memory, one can understand why Levinas took an oath never to return to Germany again.

Within the contemporary, philosophical discourse, greatly influenced by Jean-Paul Sartre and Martin Heidegger, Levinas' interest in existential philosophy was further stimulated by connections with Gabriël Marcel. He joined a study circle that focused on the publications of Marcel. His interest in existential thinking, and the awareness of the importance of relationships for the shaping of human subjectivity, as well as the place of the other in defining the subjectivity of the human "I", made him aware of totality-thinking in Western philosophy[7]. According to himself he was above all other influences, herefore tributary to Franz Rosenzweig (Levinas TO:23; TI:XVI). He was aware of the possible damage of totalitarianism[8] (centralised authority with dictatorial powers, subordinating all aspects of individual life and freedom to institutional forces) on the human subject and personal identity.

---

6   This publication, Levinas' first original contribution to philosophy, is a research on the problem of the Good, time, and the relationship with the other as a movement toward the Good. It is about moving from anonymous existence to the emergence of subjectivity. This is encountering the other who accompanies the I like a shadow of the self (a kind of duality). In the dialectics of time, the dialectic of the relationship with others is established; that is, the establishment of true dialogue. The Other delivers us and grants us existential forgiveness. With reference to time, hope is important. The acuteness of hope is about the seriousness of the moment. In hope, the very suffering of the moment becomes like a cry; a sound echoing forever through the eternity of spaces.

7   *Totality* in an idealistic sense (predominant in the dialectical philosophy of Marx and Hegel), refers to the premise that a system comprises of internal relationships, or alternatively, an entity that does not relate to anything outside of itself. It is complete in itself and grounded within its own created synthesis.

8   Totalitarianism has links with totality-thinking as coined by German idealistic philosophy.

In 1961 Levinas obtained a state doctorate on the title: *Totalité et Infini* (*Totality and Infinity*) (Levinas TI 1968). He clearly indicated his resistance against the idea of totality (completion in itself, excluding external factors) (Levinas TO:23; TI:xvi). One can even make the profound statement that Levinas' ideas in *Totality and Infinity*, became cornerstones for his academic career and design for collegial dialoguing. He also found a key alley in Franz Rosenzweig. Common between the two is the fact that they both oscillated between the Hebrew-Jewish tradition and Grecian-Christian thinking. Thus, the emphasis on "between two worlds" (*Entre deux mondes*). The American philosopher Richard Cohen wrote in his publication "*Elevations*" about Rosenzweig and Levinas: "Far more important [...] than their particular differences and similarities, is the essential affinity, the brotherhood, the proximity, that brings these two major thinkers together" (Cohen 1994:162).

After being professor in Poitiers, he moved to Paris-Nanterre. During the students' revolt of 1968, he did not sympathise with them. He opposed the fact that they acted in a totalitarian way without any form of differentiation in their mutual encounters. Even the lack of respect over against elderly (people with more responsibilities) hindered him extremely.

He lectured at the Sorbonne from 1973 until his retirement in 1976. In 1974 *Autrement Qu'être ou au delà de L'essence* (*Otherwise than Being, or Beyond Essence*)[9] was published. He devoted the publication to all human beings from all different nations that suffered under hatred inflicted by one human being towards somebody else (the other/others), resembling the suffering of Jews under antisemitism (Levinas 1974/1991). Thus, the attempt to redesign human subjectivity by means of a relational primary ethics.

---

9   Levinas, very worried about humanity, tried frequently to release us from prevailing thinking patterns. He wanted to design a new understanding of human subjectivity. It implies a paradigm shift away from Edmund Husserl's transcendent self, and Heidegger's ontological concept of being (*Dasein* – *Sein* interplay), to the link between the ethics of responsibility and human subjectivity. Levinas' move is from an enclosed form of being (what is and what is not), to a more open-ended and inestimable paradigm. He replaced a totalised sense of being, with one that was infinite. In the publication (AZ), he conceptualises an ethical relationship as one of displacement between self and Other and even as hostage.

CHAPTER 4

Human subjectivity within the framework of relational ethics

Self-awareness and the attempt to acknowledge subjectivity, are embedded in the complexity of relational ethics as primordial. Thus, the statement by Levinas: In the same moment I become aware of my being human, I become aware of my original, natural injustice. I become aware of the damage I inflict on the other, due to the character of my own ego-structure (Levinas MG:41).

The event of self-awareness is a kind of personal incarnation; the subject becomes "flesh and blood". To become aware of one's irrevocable responsibility, is to be exposed to a kind of radical metamorphosis. It is, thus, impossible for a human being to forget his/her "*avatar of subjectivity*" *(son avatar de subjectivité)* (Levinas NP:105).

In the preface to his book *Totality and Infinity*, he started his defence on the subjectivity of our being human. He explicitly does not want to promote subjectivity as merely an egoistic protest over against totality, or as a fearful reaction over against the dread of death, but as founded by the idea of the infinite (Levinas TO:20; TI:xiv).

What is subjectivity? This question leads to the following anthropological question: What is the essence of our being human and who is this human person?

In order to answer this question, Levinas will argue that subjectivity is essentially about the moral subject.

The question about the human subject in Levinas' thinking, will be dealt with in three sections:
- The concept of *perichoresis*[10] within Levinas' philosophical and Jewish writings
- The founding of subjectivity in the idea of the infinite
- The advantage of Jewish wisdom

---

10 *Perichoresis* (not used per se by Levinas but by the authors for sake of clarity and relevance) refers to a kind of interacting or playful rotation often used in theology to indicate the Trinitarian dynamics. It comes from two Greek words, *peri*, which means "around," and *chorein*, which means "to give way" or "to make room". I will use "interplay" in the English translation. The latter reflects the intention of the researchers, namely that our human experience cannot be compartmentalised (De Boer 1989:10). Despite differences the message in communication is more or less the same (De Boer 1976:79).

Perichoresis: The interplay between philosophical and Jewish writings; the ethical relation as extraordinary relation

In this section, the focus will be on the Jewish writings.

Despite the fact that Levinas' philosophical and Jewish writings were not published at the same publishers, they should be read together as a unit. Thus, the reference to *perichoresis*, or "interplay". The mutuality of an interplay refers to the fact that the one could be read from the view of the other and vice versa.

For Levinas, the Jewish heritage is very rich and about sheer wisdom. It should be viewed as supplementary (partly critical) to many other wisdom traditions, for example the tradition of Greek philosophy (Levinas AV:233-234). Levinas even referred to the Christian tradition (the Bible), the Talmud and later Rabbinic commentaries. He does not refer to these texts as evidence for doctrinal views within a religious discourse, but as true witness of a specific tradition and account on religious experiences (Levinas HAH:108; HAM:145). Our Western tradition is not merely informed by Greek thinking as in Plato, Aristotle and even the pre-Socratic worldview. One should admit that the Bible and also the Talmud played an (at least) equally important role. Therefore, one should realise that all the wisdom traditions are embedded in what can be called *a process of thinking* and wise reflection (Levinas HAH:107; HAM:144).

Wisdom thinking correlates with human responsibility within an ethical framework. Thus, the importance to turn to Levinas' understanding of subjectivity within the dynamics of relationships and ethics.

- The followings questions surface: In what way is ethics connected to subjectivity? Is it in any case possible to link ethical thinking (as anchored and connected to the subject and linked to Buber's "I-Thou" model) to a model that is founded in human responsibility? A model that even precedes human freedom; that is, a model that is founded in the thesis that responsibility is essentially a relationship of *re-spond-ability*, framed by the reality of the other.
- The following assumption is presupposed: Responsible precedes freedom. It is not a responsibility for oneself (*responsibilité pour soi*); it is not encapsulated by the existentialistic notion that you are only responsible for yourself. It is about a responsibility to and for the other

(*responsabilité pour l'autre*). This responsibility for the other is not a choice, but an existential givenness.

Levinas finds concrete evidence for this other-centeredness in Ezekiel 3:20: "When a righteous man turns from his righteousness and does evil, and I put a stumbling block before him, he will die, since you did not warn him, he will die for his sin. The righteous things he did will not be remembered, and I will hold you accountable for his blood."

With this quote from the Old Testament (the Hebrew Bible), it is clear that responsibility is shaped by a code of conduct that makes one accountable for the other. Responsibility implies accountability, thus, the introduction of the notions of righteousness and justice. This ethical dimension in the awareness of the other, implies that the other constitutes ethos in such a way that the other opens the dimension of the Other that transcends the concreteness of now and brings about a sense of infinity. Subjects thus gain access to the abstract realm of spirituality; the subject receives from the Other, a transcendent or meta-awareness, beyond the capacity of the I; that is, gaining and receiving an idea of infinity.

The founding of subjectivity in the idea of "infinity"

In meeting the other, this physical presence and concrete encounter as narrated in the Ezekiel text, brings about a face-to-face encounter. It opens a kind of gateway to infinity that supersedes totality; that is, the tendency that spoken and written words already solidify into the register of totality and lose their resilience.

Levinas links his idea of the infinite to responsibility. The idea of the infinite implies in a very poignant sense "the infinite of responsibility"; it is a responsibility for subjectivity as structured by and embedded in the being for the other (*être pour l'autre*). To defend subjectivity, is to stand up for the quality of our being human; one defends human dignity and the person of the other. Subjectivity in this sense, means that "humane humanity" implies more than the thinking of the human mind, and, thus, becomes founded in the idea of "infinity". "Infinity" therefore guides and directs processes of thinking and stimulates reflection. The infinite is not a by-product of the idea of the infinite. It is even not an object of intentionality as in the case of phenomenology. The infinite lurks in a pre-reflexive experience; it creates a yearning for the infinite due to the sublime attunement that in every minimum lurks "a more". This more represents a sense of infinite that the reflexive mind has forgotten long ago (Levinas TO:23; TI:xvii).

Gradually one realises that Levinas' philosophy is not merely about empirical observation and phenomenological descriptions on the level of sensual awareness. Life implies "more". This more functions like a kind of "spiritual more" with roots in a mode of anticipatory intuition that can be called an "eschatology of infinite impressions". In the introduction to *Totalité et Infini* (1968), Levinas gives an indication of the direction of his reflection. He calls it "the eschatology of messianic peace" that transcends an ontology of war (Levinas TO:23).

"Eschatology" has for Levinas a very specific meaning. It refers to the idea of the infinite that constitutes a thinking that supersedes the limitations of mindful thinking; it constitutes a relation to a surplus that is external to all forms of totality. It introduces a very subtle form of "*as if*" (*comme si*); the objective totality cannot really fill or comprehend the true quantum of the essence of being (Levinas TO:16; TI:xi). The source of this relation to "more" (a surplus) must not be traced back to the energy of needs (*besoins*) focussing predominantly on instant satisfaction (need-satisfaction). It resides in a yearning, existential desire (*désir*), for infiniteness that is evoked by eschatology itself. It is, thus, linked to a relationship that, although linked to the sensuous-affective level, surpasses an affective intentionality in the direction of the other, and, thus, can be called "transcendent".

Transcendence in Levinas' thinking evinces the surprising characteristic of being both a common everyday event, a relation, and, what he will call, "infinity". What needs to be understood is that "transcendence" is in the first place anthropological; a human affair in the connection with the other, for the other.

Insofar as "infinity" means "the not-finite", it refers to the non-mastery quality of human expression. So far as infinity has a positive sense, it has the affective qualities of desire for sociality, and of joy. Thus, "infinity", before it is interpreted as "God", or reify it as the highest being, is a quotidian event that takes place at the sensuous-affective level and repeats itself originally as a pre-cognitive and pre-intentional entity – an embodied memory of the flesh.

This relationship with transcendence has also the structure of an ontological awareness of divine existence in the sense of Descartes' understanding of structure. Structure does not refer to concrete content, but to an ontological predisposition, or ontic givenness, that establishes a relationship with the infinite. The latter can be contemplated by means of eschatological expectations; that is, a mode of thinking that toys with the fascinating idea regarding something (an idea) that is not limited by the outlines and confines of an object, but something that can do even more and better than the capacity of the human mind (Levinas TO:49).

The infinite, eschatology or transcendence, cannot be comprehended by the cognitive capacity of reason and reflective rationality. Not even by the correlative schema of intended significance and the meaning of matter. Intentionality cannot capture the essence of the infinite; it merely supersedes the subject-object relationship. Eschatology and the messianic peace cannot be grasped by the human reason, because the mind will disturb the spiritual character of the infinite; it will solidify the dynamics of peace into the rational constitution of totality (a controllable and all-comprehensive system).

The idea of a totality is the direct opposite of the idea of the infinite. All-comprehensive thinking is too limited to grasp the infinite. At stake, therefore, in eschatological mindfulness, is an exceeding (*débordement*) of objectifying thinking by means of "forgotten experience" that feeds eschatological mindfulness (Levinas TO:23-29; TI:3). At stake, is this forgetfulness and misremembrance of an experience that unlocks totality, keeps transcendence vivid and acute and contributes to responsible freedom.

Selfawareness as freedom within the confines of conscientiousness and wisdom (conscience morale)

The contribution of Jewish wisdom texts to the debate on the extraordinary paradigmatic background of the ethical dimension in relationships, resides in the fact that mature, religious thinking in adulthood, opens up the perspective of an external entity that grants the human self, outside the confines of that self, a profound sense of human and humane sovereignty (see *Une Réligion D'adultes*, 1958, in *Difficile Liberté, Essai sur Le Judaïsme*, 1963: 24-41; in Dutch 1978:35-49).

In Jewish thinking, the ethical relationship is viewed as an extraordinary relationship. The transcendent or external factor does not endanger human autonomy but promotes the independent free character of our being human. The philosophy of self-maintenance (self-assertiveness) often runs the danger to establish an autonomy that is absolute, excluding all connectedness to external transcendence. Jewish wisdom reckons with the fact that the human soul is not like a monad, but open to real transcendence, to a divine factor that promotes soulful being, rather than demoting our being human to an encapsulated, enclosed totality in itself (Levinas DL:31).

In Jewish wisdom, autonomy is being safeguarded in relation to Exteriority. The latter institutes autonomy and a unique sovereignty. In Jewish education and catechism, the self is not "absolute". The catechism (Jewish didactics) helps to establish the autonomy beyond the confines of a subject-object schematisation. In terms of a very paradoxical formulation, it means that autonomy is founded by heteronomy. And this heteronomy is determined by the creative word: The commandment (Levinas DL:48).

Within oneself, human beings are exposed to an inner torment, a state of chaotic confusion (*déchirement et déséquilibre*) without meaning and direction (see Peperzak in a footnote, Levinas HAM:60-61). The encapsulated self finds him/herself in a condition of affliction, a kind of soulful disequilibrium and experience of being torn apart (*déséquilibre*) (Levinas DL:31). Then, when one becomes confronted with oneself, one is immediately exposed to the fact that our being human is in fact a violent infringement on the other. Self-awareness is, thus, not a guiltless maintenance of self-assertion, but embedded in the consciousness and conscience-smitten awareness of the ethical duality: Justice-injustice. Being aware of my natural and original injustice, and the damage I inflict in my ego-structure to the other, coincide with our becoming aware of one's being human. My freedom, thus, is voluntary and arbitrary and makes an appeal on investiture. The normal exercising of the I-functions, (functions that transform everything into a me-possessiveness), becomes subjected to an existential critique (Levinas DL:32).

The interesting fact is that freedom, in order to maintain itself as being sovereign, is not freedom from any kind of direction, but freedom as exposed to judgement, and thus, subjected to a commandment: A commandment that is not violent and oppressive, but is in fact a promoting order, an order without force (*ordre sans force*).

Freedom is "clothed" in an investiture and, thus, empowered with abilities. Without the framework of an investiture, the I is without direction, meaning, wisdom and reasonable thinking; the I becomes confused, desperate and disoriented. The freedom is always a subjective mode of being free. The investiture moulds freedom into a capacity to act in a meaningful manner. In other words, the freedom becomes responsible. And this responsibility is exercised and established in facing the Other (Levinas DL:48).

The establishment of this kind of responsibility correlates with what Levinas calls a "metaphysical yearning". It is about a longing that coincides with a commitment to the investiture; it represents a mode of entrustment that eventually implies hospitality, diaconic outreach and liturgy. The implication is that subjectivity receives the other within the mode of hospitality in order to serve (*diakonia*) (Levinas EDHH:194). *Diakonia* is about a commitment of reaching out to the other without reservation; it is performed as a kind of liturgy, as "a work without reward" (Levinas HAM:70, referring to the original meaning of "*leitourgia*").

The interesting point in Levinas' argument is that righteousness and fairness are not produced by the subject. One can even not claim any right merely since every human being needs a living space (Levinas MG:42). Rights and the claim for dignity are not the result of a need for place, space and territory. They reside in the freedom for hospitality and the dynamics of generosity that emanate from the Self to the Other without any condition and demand for thankfulness (Levinas HAM:68). Hospitality resides in the right of the guest that appeals to one's generosity; the plea of Abraham in the Old Testament to step in on behalf of the Other and to spare Sodom and Gomorra.

Subjectivity explodes so to speak from a moral conscience (*conscience morale*). The moral conscience calls the forgotten past into existence – the forgotten experience. The subject is in search for his/her order; it is about the quest for the good and human well-being. But, in our moral conscience, it is not merely about a general kind of goodness (generosity), it is in essence about the quest for fairness and righteousness within the encounter between me and the other. The latter boils down to the quest for hospitality (Levinas TI:xv).

The following question surfaces: How precisely discovers the subject his/her freedom as arbitrariness? How is the moral conscience established? What kind of event lurks underneath this kind of freedom? What is the pre-reflexive experience that feeds the human mind and processes of thinking? This pre-reflexive experience must be a foundational stimulus for processes of thinking within the reflecting subject.

The hunch is that the stimulating source and instigator for a moral conscience is closely related to the discovery and breakthrough of an external factor, namely the exteriority of the transcendent factor; in the event of encountering the other; in facing the other. One becomes aware of the damage inflicted to the other due to one's own ego-structure. The face and presence of the other brings about a conscientious awareness of a command without force (*sans force*), and a setting wherein totality ruptures (Levinas TO:18). The appeal on an investiture, corresponds with a surplus within the relationship that supersedes the realm of totality.

The threat of war and violence: The breakdown of totality (detotalising)

In his introduction to *Totality and Infinity* (*Totalité et Infini*) (TI:ix), Levinas explicitly stated that it is decisive to find out whether we are not victims of a moralistic enterprise and totalitarian system. Is it possible that one can become the dupe of ethics and morality?

The discussion of this question needs to contrast morality and ethics with the hard core reality of, for example, war. In this regard, politics serves the interests of war, namely, to win and to destroy. Politics becomes the art of rationality (to convince the other). But politics then stands diametrically over against morality. It is the same with philosophy: It is contrary to naivety (Levinas TO:13).

War poses an order that transcends all modes of order. In fact, it extinguishes morality. In war everything becomes lawful that the divine forbade. To exercise force, becomes proof of what being is about. War is in fact the exercise of violence with the eventual aim: To win and to destroy; it destroys oneself, as well as the other.

War is an example of brute totality. Eventually it destroys the dignity of subjectivity and violates morality. Thus, the reason to attend first to totality and the quest to demask totality: the breakdown of totality. Afterwards, attention will be given to the meta-realm of life (metaphysics); the quest for home and place in this world, and the subject in search of authority – his/her master.

It is the contention of Levinas that the concept of totality in Western philosophy, displays features of warlike behaviour and destructive violence.

The basic problem is that individuals in totalitarianism[11] lose their unique identity, and become reduced to mechanistic carriers of forces that control their lives without their personal consent: artificial freedom without insight and choice. One becomes dictated from the outside.

Levinas' concern is for the dignity of the individual; for the identity of separate entities and subjective integrity. In this sense, Levinas' critique on Western philosophy is directed to a conceptualisation of totality wherein the separate parts are reduced to merely mechanistic carriers (robots, gears) of external forces that control and govern without personal consent. With Western philosophy is then meant not merely one kind of philosophy in Western thinking, but a generalisation that refers to positivistic rationalism – the whole becomes a rational endeavour without space for meta-perspectives. Social dynamics and political actions and management are then determined by a collectivity that is to be justified *a posteriori* (subsequently and afterwards); the many are reduced to the one explanatory and rational principle (causative reason). The abstraction of the logos (rational concept of the human mind/intellectuality), or the highest form of being/Being, become the solution to the mystery of being.

Due to methodology in science, verification of facts becomes the norm. Rationalistic theories mould truth into intellectual principles that reduce social dynamics, and the unpredictability of life, into a collectivity of, for example, "nation" (national enterprises). Global collectivity becomes the explanatory narrative that absorbs history into systemic rationalism. The ultimate becomes the collectivity of a dominant "whole"; a kind of collective myth for the unpredictability of historical, life events[12].

---

11 The whole becomes an authoritarian threat and powerful dictatorship that dominates and manipulates the parts in such a way that the system becomes exterior to the individual concerns and humane quest for subjectivity and meaningful identification. In this process, responsibility is transformed into mechanistic cooperation. The external powers in the system oppress the integrity of personal choice and freedom (Note of translator).

12 In terms of the broader scope of the research project, one can understand why Nagy can be connected in one way or another to Levinas' thinking. For example, Nagy's notion of a family as a system of loyalty wherein the loyalty of the group is seen as a prevailing cohesive factor "above" (exterior to) the individual, can perhaps be interpreted as such a (mythical) totality wherein members are subordinated to the whole. It could be viewed as a kind of strict systemic collectivity. However, Nagy is sensitive to the contribution of individuals (individuation), and the threat of psychotic confusion interpreted as ethical entanglements. Nagy's approach differs in this aspect from sheer totality.

Back to Levinas' critique on totality in Western thinking. Epistemology in many scientific approaches to methodology, is about rigorist control of reality. An example is the subject-object split that transforms truth into the conceptual constructions of the human mind. The reflecting ego, the analytical dominance of rational analyses, exercised by I-functions, became the dominant factor. Thus, the reason why achievement ethics prescribes human behaviour and unique subjectivity (Levinas MG:42; DL:32).

In modernity, the epistemological question regarding the relationship between the knowing subject and processes of knowing in the observation of the object, corresponds to a large extent with the quest for truth in antiquity (Levinas NP:29-30). However, the difference with antiquity is that the cosmic whole of the universe in, for example Hellenism, disappeared and collapsed before the force of analytical reasoning. The hierarchical order of antiquity is replaced by an order created and designed by itself – the order of intellectuality/knowledge (*savoir*) and knowing. Consciousness is about the order of knowledge: the rationality of interiority (the Self within circular sameness). The act of knowing (epistemology) attains hereby a violent character, namely, the force of the Self that seizes everything it can control. The eventual effect is that even in the encounter with the other, the other is transformed into the characteristics of the self and becomes a replica of that self; everything is then moulded into sameness without critical differentiation. In this way, theory formation becomes a violent exercise; the act of knowing (epistemology) becomes violent in itself and, thus, destructive to the unique subjectivity of the other.

In a relatively early article, *Ethique et Esprit*, Levinas clearly sets his philosophical agenda: a protest against violence. With violence is meant all human actions performed as if one is the only entity that acts. It projects the illusion as if the whole of the universe is there to be subjected to the acting self and, thus, to be manipulated by this act. The further problem is that one performs the act without realising that one is the acting agent and, in this sense, a co-actor and co-role player (Levinas DL:18).

The wonder of speaking and talking to one another, this unique and wonderful order, can conquer violence. For the speaker, the other does not appear in the nominative, but in the vocative. The other is not a correlate of my image of him or her. In fact, the I does not even think of him or her; *I am there for* him or her. This is not about knowing the other, but about being "en société" (Levinas DL:23). Being in a discourse and in companionship, morality and ethics are not deferred. On the contrary, violence is adjourned.

In speaking and narrating by means of language, one abandons any mode of authoritative domination and control. In fact, speaking and listening are intertwined and in this sense one. The content that is articulated in speaking is only possible to be transferred in a face-to-face encounter. Without even knowing the other, the other is acknowledged in such a face-to-face event. Thus, the thesis: Speaking establishes an order of equality, and in doing this, recognises (*reconnaît*) justice accordingly (Levinas DL:20).

Already in the possibility of speaking, lurks the possibility of justice; justice not as a characteristic, or a kind of deposit, but as the potential and possibility to do justice, and to act in a just manner. Justice then becomes a consequence of a commandment. The question: What is right? emanates from: You shall not kill (*Tu ne tueras point*). It is a commandment flowing forth from a face-to-face countenance; it is about a position of watching –others look at me and watch (*Autrui me regarde*) (Levinas DL:20).

Speaking as origin of doing just, is in fact also the starting point of sound rationality. One starts to reflect and think. It is about a kind of recoil. But to hesitate, is a mode of respect. Negotation is based on this authentic speaking (and not the other way around). In this event, the act of speaking, reveals the authenticity of ethics. In the moment of seeing the other, I cannot pretend anymore as if I am not seeing him/her. Then, in that moment, I must speak. As I look, I am watched; watchfulness aims back towards the looker. It does not give itself up, facing the face. Looking, to gaze and to watch are predominantly about the complexity of being watched by the other without any attempt to surrender; one is forced to become engaged in the moral framework of the situation. The latter precedes all forms of theory and sets the condition for reflecting and mindful thinking. Conscience conquers the world not by force but by speech; it creates a kind of ethical resistance over against dominating possessiveness and destructive control.

The notion of countenance or visage, a face-to-face encounter, needs special attention in the breakdown of totality. Contact with countenance, does not refer to contact with something. It is about a kind of leaving oneself; a movement of stepping out of oneself (*sortie de soi*). One is approached by another entity, and is, thus, not merely bounded to a mode of isolated self-experience. What one experiences is, in fact, an ethical resistance that penetrates all modes of exclusive totality. Thus, the command not to kill the other, but to save the other, and thereby, at the same time, oneself.

The face-to-face encounter with the other is like a trade. This trade with beings, starts with the command: Thou shall not kill. It is indeed a strange trade, totally out of step with the patterns of usual relations within worldly encounters (Levinas DL:23). Relational ethics transforms and supersedes the so-called normal experiences.

When one turns again to the notion of war and violence, it seems as if war and violence suspend ethics. However, the truth is just the opposite: Ethics defies and adjourns violence. It is therefore decisive for true freedom to discover that freedom is in jeopardy. This knowing of danger creates space in order to avoid the moment of inhumanity; it should in fact prevent inhumanity. This continuous postponement of the hour of betrayal, presupposes the unselfishness of goodness and mercy; it points to the yearning for the absolute Other. This yearning assumes *the dimension of metaphysics* (Levinas TO:31; TI:5).

The metaphysical dimension

The attempt to deal with the outline of Levinas' thinking, is to always come back to his hunch that there is always "more" in the dynamics of intersubjectivity, and that the encounter with the other exceeds the realm of sheer rational analyses. "The more" (surplus) even exceeds the comprehension of analytical theories. Life is framed by a meta-dimension: transcendence.

From a philosophical point of view, the relationship with transcendence, a relationship with something that cannot be comprehended fully, and exceeds the capacity of analytical thinking, is to probe into the realm of differentiated otherness. One should understand that the relationship with transcendence is not in the first place about rational thinking for the sake of intellectual reflection and rational curiosity; it is about an ethical relationship. The challenge is to grasp the ethical relationship. Step number one is then to understand that ethics is not originated by ontology: the theory and thinking about the essence of being. It originates from something that is more original, and also profoundly different than being/Being. This is the reason why one of the earliest articles of Levinas wrestled with the question: *Is ontology fundamental*?

(Levinas TO:13-24). His answer to this rhetoric question: "No". But what is then in fact fundamental? Levinas' answer: *the ethics or metaphysics*.

A metaphysical relation is about a relationship with a being or entity that is outside my framework of reference, and, thus, exterior. In this respect, one should again remember Levinas' Jewish background. In Judaism, the ethical relationship is an exceptional relationship. Without compromising our human sovereignty, the contact with an external being is an advantage: It is both a connection with a source that institutes and invests (Levinas DL:31).

The external being (*être extérieur*) refers to an "Other". It is essentially about a relationship with transcendence. Being exterior, means that the Other's otherness (fact of differentiation) resides in the fact that the otherness of the Other is exactly at the same time its content. The question can, thus, be posed: But is this exterior being, God? That is not necessarily the case. God rather comes to the idea (*Dieu vient à l'idée*). This coming of God opens up different dimensions, and a variety of hermeneutical options as well. The other can also become the other human being in its poverty and nakedness (without context).

Levinas sometimes write "the other" (*l'autre*) with a capital: Other (*L'autre*). In other cases, he uses only other (without the capital). The implication is that even Other (*L'autre*) can be translated as "the other" or an "other". Sometimes he even uses the older form of "others" (*autrui*). Others then means, specifically, the other human being (the other person), or fellow human being.

The further implication, is, as in the case of other/Other, even the notion of "transcendent" has many layers of meaning. In the first place, "transcendent" refers to a relation with an end term (an ultimate entity) that cannot be reduced to the inner dynamics, the playful dynamics of interiority (*jeu intérieur*). Transcendent does not refer to the inner realm of human mindfulness. Also, it cannot be reduced to any kind of representation within the realm of observational facticity. The metaphysical movement represents a yearning, longing and desire for something invisible. In other words, it is about a yearning and urge that are not the result of a mere theory, thesis or hypothesis. It is also not a mere regressive longing for a birthplace or fatherland. It is about a metaphysical desire for "invisiblity". The yearning for something invisible describes a metaphysical movement towards what is indeed transcendent and outside the grasp of mere intellectuality. The transcendent as longing is an inadequacy (the insufficient ability of reason), and, thus, essentially and necessarily a transcendence[13].

Transcendent also refers to movement; a movement of transition as for example to move beyond and exceed the limitations of existential being – a kind of trans-*ascendancy* (movement beyond supremacy, domination, control and therefore exterior). The term also demarcates a kind of inadequacy due to limitations between "I" and "other". In the relation between "I" and "other" there is always a strange non-descriptiveness that refers to exteriority. Even in the most intimate dimension of relationships, the erotic relationship, there is always something "exterior" and "outstanding" (some dimension of "future"). The relation cannot be captured in terms of "totality" (under control), or in terms of "I possess" (possessiveness). Even when one gives oneself to the other (surrender in terms of the intimacy of cares), this act does not imply to capitulate before a kind of force, and eventually, become overpowered. Caress as surrender is about entrusting. Because in entrusting there always looms the dimension of a promise of something still to become – a future prospective. Therefore, the reason why subjectivity (the "I") and "other" (as subject) are always clothed in the mode of passivity (still to become) (Levinas TA:55).

The fact that the relationships are characterised by inadequacy, all modes of encounters refer to asymmetry. The Other who is exterior, is inadequate in terms of each conception, presentation or image.

At stake, is a relationship with exteriority that does not violate human sovereignty. On the contrary, it institutionalises and establishes our being human. This is only possible when a human being can be empowered as an "I" and is an independent entity in itself. If not, sovereignty/autonomy is merely a fake. The term "I", can only be maintained in an absolute sense as an "I" within a relationship, due to the dynamics of asymmetry. It is only then that it is possible for the "I" to get access to a relationship with the Other. In the same way as the Other has its otherness as content, my identity is my unique content. Identity is about the identification of the "I" with "it-self". Metaphysics can only be established and maintained in the first person, from the one pole of the relationship of the self to, and with, the Other.

---

13 What makes it so difficult is that due to the many layers of meaning, transcendence can refer to "height"; even to "Master" and "Lord". See Levinas' letter to Martin Buber in 1963 (Levinas NP:53-54).

About the social dimension of relationships

The outline of Levinas' basic philosophical stance, may leave the impression as if ontology, and, therefore, the notion that the essence of Being (German: *Sein*) determines the whole web of relational networking, even the character and identity of all forms of our being human (existential orientation) (German: *Seinde/Dasein*). It leaves the impression that social relationships are predominantly compiled and determined by the interaction between "I" and "I"; between "I" and "others". Social relations are then subjected to the structures of Being (Levinas TO:18). It seems as if thinking starts with what "is". From the comprehension of the whole of being, one can then derive the understanding of every component, that is, the particular differentiation of being.

But this is not Levinas' intention. The appearance of the other cannot be reduced to ontological categories. Without any doubt, the other should and must be understood. However, the relationships supersede the capacity of analytical understanding (Levinas TO:18). The reason is not that the "I" cannot understand or grasp the other, but because the other does not really touch me and encounters me by mere understanding and conceptualisation. The other is a unique being, a separate category (individuation) and does count due to its special, separate identity. The other is not the by-product of any form of understanding; it is not conceived as being exemplary of a specific kind, group or class. The other is called into being by means of an act of speech.

It is at this point that one must understand why Levinas introduced the concept of metaphysics. The interaction between the "I" and the "other" is embedded in *meta*-physics – the exteriority of transcendence. The metaphysical relation is not a relationship conceived by understanding; it starts with speaking, processes of verbalising. To formulate more precisely, it starts with the act of speech wherein one addresses the other. The speech of addressing is not the result of an a priori that already exists in a mode of awareness, in fact, speaking as a mode of addressing is the precondition for processes of conscience (*pris de conscience*) (Levinas EN:19).

The relationship between the understanding of the other *and* the other as interlocutor (*interlocuteur*) are inseparable. Understanding the other cannot be separated from addressing the other (Levinas TO:19). "Being inseparable" is from a different order than the order of sheer understanding. In other words, inseparability is different from the mere attempt to understand by means of words, because it deals with an interconnectedness and mode of being that I share from the start with the other.

Therefore, the ontology, the presupposed inseparability between understanding and being, is not fundamental and not the starting point. Fundamental, and, thus, the starting point is ethics. Ethics is the most primary form of philosophy: It is foundational and comes first (*prima philosophia*) (Levinas in Peperzak 1995:xi).

The title of a lecture held in 1984, is in fact an introduction to his basic premise for doing philosophy: *L'Ethique Comme Philosophie Première* (*Ethics as First Philosophy* – the primary starting point of reflection and wise thinking). More or less in the same way as Aristotle's viewpoint that philosophy and the interplay with ontology is first, so philosophy within the interplay between ethics and ontology is first. The first of ethics cannot be separated from Levinas' ideas on the *meta*-dimension of life; the interplay between the infinite and "the between" in the I-Thou encounter; the "more" of transcendence. In terms of methodology, in all these concepts (encounter, subjectivity, relational interaction, other/Other/others) a many layered hermeneutics should be applied. To interpret Levinas' thinking, one should always keep in mind that "first" refers in the first place to prior in Jewish thinking (with the transformation of praxis as its primary concern, instead of the cognition of truth). It is about the origin of his philosophical agenda, namely, to construe a very special relationship between the "other" and "Other". "Face-to-face with the other person, the command of the other person comes 'as though' the I was commanded by God" (Richard A Cohen 1994:271). Due to this primary premise, the interplay between ethics and ontology is the key to what can be called a "*Levinas' mystique*".

In the prior of ethics, ethics appears as a kind of "*ethical strangeness*", because the appeal to our being human, the quest for a humane anthropology (the humanity in our being human), seems to reside in an ontological disruption, a disturbing *rupture of being*. This *strangeness* appears as a kind of messianic (even eschatological or utopian) interlude in the landscape of philosophy. "*Strange*" refers to the "other" as stranger. Nothing is stranger, more foreign and more exterior to the "I", as this "mystical and begging other". It is due to this strangeness, that the exposure of "*infinite responsibility*" becomes an ethical appeal, preceding all initiatives and choices.

In Levinas' outline for a methodological programme to detect the first factor, a primary starting point for a philosophical interpretation of the order of justice, ethics becomes a point of origin from which wisdom thinking departs. In this *"fundamental first"*, the paradox between "doing" and "viewing" is not yet possible and at stake. This "original first" (fundamental and primary starting point) of ethics, precedes even ontology (Levinas DQVI:143); it emanates from *the act of wording* wherein the *creativity of verbalising* and *the speech of dialoguing* calls being into existence; it invites the other as *strange guest* into the intimate space of hospitable being-with, the humane intimacy of co-existence, meaningful intersubjectivity, and graceful receiving. "Speaking" then refers to a primary mode of appeal and summoning to responsibility, as well as addressing (the imperative mode); it is about sensible, prudent understanding and accommodative, hospitable agreement.

"The first" provides identity to the "I". Within this metaphysical and ethical relationship, the "I" is positioned as being summoned to opt as an existential first. The dimension of metaphysics is therefore in the first instance not a dimension of "between", neither of merely intersubjectivity. It is fundamentally about a *foundational dimension of subjectivity*. The metaphysical relationship is about a radical different order than the epistemological knowing relationship of a theoretical endeavour. The other is exactly within this realm of "first", not "knowable" in the sense of a phenomenological transcendental process of viewing (Husserl). As subject the other cannot be objectified or be reduced to merely a thematic entity for scientific positivism and rational analyses.

The previous outline is an attempt to explain why the dissertation wants to clarify Nagy's prevalence for ethics, rather than to outline merely a psychotherapeutic approach to human well-being or describing a strict ontology of being within the field of helping and caring. Ethics is not the outcome and result of the "realm of the between", compiled by merely psychological and transactional data and factualities. In family therapy more than merely a psychic disposition in intergenerational networking and systemic interaction is needed. Due to individuation, as well as the concept of multi-directed partiality, Nagy conceived every separate self as a unique "I", relating to a "Thou" in order to prevent the "I-Thou" interplay of becoming an abstract, illusive event.

Responsibility is not a precarious and accidental happenstance and psychic disposition, but about a substantial contribution of every individual to the human whole, and the order of intersubjectivity (family, group, institution). The order is always a construction a posteriori. For children, therefore, when they start to speak, there is not a causative pre-order, but the other as the original pre-other. In this pre-order (the foundational relationship with a pre-other, before me), the subject starts to address the other. The subject makes an appeal by means of "verbalising speech", wording and talking (*language*-ing). Speaking is, as prior, an invitation to the other.

Due to this word-event, the "I" becomes aware of the other, as well of him/herself. It also demarcates and underlines the fact that both the "other" and the "I" are not smothered into a kind of sameness. Co-existence is exactly about the fact that the "I" and "Thou" are separate entities, and, due to individuation, different. The relationship is, thus, to be understood ethically, and is therefore universal. Perhaps, the reason why Nagy could claim that his concept (thesis) of "a justice order" is "universal" and primary.

Back to Levinas' notion of metaphysics. In a metaphysical interpretation of the "I-Thou" intersubjectivity, the advantage is that the "I" is "saved" from "totality". This advantage constitutes the independence of being and the free dynamics of "self": One *is* one-self, but, at the same time, "leaves one-*self*" (*sortie de soi*).

In being one-self, one discovers an interiority and distinctiveness that is different from the prescriptive totality. It reveals the interiority of an inner space wherein one can operationalise care and responsibility for oneself. One discovers an embodiment of unique potential: "I can, and, I am able". The power of knowing of the self, becomes a meaningful web that could be spread over all phenomena that appear to the knowing subject. The inner power as an identification between "I" and "self", is not the monotone tautology and sterile monadology of A=A. The identification between "I" and "self" is also not a reflection on the abstract prefiguration of oneself by oneself (Levinas TO:35). What is in fact taking place, is the concrete relationship between "I" and the world. It is not about an abstract or theoretical relationship. This concrete relationship between "I" and "world" wherein the "I" manifests or reveals itself, as a "self", establishes itself as a sojourn and place to stay in this world. The world is then the "other" that "I", in my concrete embodiment, inhabits. Inhabitation is not the possessiveness of totality, but the necessity of separation (*se-paratio*) in order to create a safe space of home and intimate hospitality.

Habitational enjoyment: Being at home in worldly spaces and embodied encounters

For Levinas, there is no reason to view embodiment and our being in this world as a mode of being in exile. Existence should essentially not be viewed as inauthentic and deprived from meaning and enjoyment. In fact, we live from the gifts of this world. The world is a givenness and to receive all its gifts gracefully, contributes to human well-being. Thus, Levinas' emphasis on enjoyment (*jouir* – to enjoy). We bathe ourselves in the wind, the rain, the water and the sun. All daily activities and bodily functions like breathing, eating, walking, working, reading or making music, are embodied expressions of sheer joy. Even our inputs and exposure to possible stress, is not to be separated from enjoyment. They are expressions of the embodied fact that one is in contact with the authenticity and truth of being human; they are modes of being at home in this world, and the fact that life is pleasant and brings about fulfilment.

Being at home (*chez soi*), is about a kind of interiority wherein the inner being is a safe space for being independent and differentiated from the smothering whole of totality. Here one is "saved" from the non-personal threat of massification and global collectivity. Being at home, creates a sense of belongingness wherein one can become wholly connected to oneself; saved from just "being there" amongst things without being acknowledged as a unique, human being. The interiority of inner enjoyment, and the sense of "I-am-at-home", become a hospitable space for becoming engaged in the exteriority of the world. It creates a reasonable hermeneutics for self-understanding and helps one to adopt and conform to basic needs. Everything becomes a kind of "other", but, at the same time, an invitation to assimilate the advantages of life into the being of oneself within the acute and alerting awareness of the sameness of things.

Habitational enjoyment, our interiority, is structured around four basic aspects of our being in this world (with existential others): Finality within need-satisfaction (desires); embodiment; dwelling; possession and labour.

The finality of need-satisfaction – existential, embodied hedonism

Eating and nutrition are biologically speaking, part and parcel of finality. In terms of biological needs, in eating and need-satisfaction we transform the other into nutrition and food: Food should serve basic needs for living in time and worldly spaces (finality of need-satisfaction). Luckily, human beings live not primarily by this necessary mode of finality. Basically, what is at stake, is that humans find pleasure in nutrition and dispose over it; one starts to like it, and in this sense, one can gain power over it; one starts to enjoy it (*jouir*) – the finality is overcome. What happens now, is that within human beings, an "inversion" of biological needs takes place (Levinas TO:154). In other words, the need for food is not bounded to the basic concern for beings to exist. Differentiation takes place.

The "need for food" is not determined by the concern and goal to survive and to live. The goal is merely the food in itself. In this sense, human beings dispose over "*other*-things" so that Levinas opens up new perspectives on the "*hedonistic morale*". The latter does not look beyond need-satisfaction for a higher goal, or order, to attain meaning to the graving and need-satisfaction, even to discover its value and utility. The value resides immediately in the substance. Enjoyment of needs, and the fact that need-satisfaction can be pleasant, become an indication of the fact that the deadly finality of "one-only-lives-by-bread", is overcome – "existential hedonism", thus, prevails and attains the positive value of enjoyment.

The realm of sensuality and affects – human embodiment

One lives life by means of sensual qualities. These sensual qualities belong to the realm of feeling. Levinas formulates as follows: Our ego-qualities vibrate due to the affective (Levinas TO:155). But the realm of the affective, and the resonance of sensuality, are not a pre-developmental stage for thinking.

Our body inhabits the world. Sensuality is pleasant and can be enjoyed. However, within sensual enjoyment, we are confronted with a disturbing "*unrest*". The most elementary components of embodiment are never wholly trustworthy, because they are part of the "other". The "I" is indeed dependent on the elementary qualities of our body. However, as interior, I transcend immediately these qualities and can act independently. Thus, the paradox of being dependent, but also being independent. This paradox is enough reason for concern.

The fact is, that in life, we are never free of any form of concern. We don't exist carelessly. It does not mean that we are delivered to fate and dread; it is not about a kind of depressive concern. It is care that emerges from a foundational connectedness with a zest and love for life. We live with commitment and an eagerness to be engaged; therefore we care.

This mode of care should be differentiated from the absurdity of nihilism, and the abnormal situation of violent exploitation. The latter is a setting wherein the messianic awareness of hope and peace (the peace of the *Sjabbath*) is absent and being violated.

Dwelling: The interiority and intimate place of refuge for contemplation (recueillement)

Dwelling and the experience of being at home, need to be understood as a kind of internal introspection; a coming back to a place wherein one becomes free to contemplate. One experiences anew the outer world (exterritorial) (Levinas TO:199). It is about a safe haven or intimate space wherein one regains an impetus to move outward to the cosmic dimension of our being human. This safe haven is a precondition for meaningful activity. The intimate, interiority for meaningful inhabitation is not constituted by the subject. Nevertheless, this dwelling place is indeed a precondition for the sound cooperation and constitutive functioning of the subject. It is a resort for further operations. Before the subject "sees" or "views" the world, one is at home in this haven of intimacy.

For Heidegger, one experiences the world as a foreign place without any guarantee (*Unheimlichkeit*). For Levinas the world is primarily a dwelling place to be inhabited. Due to this sense of "*at homeness*", one can act and labour (Levinas TO:178-179). To turn back to the intimate space of home, is to suspend enjoyment temporarily in order to reconnect with an inner freedom. In this sense, one receives anew confirmation of being. It coincides with an appealing awareness from elsewhere (transcendent dimension). One regains confidence and a sense of well-being due to this intimate familiarity, and the empowering experience of being confirmed as a subject: "I" am indeed "I". This coming back to oneself, is about an intimacy with *somebody*, with an "other".

Internal introspection is like experiencing an entertaining reception. One is welcomed by the "discrete other"[14]: Hidden, but still present as the always-present-other (host). The implication is that this intimate space of home (the intimacy of humane humanity) had already been inhabited before, even before I discover this safe haven of refuge.

Without any doubt, introspection exposes one to loneliness; the loneliness of the individualised "I", separated from others. However, the comfort in this loneliness, is that it is always a loneliness in a human world. Dwelling is a transcendent condition for our being human, and for authentic subjectivity. Due to this phenomenon of dwelling, there is a kind of distancing and break with our natural existence. One, thus, gains a form of possession and control.

The economy of communality: Possession and labour

It is characteristic of our being human, to master the elements, to incorporate them and to transform them into some-*thing*. Humans do not start first with a portrayal, in order to operate afterwards from this imaginative depiction of things. In the act of operation, the human hand produces and call things into being. The thing/matter (*la chose*) is a form of existence wherein independency has been lost. In fact, it had been reconstructed and moulded into what one can call: the obtained status of "*have*"; it becomes a kind of being. This process of becoming can be called "labour".

Labour then means: The power of the human hand intervenes and grasps. In this action of intervention, the human hand takes possession of matter; it connects the elements to a kind of achievement and goal that have been prescribed by needs and the concern for need-satisfaction. The hand becomes a useful and inventive tool. Metaphorically speaking, this aggressive intervention is like a Prometheus act (Levinas TO:187); it changes matter into possession.

As possession, things do not exist on their own. They exist as property, as "haves", as money. It is therefore possible to dispute things and to compare them. Labour changes things into commodities. This is the reason why possessions refer to a more fundamental relationship; to a metaphysical relationship.

---

14 This "discrete other" is for Levinas an exponent of femininity (womanhood) due to the notion of care and intimacy. It does not imply, that Levinas excludes males, and that it should become a gender issue (see Levinas EI:61). For Levinas' view on femininity and being a woman, see Brüggeman-Kruijff 1993. About the "discrete other", see Levinas TI:145; TO:199.

The irony is that things show no resistance to this intervention. The resistance is performed by others who also possess. The "I" cannot possess them. They act independently and can start to dispute possession. But in doing so, things are being ratified. Eventually, the possession of things results in dialogue. It becomes a conversation about things (De Jong 1989:120).

In this conversation, the world becomes communicable. The implication of this verbal communication is that things become a "community of goods" (De Jong 1989:120). The communication of goods implies a kind of economy, literally, the law and regulation of dwelling. In economy things become communicable and communal; it is about sharing and receiving. Labour, thus, creates possessions and stands in service of goods that become communal. The intriguing question now is how to establish a fair economy, based on justice and a reasonable contract that regulates honest receiving and trustworthy sharing. In this respect De Boer (in Peperzak 1995:163), poses the question: "How does the good faith originate with which one concludes the contract?" The obvious answer: Only through the dialogue that precedes all other forms of dialogue, namely, the primordial experience of the "Countenance/Visage": the absolute form of ethical resistance. The face-to-face confrontation with "Countenance", summons and interpellates me in an irrevocable manner; it summons subjectivity to signify and to instil meaning in inhabitational living.

Encountering visage in the quest for meaning (sense): *The subject in search of his/her master/mistress*

The finding of a dialogue in order to establish authentic dialoguing and to establish meaningful dialogical encounters, are some of the core challenges facing our being human in worldly spaces (Levinas DQVI:211-230).

It has already been pointed out that subjectivity is founded in the idea of the infinite. The implication is that subjectivity is founded in something exterior to the normal order of things. It is evoked by a yearning for a messianic moment, and a longing for eschaton. It is about a longing for eventual and authentic truth, and a mode of justice that will always be future and never be factually available. The meaning of being (*sens*), never resides in being itself, neither in nature, nor in history. Meaning is exterior; it approached me from the outside and judges me. Thus, the reason why a theological mode of speech always refers to the fact that only God can be the judge (Levinas MG:49).

Meaning starts with the experience of being visited by countenance/visage (face-to-face-encounter). In this sense, subject is defined by passivity. Of this passivity the desire with its needs (*désir*) within erotic relationships, become an example; the desire disconnects the intentionality.

The erotic relationship as foreplay

The interplay between power and the relationship with the subject and the other, become complex when the relationship is, on the one hand, personal. On the other hand, it is not established by the "I can", or "I know". The point is, the relational dynamics as exponent of ethics, should not be about the power and force of the subject. The subject is not summoned to dominate and exploit his/her world and environment. The finding and establishing of a very exceptional relationship, namely sexual intimacy, is often exposed to the abuse of power. Thus, the reason why erotic connections, become problematic indeed (Levinas TA:73-84).

The outline of the erotic relationship is described by Levinas in *De L'existence à L'existant* (EE 1986), very specifically in *Le Temps et L'autre* (TA 1979). The "I" is in fact always moving out; existence transcends into the direction of the other. This movement of reaching out, and attempt of going out towards the other, are problematic, because the other is in a very special way always out of range and alterative (Levinas DTA:55). When sensuality (*eros*) comes into play, the movement to the other becomes even more complex due to the fact that Levinas uses terminology that refers to a feminine dimension (womanhood): The dual connection *eros* – feminity.[15] In the description of the erotic relationship (Levinas in EE; especially in TA), the "I" reaches out to the other, approaches the other, in terms of "the feminine component of life"; it is a movement towards the other that is always out of reach and sign of what is always fundamentally absolutely exterior.

It is for Levinas indeed difficult to define subject if the latter resides in passivity. The intriguing question is whether there is in the human being another "master" possible (*une autre maîtrise*); a master that is not merely about a virile force (*virilité*), or the ability to produce and to conquer. Thus, the

---

15 The problem here is that in the connection between *eros* and the femininity, women can still be assessed in terms of gender issues and existing cultural connotations about womanhood, fed by hierarchical paradigms. See Luce Irigaray in Bernasconi & Critchley 1991:109-118. See also Brüggeman-Kruijff 1993:101-118.

intriguing question: Is it possible to deal with a mode of subjective passivity wherein the intimate personal realm is still intact and retained? If possible, this kind of relationship will be remarkable indeed: The person should stay intact, but at the same time, the Other cannot be grasped and reduced to merely a phenomenon; the Other then as constituent of an intentional subject.

The further implication is that, if it is possible to identify a passive "I" (subject), one should realise that the relationship with the other should not be described in this case by means of spatial categories, but merely in terms of temporal categories. The other is then first, due to time, not due to his/her psychological makeup, character or appearance. The other is neither an "alter-ego". For example, the other becomes the weak, the vulnerable, the widower, the orphan or poor. And, in this case, the "I" can be the rich/the wealthy, or the most powerful (Levinas DTA:53).

In his attempt to find an original form of pure relationship, Levinas poses the question, whether one can find traces of such a mode of relationship in culture. It should be traces of a relationship towards the other, wherein the otherness of the other in its unique differentiation, is still intact and an ingredient of the content that determines our being a person. In his earlier writings, Levinas calls this kind of alternative, "time and the other"; "the feminine dimension" (the metaphoric function of female and womanhood).

Levinas does not want to describe femininity in terms of a gender issue as connected to the description of masculinities; that is, not as complementary to masculinity. The sexual differentiation rather refers to an ethical differentiation. In other words, it is an indication of original differentiation that is ethically based[16]. The erotic relationship is as such not ethical. The ethical dimension comes into play in the failure (*échec*) that makes an appeal on communication and becomes the starting point of speaking. This failure (*échec*), is about a very strange paradox: It underlines the limitation and end of "I-can". At the same time, it does not destroy the person. The hand that caresses, does not know beforehand what it is looking and longing for; it does not want something per se. The specific character of eroticism is that it is

---

16 One would be careful not to read Levinas' remark on the link between *eros*, ethics and femininity in the same paradigm of Jean-Paul Sartre's interpretation of the male-female relationship wherein love is a kind of "disguise" for conflicts between two modes of freedom, and that on being a female (femininity), should be constituted and interpreted from the viewpoint of current views on masculinity. This interpretation is possible, but not to be recommended.

not focused and instigated by becoming one (copulation and intercourse as fusion/unification), but an expression of authentic longing and intimate desire. Copulation can steer the longing and desire in a wrong direction; it then leads astray. It misleads, due to the fact that it is a desire for unification, and not fundamentally directed towards the subjectivity of the other. Eroticism, thus, needs a *meta*-dimension wherein transcendence grants erotic desires an external meaning.

Levinas calls this exteriority, the metaphysical dimension of erotic desire: "*Désir métaphysique*"! It means that the erotic relationship becomes a sign of the original asymmetric relationship. Sexual differentiation becomes a trace and sign of ethical differentiation. Desire and longing are on a more fundamental level; the longing and desire are about a "trace" of the "Other" within the Self. In fact, it becomes in this sense, a heteronomous experience (See Levinas EDHH:190). An experience of the absolute exterior seems to be very strange indeed. In fact, this heteronomous experience seems to be a contradiction in terms[17], but this is precisely what a metaphysical desire is about.

Existential embarrassment: "The me" (*en moi*) as anchorage of ethics

Finkielkraut (1984:141) once said that the moral awareness in me does not come from me (*La morale en moi ne vient pas de moi*). For Levinas, subjectivity is unique in the sense that the ethical perspective took root in the "I". The ethics of the inescapable, and non-indifferent being, found an anchorage in me (*en moi*). For Levinas, this notion of anchorage is important, because if ethics did take root in anything else, for example, in a relation that preceded all modes of established relationships, or in a social entity that preceded the individual, ethics would have been a derivation of, or even an appendix to the general order of being.

But ethics is a moral principle in me (*en moi*); it is about a "me-perspective". In this regard, it starts as an interior perspective. The metaphysical relationship starts within me; from within the heteronomous relationship. The metaphysical desire is then merely "my desire". But the important point is that the "metaphysical desire" should not be shaped by me, by my needs. It

---

17 "*Peut-il y avoir quelque chose d'aussi étrange qu'une experience de l'absolument exterieur, d'aussi contradictoire dans les termes qu'une experience heteronome?*" Levinas in EDHH:190.

does not reside on the level of need-satisfaction; it is "in me", but not "from" and "by" me. In fact, it is about a desire and longing that can never be satisfied (insatiable compassion). It is about a desire for the Other, and within this metaphysical desire, ethics finds (by means of this desire) a subject.

The metaphysical desire presupposes a subject that dwells in this world, is at home in the existential dynamics. The deep yearning and desire for the "Other" are born in an entity (Being) that lacks nothing (Levinas EDHH:193). This metaphysical desire is actually an embarrassment, in the sense that the subject becomes obsessed with it; it is indeed about a very strange intrigue, namely I become involved in something that does not really touch me. From the perspective of autonomy, the metaphysical realm should have made me indifferent. However, that is not the case. It is exactly due to the metaphysical desire, that the subject cannot respond with indifference; the subject is overwhelmed by the Other. The latter demarcates the predicament of subjectivity. Thus, the reason why this predicament can be called an embarrassing position indeed. It is about an irrevocable and strange event; it comes as a great shock that fills one with "insatiable compassion".

The otherness of the "Other": Countenance/visage

Due to the fact that one is overwhelmed by the Other and cannot ignore the awareness that one is fulfilled with this "insatiable compassion", it becomes imperative to analyse the concept of "the Other". For the further outline it is necessary to get clarity on what is meant by this concept in Levinas' philosophical approach.

Firstly, the "Other" as source of the metaphysical desire, specifically the "Other" that calls this desire into being (not like a wakeup call), does not belong to the totality, also not to the realm of the "Self". The Other is no manifestation. Manifestation is about phenomena that are dependent for their meaning on the "I"; that is, the awareness of the "I" in its observation of objects (objects in their appearance as phenomena). The "Other" (*Autrui*), also the others (*l'autre*) are in fact immune and cannot be defined by the game of meaning-giving or captured by phenomenological observations performed by the "I". If the "Other" is subjected to a system of significant signs and be rendered meaning by the "I", both will lose their unique being and identity. The Other has its alterity as content in itself.

The Other does not manifest itself, does not appear before an "I" in the sense that it is dependent from the "I" for its position in a cultural setting or in an embodied form. The Other is not a phenomenon (accessible to the question: What is that?) (Levinas AZ:45). One encounters the Other in a face-to-face meeting; one engages with the Other as Visage/*Countenance*[18]. Levinas also refers to "Countenance/Visage" as "presence in itself". It is about an epiphany of countenance that has a proper meaning in itself, independent of any other form of meaning rendered by worldly associations (*comporte une significance propre indépendante de cette signification recue du monde*) (Levinas EDHH:194).

In the previous paragraphs the notion of face (*visage*) was translated with "countenance" as well. At stake, in visage is the actuality of a meeting with the other: face-to-face. Within context, face/visage implies more than the facial features or expressions. Face/visage is about a direct appearance wherein one is exposed to the dynamic presence of the other. In his translation of *Autrement Qu'être ou au delà L'esssence*, Ab Kalshoven pointed out that the French term "*visage*" should be read simultaneously with the verb "*viser*"; it means to eye a person, and to focus on that person personally (See Levinas AZ:270)[19].

What one should take into consideration, is that countenance/visage implies a temporal dimension. The epiphany takes place irrevocably in time, in the here and now. It refers to the presence of the Other. In this now, autonomy is transformed into heteronomy and arbitrariness into freedom due to the investiture: the humanism of the other person.

Due to the well-being implied in the "presencing countenance/visage", it becomes possible to toy with the idea of "healing through meeting". One can

---

18 The appearance or expression of someone's face; it also refers to approve of, or to give support to something within a face-to-face encounter; the look or expression of the face. One can also use "visage": Referring to seeing, countenance and appearance. Visage is the term used by Levinas. In the translated text, visage and countenance will be used as two interchangeable terms, supplementary to one another. Countenance represents more the event and form of encounter, while visage refers more to the event of presence and communial facing. See also note 59 by translator.

19 It is indeed a question how to translate "*visage*". Instead of "face"; or "countenance" the English "visage" can also be considered. In Hebrew, face of the Other, Countenance, refers to both the whole presence of the other. It includes welcoming, greeting, peace, blessing and even a kind of benediction – the Other looks at the one in front, with grace, compassion and mercy. One is enriched and empowered by the looks of the face (appearance of face – *prosōpon*); face implies a gracious turning towards man and the establishment of communion, fellowship and a relationship of trust. When God hides or turns away his face, it implies withdrawal of grace. Note by translator, DJ Louw.

even consider the notion of "a healing dialogue". But then it is important to understand that the dialogue does not start with the mutuality. Dialogue as such cannot bring about healing. If healing is in one way or another possible, it is because of the asymmetry, a diachronic understanding of time, and the importance of the non-totalising transcendence.

The Other carries an own unique significance that is independent from any worldly connotations associated with the concept. The "Other" does not emerge from the context, nor does it appear by means of any form of mediation. The appearance is from itself and carries its own significance (Levinas EDHH:194). The "Other" signifies itself; it is not absorbed by the world but enters the world of being and awareness belonging in fact to "my world". In this sense, the "Other" visits my world, and encounters the self.

The coming of the "Other" as a strange visitation, is not about the appearance of phenomena that can be observed; intentional observation cannot portray the "Other". Furthermore, the "Other" presents itself in terms of a command/order (*une ordre*). The order is a disruption of egoism and selfish smugness. However, this order does not destroy freedom; it promotes and establishes freedom and its unicity.

The order is not "my creation", but an interpellation, a directive and summons; it constitutes the fact that the "I" is unique, irreplaceable.

The fact that the "Other" constitutes the "I", does not mean that the "I" is directly identified with the "Other". One is identified with the order or command so that I make the appeal to the "Other", with the intention to mirror back to me; the Other should focus on me personally. This is how responsibility is being brought about. This kind of responsibility posits and investitures my freedom. In fact, it overpowers me, but at the same time, empowers the other as well (Levinas EDHH:197).

What is quite exceptional to this visage, is that one cannot ignore the appeal to act in a responsible way. The visage is so vivid that one cannot forget it, or one is just too deaf not to hear the appeal. It comes to me as an urgent warning that needs immediate attention; one is encircled from all sides so that the human being itself becomes a whole web of responsibility (*Il est dans sa position méme de part en part responsabilité*).

In terms of Isaiah 53, responsibility gains the spiritual status of service, a kind of *diakonia* (Levinas EDHH:196). With reference to Jewish spirituality, it is not so farfetched to assume that the "I" in Levinas' thinking, eventually attains the character of a *diakonos*, a kind of *èbèd JHWH*. To serve vicariously, becomes characteristic of our position and *habitus* in this world. We are not here for ourselves, but position ourselves as being there, for the Other, to the Other, and for others as well.

Position in Levinas' thinking, indicates an attitude that cannot be reduced to a rational category of the human mind (Levinas EDHH:196). The position is not the result of a phenomenological intention. As said, it is irrevocable, so that one cannot simply leave your position like a deserter. The position is about morality and an existential movement that precedes all forms of intentionality. The movement is instigated by this metaphysical desire (*désir métafysique*). The result is that I am immediately moulded into a responsibility that leads to a vocation, representing the "countenance/ visage" of the "Other" in the mode of authentic solidarity with the weakness of others. In my position, I am here, available for the other – a manifestation of substitution (Levinas AE:125; AZ:146).

The outline on the meaning of countenance/visage boils down to the following: The visage is a kind of command, petition and instruction; it is carried and empowered by the transcendent. The terminologies which Levinas used (such as "entrance", "epiphany" and "visitation") are all indications of exteriority – it comes from beyond and is thus exterior. All these categories should not be rendered as merely ontological categories (being functions). They surpass all forms of comprehension. They are also not the result of ontic analyses, or the consequence of subjective processes of signification. They are much more operational, in the sense that they establish significance, and put all such functions under judgement. They establish, confirm and transform the "I-operations" into:

- *Liturgy*: An investment in the infinite without reward; an expression of the ethics of patience – Levinas HAM:69-71).
- *Diakonia*: An expression of service and demonstration of the "servant of the Lord" – vicarious reaching out.
- *Substitution*: Solidarity as expression of deep concern – on behalf of the other, for the benefit of the other; it is about a passion without any a priori (Levinas AZ:150; AE:130). This passion is established as an allegiance (*allégeance*) – a kind of loyalty – of the self, to the other; the other as an uneasy disturbance (*inquiétude*) (Levinas AE:32; AZ:48) of human smugness.

The dynamics of paradox within the intriguing interplay: Desire – visage – trace

The three concepts: desire, visage and trace (significant footprints/traces) play an important role in Levinas' paradoxical methodology of philosophical reasoning. Within this trilogy of foundational thinking about the embeddedness of subjectivity in exteriority (transcendence), and the networking relationship between "I" and "Other/other" as an ethical relationship, one discovers the gist of Levinas' reflection on the framework for humane and responsible being. While the metaphysical desire frees the subject from totality, the notion of trace/footprint/marking functions as conscientious memory and remembrance of lost, forgotten experiences that keeps thinking going.

As already argued, it seems as if the term "metaphysical desire" sounds like a contradiction in terminus. How can one describe human ability (the capacity to become operational) in terminology that indicates the passivity of activity (being functions) with its point of control (appeal, commandment, imperative) in the exteriority of a different "master"?

Subjectivity is about a vivid mode of authentic being. The strange element in Levinas' argument is that subjectivity is moulded by passivity. The question surfaces: How is it possible to define the subject's being functions by means of a concept that refers to sheer passivity? (Levinas DTA:52). Furthermore, the reason for this passivity is Levinas' attempt to link the passivity of an erotic experience to a desire and need that does not have unification as goal (*eros*; longing, manipulation of the other), but "femininity" (Levinas DTA:65) (promoting the other).

Eros is about longing, desire and need. But in authentic erotic desire, the other is not the object of *eros*. Objectification of the other/others destroys the trustworthiness of the erotic relationship. Objectification is counter-parted by a *meta*-dimension of transcendence. This is needed in order to take care of the unique identity of the subject, and to safeguard subjectivity against the violence of totality. It is within this background, that Levinas imports the notion of desire and its connection to *eros*.

Desire is essentially structured by intentionality. Desire is an intentional act that is directed towards the appropriation of objects; it is steered by its attempt to annexe things and the world. Desire represents being as an existential endeavour that wants to satisfy needs and cover all forms of deficiencies. One can even describe it as an organismic dynamic that wants to complete and overcome all forms of insufficiencies and lacks. Human need can be understood as libidinal energy: that is, in search for satisfaction. It is like an existential imperative and urgent attempt to persevere (*un être persévérant à lêtre,* with reference to Spinoza) and self-maintenance. In terms of Ricoeur (1965:55-56), needs are existential efforts (*effort pour exister*) to live and to survive. The desire is like a craving, and is, thus, focused on objects that could satisfy these cravings. It represents the original ontic starting point of human existence and being functions. It is as if the ontic desire tries to grasp the essence of being in order to cope with the excessive longing for existing in a meaningful and significant way. The desire, thus, appears as a basic feature of our being human. In this respect, Freud's psychoanalytical model with its emphasis on libido, renders a steering function to the ego in order to direct excessive desires into meaningful tracks, preventing the super-ego of destroying I-identity. The "I" should be protected in order to perform its acting capacity within even "object-related" relationships (see about Fairbairn in ch.2, and Rouppe van der Voort 1991:61).

Many thinkers have tried to describe the "I" (the dynamics of the ego) in terms of impediment-theories designed around different theses on desires and the urge for need-satisfaction. But it is exactly within these paradigmatic approaches, that the burning question arises: How free and autonomous is the "I", the subject, to manage needs in a meaningful way?

The heteronomy of responsibilty as re-spond-ability

To deal with this question, attention should be given to the notion of responsibility as a prior factor in the establishment of loyalty and trustworthiness.

It seems that one has to replace the Cartesian formula of "*cogito ergo sum*" (I think therefore I am), with "*amo, ergo sum*" (I love therefore I am), or with "*respondeo ergo sum*" (I am re-*spond*-able and responsible; therefore I am). Perhaps even with "*non concupisco, ergo sum*" (I am more than desire – being merely covetous – therefore I am). But in all these formulations, the "I" is portrayed in terms of its right to maintain itself, and to focus on self-development and self-assertiveness.

It is now necessary to pose the question whether it is possible for the "I" to determine an ontic shortage in itself and then to decide afterwards how to overcome this shortage, and eventually, to satisfy all basic existential needs within the parameters of self-autonomy? Or does the shortage come into being due to heteronomy?

The notion that the self needs the other in order to become itself, is a perspective that often surfaces in many relational theories within the framework of dialectics. In this regard, the Hegelian dialectics in existential philosophy plays a role indeed. We have already referred to Freud's theory on the libido and the need of the ego to find an "Other self". In the formulation of Lacan (in Mooij 1977:124): The desire of man is the desire of/for the Other (*Le désire de l'homme, c'est le désir de l'Autre*). Being directed and aligned to the other, or an object[20], both are established from a psychological point of view within the triangular structure of relational events. The "I" muffles the other/others out of its way. It then transforms their needs into own needs with the claim: I am first. The subject, the ego, thus maintains his/her first rank position. In principle, the other then becomes an enemy. In this scenario, "morality" becomes the false masquerade of enmity. It is not any more authentic morality, because the so called "morality" alienates, suppresses and becomes artificial. The further dilemma is that the "I", as moral subject, becomes the trace of indirect enmity and merely a sign of suspicion as in the theories of Marx, Nietsche and Freud (See Ricoeur 1965:42).

Disproportion: From neutrality to the lament of significant being

The introduction of transcendence and the connection between the "I" and the metaphysical desire are complex. The metaphysical desire is about the reality of transcendence, but the latter cannot be transformed into the object of an intentional analysis as in phenomenology. The desire is not about objectified being and an existential shortcoming. The metaphysical desire is from the start an existential longing for the other – being-for-others (*l'être pour Autrui*). In this yearning for the other, the "I" is the only component that can be described as subject, namely in terms of an "insatiable thirst". But it is precisely here that the "I" is challenged by a dilemma: On its own the "I" is exposed to the dilemma of "being torn apart", without equilibrium (*déchirement et deséquilibre*). The further problem is, that the other, as term, cannot be described in terms of being. The other is a disproportionate entity and fully

---

[20] See René Girard's writings: Desire is informed by the mimetic character of needs. In this regard, the other functions as both model and obstruction.

inadequate. The other is neither a dominating totality, or kind of master. The other is a guest and not a correlate of my desire or consciousness.

It is against this background that one needs to understand Levinas' critiques on Western philosophy. Western philosophy starts with the primordial position of self-consciousness (*conscience de soi*). The primordial self dominates the thinking (Levinas Trl:11). It is about a very exclusive approach that abandons the other from the realm of the self. In fact, one can formulate it much harsher: The other is destroyed by the monadic smugness of the self. There is no space for the other in the prison of the self, because where the self is in control (I, my-self), the other is a non-entity. The Other also becomes non-existent. Thus, the reason why Western philosophy finds itself in the cul de sac of a sterile, ontological unity of absolute totalities. Even the unknown is transformed into the realm of the known; awareness is always a consciousness about some-*thing*. This tendency to translate everything into the rational categories of the well-known, is called by Levinas the "pretention of the spirit" that proclaims everything by means of the kerugma of language into the "it" of explanatory words. The pretention of mine dominates all forms of epistemology (Levinas EDHH:218).

In epistemology, knowing becomes the exclusive act of consciousness. A consciousness that is established by the idealist concept of logos (Levinas AE:125). The predicate, what has been said, becomes the main topic, because "the specific this" is moulded into "a general that", and, eventually becomes the topic of scientific discourses. People starts to talk about some-*thing* with one another. For example, now they can talk about commerce, philosophy, science and technique. Particularity becomes generalised so that general concepts precede all forms of particularity (Levinas EDHH:222).

The idealist transformation of the particular into the general, in order to explain by means of logic, is in fact a cunning detour:
(a) The "I" that identifies itself as "I", performs in fact a detour. It is done by means of a discourse: the comprehension of the "logos" via rationalisation. Everything is about self-illumination and self-understanding. But this self-understanding is always an understanding in terms of some-*thing* else. The irony is, that in this vigorous process of self-understanding, the "I" makes it-*self* into a topic and object (it). This is exactly the same with the otherness of the other (Levinas Trl:14).

(b) The identification of an "it" as "that", requires a kind of "mediation" that implies an appeal on neutrality. Furthermore, this appeal is in fact about a retreat into a "resort of neutrality" (*recours aux Neutres*) (Levinas EDHH:168). Epistemology becomes the power of generalisation: Everything can be explained in terms of the one logical principle that becomes the cornerstone of scientific reflection and explanatory hypotheses. Rational clarification becomes the epistemological motto for being scientific, and, thus, verified knowledge. Furthermore, communication becomes a commodity. Significance is reduced to a neutral entity: The one explains the significance of all the other. What eventually can be accepted as truth, is what is explainable in general terminology: the collectivity of verified truth (Levinas EDHH:168). Justice becomes eventually subjected to a totality of truth wherein ontology dictates validity, and not ethics.

In the light of these positivistic detours, one should understand Levinas' vigorous programme to find a way out of this epistemological dilemma: A horrible neutrality that dominates the quality of our being human. There should be a way out of the discourse of general collectivity (the totality of being), back to the particularity of being human. It should be a mode of being wherein justice is not an accidental by-product of rationalised knowledge. It should be a way how to temper power in order to promote meaning and significant direction.

For Levinas, there is indeed another wise tradition and informative paradigm. It is the paradigm of wisdom that resides in the wisdom of the heart; a kind of knowledge present in myself (Levinas MG:145). It is about a tradition of reflection, that "hears" and understands the other. This mode of wise reflection is often verbalised in the mode of a lament: The injustice of oppression is being articulated as "crying aloud to high heaven". In this lament the other is profiled within the tradition of justice. The latter acting as trace in the conscientiousness of self-awareness.

Justice originates from disproportions in relational networking with others and myself. In such a case, the logos of a commandment dictates: "Thou shall not kill". This commandment links one with the presence of the Other. It connects being with transcendent visage; it is about a presence that precedes all other modes of representation. Levinas calls this presence "countenance/

visage"; a "countenance/visage" that is at the same time "epiphany" and "visitation". In a nutshell: Before I "see" and even "know" that I am seeing, I have already been seen. Before I become aware of my differentiation, I have already been differentiated and summoned.

It means that the "I" can never rest in a kind of totality of self-smugness. The subject is not encapsulated by self-knowledge, nor by rational attempts in epistemology, projecting its findings into general statements and theories that explain particularity. Subjectivity, stirred by its metaphysical desire, is always delivered out to an "ultimate agitator", or "*meta*-physical trouble-maker" within the realm of ethical relationships, namely the mysticism of a trans-factor: the Other/other.

The many layered meanings of a meta-agitator/trouble-maker

In Levinas' thinking, the many layered meaning of three basic terminologies, namely the "Other/other" and others, visage or countenance, and mocking presence, operate like traces of exteriority and transcendence.

The alterity of "Other/other"

The terms "Other" and "other" are used by Levinas in a fairly arbitrary way. In some cases, the reference is merely to other; in many other cases it is with a capital: "Other". It can become confusing indeed. However, it refers basically to the other in his/her alterity.

Visage: The dynamics of an oppositional beyond

Visage or countenance is the óther in opposition to a form of being, derived from totality, or a kind of neutral, anonymous understanding of the essence of being/Being. Visage is a dynamic concept with its own unique operation. It indicates a kind of "beyond" within a *meta*-realm (coming from elsewhere). Nothing knowable can explain its origin and character. It is indeed about an "expression" (Levinas TO:51). It does not refer to an expression of "some-*thing*", lurking behind, but an expression in its own right and terms; an expression of itself, from in itself: *Kath'auto* (Levinas EDHH:197). It is not an artificial mask that covers a secret or hidden kind of personal entity; it is about a direct encounter.

In one of his last interviews, Levinas explained the term "visage" as follows: Visage is an indication of the unique I-dynamics within the other, concerning my being human. As with a portrait, it displays what takes place behind the attitude in terms of his/her lonely forsakenness, vulnerability and mortality. This subtle backdrop of being, makes an appeal to my original responsibility to *some*-body in his/her unique being in this world. The other in this sense, is in fact "the loved one" (Levinas TO:299; EN:257). The visage makes an appeal upon me, even before I am factually connected to him/her. In the appeal of the other, the other becomes my "original" or "ancient" responsibility. He/she becomes "my predestination"; I am predestined to be with the other in co-existence with others. "Ancient" then refers to a pre-responsibility that is older than my existence in time, an appeal (*à mon antique responsabilité*).

The presence of visage: the mocking of conscious representation

The presence of visage is actually about being-there. However, this presence is different from all other modes of encounter, because it has got a kind of mocking effect. It is an unmasking mockery on every conscious attempt of representation and comprehension. The irony is, that the "I" is always "too late" for this presence. The "I" has got an untraceable backlog. In order to explain this handicap of always coming too late, Levinas illustrates this backlog by using a text from Song of Songs 5:6(a) in the Old Testament: "I opened for my lover, but my lover had left; he was gone" (Levinas AE:112; AZ:133).

The moment when the visage breaks into my order, I lose its image and significance. It disappears not because I am not watchful enough. Even when I am wide awake and quite alert, I lose its image. The visage comes and goes like a thief during the night; you cannot see it because it is not some-*thing*. I can only see its traces. This is why Israel was summoned to do, to act and to obey the command, even when the doer will hear later: Doing precedes hearing. According to Levinas, the rabbinic commentators ascribe this very strange order to the fact that "good" is primordial. Therefore, the existence of a primordial adhesion to what is good. This adhesion precedes the freedom of choice, and the attempt to distinguish between good and evil (Levinas, *Quatre Lectures* QLT:95). The act of obedience is not about a controversy: Praxis in opposition to theory; it is rather about a way of actualising, without starting first with the possible (Levinas QLT:95); it is about an original attachment with the property and instigating factor (*attache originelle avec le bien*) (Levinas QLT:96); it is about profound integrity – the deep structure of subjectivity (*Une structure profonde de la subjectivité qu'est la Temimouth*) (Levinas QLT:93).

The previous outline explains the in-depth structure of subjectivity. It also clarifies the character of responsibility as an ethical concern in relationship with a command. This structure is about the prior experience and exposure to the Tora (*l'experience préalable de la Tora elle-même*) (Levinas QLT:83)[21]. The first and last in human existence is not death and fate, but commandment and *diakonia*: The compassion for the vulnerable. The predestined infinite responsibility is an ethical concern.

Levinas' visage, and its connection to words like "obligation", "merit", "earning entitlement", "self" (inclusive of "self-delineation" and "self-validation"), "legacy", are linked to responsibility and receiving. In the case of Nagy's psychotherapeutic discourse, they are exponents of "being", "achievement" and "having" (possession). With Nagy's theory formation for psychotherapy in mind, it is perhaps understandable why these terminologies are indeed essentially ethical, they could only be interpreted within the perspective of "visage" – the birth right of the other.

The other is in fact like the presence of a fleeting mirage: One cannot see the visage in person; it has no definite depiction or form; it precedes all forms of portrayal; it is there (present), but always absent in the sense that nothing represents this presence visually. Due to absence of any form of portrayal, it is virtually impossible for memory and conscience to grasp this presence in rational and comprehension terminology. What one becomes aware of is merely a trace. The visage does not appear as a "face" of another person. It is just a momentary flash of difference that breaks into the realm of the selfhood and penetrates the self; it infiltrates immanency. Like a bolt from the blue, the visage presents itself as a strange form of "presencing", irreducible to an epistemology of self; it resists any form of disclosure. It cannot be identified and is incomparable to any existing entity.

---

21 Levinas' prior is different than in the case of existential philosophy in general. For example, for Heidegger the prior factor is death. For Levinas, the first and the last is not death, but the visage of the Other. Instead of death, and the fate of nothingness (Sartre), the other as commandment and significant meaning-giving factor with the emphasis on the fact that we are predestined for infinite responsibility. Care is not about one's own being, but about *diakonia* – the compassion for the vulnerable. And this is exactly what the ethical relationship is about (Levinas EN 1991:255; TO 1987:297).

The trace of the other is ontologically speaking, total insignificant, and, therefore, also totally absent in terms of an ontology of to be. It is hidden, and totally ulterior. Before I even realise it, the other speaks to me, becomes audible and sensible. But it is totally different than being. So different that even the language of dialectics cannot capture its meaning; it operates beyond the dialectics of being and non-being (Levinas AE:10; AZ:23). Its trace indicates and describes merely perspective. But this perspective is not conceivable for the human mind; it merely opens up a peephole into being through which I become aware of the fellow human being (*prochain*), appealing to my responsibility. In this sense, the other leaves a trace that makes me feel uncomfortable. One can put it harsher: The trace makes me restless and "inquiet" (*inquiétude*). The "inquietness" penetrates my very being and consciousness; it disturbs my self-image. In such a case, it is not the "normal self", but the self that has been problematised by the other, even before it struck the self. The self that has become a question for him/herself, becomes in response, the trace of the other. In this sense, an alliance (*allégeance*) has been established with the other (Levinas AE:29; AZ:45), even before I have become aware of the other, or of myself.

The trace of the other in human awareness should not be confused with the psychoanalytical unconscious factor and the appearance of an "It" within the realm of consciousness. The term "trace" also does not refer to a defect in awareness. On the contrary, it refers to an excess not to be disclosed, but as trace, still operating as a directing factor: One to and for the other.

The emerging of the "I" from the *Illeity* of He (*il*)

In a strange formulation, Levinas refers to the fact that the other also emerges out of the illeity of a He. That is the reason why the "I" falls into infinite debt, vis-á vis the other.

Illeity is a term derived from the Latin: *ille*, meaning "He". It refers to that which is other than being. This differentiation is necessary in order to connect the "Other" to a beyond that operates on the *meta*-realm of transcendence within the sphere of the ultimate and undefinable absolute (it is neither being, nor non-being). *Illeity* evokes a He-factor that even leaves the "Other" in the trace of his immemorial past. "He-hood" is in fact incomprehensible for reason. It (*Illeity*) is introduced by Levinas to emphasize how difficult it is to explain the "Other" by means of pronouns or personal categories. It is merely a trace of visage and cannot even be captured by divine terminology like "God".

Traces are not about signs nor symbols. Signs signify and call meaning into being. It helps the mind to decipher meaning within contexts. If the trace is about a symbol, the implication is that the "it" refers to the comprehension of some-*thing*. The other is then reduced to an ontological realm wherein being is detectable and translatable into descriptive theories. The other cannot be converted into an "It"; the other is non-descriptive. In this sense, the presence of the other is in fact about "absence".

The point in Levinas' argumentation is that the trace of the Other in the self, is in terms of ontological description, sheer absence. The visage is from "elsewhere" so that the trace only refers to exteriority, transcendence and the ultimate other, the absolute other that is "more real" than Being. The only way to articulate this strange, peculiar other, is to call this kind of "Other", "He" (*ille*). This "He" presents a unique kind of "He-hood" which never had been, is *passé*, and cannot be experienced empirically or ontologically on the level of being.

Even the Being of being, is not the assignor of significance. Being cannot be derived from Being. The eventual and authentic assignor that can grant meaning and significance, is a "He" (*ille*). In his trace, the other is situated so that transcendence, (one can even say "God") comes to the idea (*Dieu qui vient à l'idée*); transcendence emerges in the idea without being grasped by the idea and absorbed by the idea. This is why Levinas proposes "He" instead of "it"; speaking precedes being. "The He" then refers to a mysterious puzzle, because it is connected to transcendence, and transcendence disturbs being; it disturbs all forms of classification and systemic orders installed by subject; it intercepts, interrupts, and distresses consciousness (*une diachronie, qui affolle le sujet*). Furthermore, the transcendence is an *anachronism* (*un étranger, venu certes, mais parti avant d'être venu, ab-solu dans sa manifestation*); a strange entity that is gone, even before it came, even the manifestation abolishes its coming (EDHH:210-211; MG:200). This is the reason why transcendence is a *puzzling enigma*, and impossible to be integrated in any way to the order of the autonomous subject. This is about a kind of "spiritual trauma" within soulful subjectivity.

The function of "trace" in Levinas' thinking, is to bring about a constant awareness and sensitivity for the visage of the other. The alterity of the other, is a trace of the authentic trace that correlates with the idea of the infinite, escaping every form of memory. This is the subjectivity that Levinas wanted to defend: subjectivity as representation of humane and responsible being-with; as subject to the other. It is about a subjectivity that the other, at the same time, already has been granted, even before the subject knows about it.

This subjectivity operates as exposure to the predicament of the other in his/her vulnerability. In this regard, Levinas refers to Matthew 25:31-46. God is present in the nakedness, hunger and captivity of the other: They are there, they are present in a eucharistic sense, before the subject even existed (*au sens eucharistique*) (IKON-*Interview*). It is about a eucharistic "*presentia realis*", indicating a presence and visage that is more "real" than being[22].

Subjectivity as animated mercifulness (Levinas)

With reference to the purpose of the research project, namely to detect the value of Nagy's contextual approach for healing and human well-being within contexts, it is necessary to highlight some of the main perspectives in Levinas' meta-model on subjectivity. Therefore, the following question: Is it possible to link Levinas' emphasis on the interplay between visage/transcendence/Other and the prior of subjectivity to the ethical basis of relational dynamics, "the human order of justice"? Can Levinas' encounter with visage, be merged with Nagy's dialoguing understanding of the "I-Thou" encounter?

In order to conclude, what is meant by the notion of subjectivity in Levinas' thinking? The outcome of the previous exposition on Levinas' thinking, can be captured by the following brief remarks.

1. *Subjectivity is about a metaphysical desire.* The basis for this desire is not merely existential needs with the focus on need-satisfaction and having. The desire presupposes a sound "Self" that takes interest in life and finds all modes of relational and existential dynamics decisive and most pleasant. Our being human should not be derived from a hiatus like need-satisfaction, hunger, thirst, displacement, suffering, nihilism (hopelessness and meaninglessness). The implication will be that our

---

22 For the terror of the Shoah, and how the ideology of corruption and violence tried to extinguish the traces of the other's suffering by killing the other, see A Herzberg 1950:31.

being human is then derived from a disrupted, dislocated, violent, and, indeed absurd world (Levinas TO:169).

Désir métaphysique is a longing that represents the quest for peace; it wants to instil peace to the other; it is about a nostalgia for something strange, even for an opposing and disrupting factor (meta-factor) that can penetrate our daily existence as exposed to self-smugness and the totality of power abuse. The name of this penetrating factor is justice. Desire is not a longing for the "being of the other" in order to manipulate and to take control over the other: the threat of mastering. It dislikes war (ethical aversion) and is summoned without any form of force (*sans force*): Thou shall not kill (*Tu ne tueras point*) (Levinas TO:67, 68). It is not about "mastering" but about "serving".

2. *"Désir métaphysique" operates within the realm of the infinite*. It is about a meta-relationship with the other; it is about the relational dynamics between a subject and the other/Other. The relationship is not about relativity, but, due to its *meta*-character, "wholly different". In fact, it is infinitely different, infinitely other: *Ab-solute Other*. Facing the Other, encountering visage, is an event instigated by visage itself: The Other looks at me, stares at the subject – *Parce qu'il me regarde* (IKON-*Interview* 1995). The reason for this penetrating staring, resides in the fact that the Other is a human being, therefore the "I" is important for him (*ille*) and exists in "his presence". The reason for the penetrating gaze of the Other, resides not in my own being human. It is the humanity of the other, that evokes the staring. It is not Being, that looks at me with benediction, but the visage of the Other that illuminates being and blesses "his people" (see the Aaronic blessing in Numbers 6:24-26 – The Lord makes his face shine upon you!). One is summoned by a "joyous force" emanating not from "being" (as in the case of Heidegger) but by the light of Visage/Countenance.

3. *The interplay between relational encounters and guilt*. The subject is always connected to the other by means of a relationship. This relationship is determined by guilt, because in being guilty (*culpabilité*), I owe the other justice. One is summoned to a calling and work of justice (*oeuvre de la justice*). This calling is not about one's own benefit and self-maintenance but directed towards the advantage of the other; it is totally unselfish and even stretches beyond death (*pour au delá de ma*

mort) (Levinas HAM:69). It is an impulse and desire to do justice; it is about a kind of liturgical labour without any gain; it is qualified by patience and *diakonia*.

4. *The significance of subjectivity is directed by a Footprint: The speech of Trace*. The Self with whom the "I" is identified (in self-identification), is the Self wherein the other already partook. It is present in the Self as trace; as trace that renders meaning by means of speaking: To introduce oneself in meaning, is about speaking (*Se presenter en signifiant, c'est parler*) (Levinas TI:37; TO:71). Speaking is about entering relationships without giving your identity away. Language presupposes the transcendence, the separation, strangeness of the conversational partner, the trauma of awe (Levinas TO:80), wherein the total collectivity is absent: The other is like an immigrant.

5. *A face-to-face encounter demarcates a primordial event for constituting righteousness.* It is not about co-existence as such. It demarcates the primordial realm which Levinas calls "Self" or "the Same". This Self or Same only turns to the ab-solute Other, The Other, due to the appealing presence of the Other. The other is not about a psychic alter-ego projected by me due to the idea of co-existence. It is about a discovery that the Other, fellow human being, is like me, and not the result of introspection due to the intra-dynamics of a reflecting "I". The fellow human being is not constituted by me. A face-to-face encounter announces fellowship, accompaniment and social communality (*Le face-á-face [...] annonce une société*) (Levinas TI:39; TO:73). There is no general or abstract "we", or neutral entity, that precedes this announcement. The social accompaniment starts in the truth; a truth that speaks and constitutes righteousness (*droîture*). Speaking is in fact to relate, but keeping one's dignity. Speaking does not presuppose a general collectivity but makes it possible: The generality is founded by generosity (Levinas TO:83). "Flesh becomes word" (verbalised embodiment) in the face-to-face encounter; close rapprochement that nurtures and signifies (Levinas AZ:140; AE:121).

6. *Visage or countenance is about no veil; it is uncovered and bare due to the gaze of the stranger/outsider.* To acknowledge the other, is to acknowledge his/her "hunger", and, thus, simultaneously about giving

to the other. The other in his/her state of humility and humbleness, does not refer to a state of minority/inferiority. On the contrary, the other is in fact my superior and in time first. The exteriority is the look and gaze of the stranger, the outsider, the widower and the orphan. In giving one speaks; in speaking one gives. To acknowledge the other, is to reach out to the other through and by means of the "it" in the world; by means of eating and making home for the displaced. To say: I was first, presupposes that the other was there before me. To negate the other, is to rob him/her of his/her right of birth. Denial of the other, can be called "murder".

7. *The "I" exists in the world by means of embodiment.* The "I" is in this sense self-sufficient, without "deities", endowed with an *a-theistic will*. The "I" is not a by-product or result of a "causative factor" but constituted by a face-to-face encounter with transcendent exteriority. Transcendence cannot be thematised or conceptualised in rational categories of phenomenological observations. The topic and concept are always a posteriori. The moral awareness transcends itself, while the theoretical awareness is limited to the interior. In transcending, the "I" is exposed to an experience that is not under the domain of its own freedom. Even self-criticism, starts as a critique on one's own freedom, outside the realm of "topic" and "concept" (see Levinas AE:29). A true and valid theory takes care for the respect of exteriority with as resource, the moral conscience and criticized freedom. A true and valid theory is open to all possibilities, even to the infinite order that discloses well-being (the good) (Levinas TO:115-117). This infinite order resides in the concrete reality of the society. It attains meaning and significance, outside the dominance of being and existential facticity. The surprising fact is that Levinas calls this realm "*the resort for the eschatology of messianic peace*".

8. *The "Self", the corporeality and interiority by which the "I" is identified in self-identification, is already connected and entangled with the other, even beforehand.* This connectedness and entanglement precede the awareness of this connectedness. The "I" in self-identification, grasps this entanglement of before, within the appeal that it is exercised by the other in ethical encounters. The surprising discovery is that the

other was there in the past participle – the infinite past before memory. The "I" carries the other in the womb of itself; it is obsessed with the other. In this sense, subjectivity is a relationship, as well as a term in this relationship (Levinas AE:108; AZ:129). As self, subjectivity is essentially moulded into being; it is, thus, connected and touched by the other. Therefore, the reason why subjectivity is defined by passivity: Being touched and summoned by the other. Of this summoning, the erotic relationship is a prelude (Levinas TA:73).

9. *Responsibility precedes freedom.* The "I" is, thus, a substitute and alternative for the other. The substitute implies a kind of hostage: The one who stands surety and sponsors, is also the one who pays bail for the other (*Bekol me'odeka*). It becomes clear that being free for the other, is not "normal" and "self-evident". However, it is also not abstract. It is concrete, anchored in materiality and human embodiment. Levinas calls this material concreteness, "the ensoulment/animation of the body". Embodiment (corporeality) and materiality are the locus of the principle: one for the other (*l'un pour l'autre*). From a Cartesian point of view, this statement of Levinas, is logically impossible: How on earth can "*res cogitans*" (thinking, rational substance; mindful thinking) ensouls and animates "*res extensa*" (extended thing, corporeal substance)? But exactly, this paradox signifies the self, the one for the other (*L'un pour l'autre*). Subjectivity articulates the animation of the body in all its vulnerability. The further implication is, that what Levinas wrote about the ensoulment/animation of the body, can also be transferred to the hermeneutics of the phrase: "The soul that emanates from and stretches out to God" (Levinas DL:31).

10. *The "I" as animated with compassionate mercy and pity.* The notion that the soul ensouls (animates, inspires), must be interpreted from the notion of tenderness and sensitivity (pity). In other words, the fact that I am touched by the other, even beforehand, is an indication of compassion/tenderness and a modification of the concept of motherhood and pregnancy (Levinas AZ:115; AE:95). It is pre-natal, pre-natural; it is the nearness of a membrane; near as labour pain and motherhood (*Rachamim*) (Levinas Sas:158). *Rachamim* is about the relation of the uterus to the other; it is motherhood in itself. In this

sense, one can even define God in terms of motherhood.[23] Here we find ourselves in the realm of subjectivity as subjecticity[24]. Subjectivity then as an identity, articulated from the start as an accusative: Here am I (*me voici*).

Subjectivity within the familial paradigm of intergenerational dynamics: The asymmetry of reciprocity (Nagy)

The following group of research questions need to be posed.
- Is it possible that Nagy's contention about the subject, could accommodate ethics in terms of a command that cannot be derived from something else? Is it therefore possible to maintain the asymmetric structure of responsibility (responsibility that does not start with reciprocity)? Furthermore, can the interpretation of the "realm of between" in judicial terminology be regarded as appropriate within the context of psychotherapy and human well-being?
- Is it possible to maintain the identity of the entities in the relationship, or is the critique on Buber's "I-Thou", namely that the "I" and the "Thou" become endangered in the mutuality and run the risk to become negated by the dynamics of the relationship, valid indeed?

For Nagy, it was important to emphasize that his approach implies much more than Buber's dialogical model. The difference resides in the way Nagy introduced the notion of intergenerational relationships within the paradigmatic framework of dialogue. The intergenerational relationship was not explicitly explored by Buber[25] (Van Heusden & Van den Eerenbeemt 1992:18). It is therefore decisive to give attention to the intergenerational background of dialogue.

---

23 *Rachamim, c'est le rapport de l'utérus à l'autre, don't, en lui, se fait le gestation. Rachamim, c'est la maternité même. Dieu est misericord-dieux, c'est Dieu défine par la maternité.*
24 See also M Schneider in Levinas, *Cahier de l'Herne*:505.
25 Gershom Scholem (1982:49-50) made an important remark: Buber was not aware of the fact that the dialogue between generations, formed the basis for many of the dialogues in the writings of the rabbis, the narratives and explanations in the Talmud. In this sense, Buber was blind for the Jewish tradition of intergenerational dialogue.

The intergenerational dialogue

Within the Jewish wisdom tradition, instruction from the Talmud was continued from one generation to the following. The learning process was dialogical and intergenerational. The Tora was the continuum and created the culture and community of: From generation to generation[26]. The notion "from generation to generation" provided continuity, but, at the same time, one should reckon with discontinuity. Discontinuity is an exponent of dialoguing. This is an important perspective due to Levinas' contention that dialogue is about a relationship between separate entities (asymmetry). This will also be the view of the researchers.

We come back to the connection between Nagy and Buber. The fact that the intergenerational dialogue is not taken into consideration by Buber, is for Nagy a shortcoming. As therapist, the familial intergenerational relationship is for Nagy special and prior. The existential interconnectedness between parents and children, points in the direction of what Nagy called "indebtedness". The latter is not determined by emotional or strategic incentives.

In the first chapter of IL, Nagy wrote about Buber's definition of dialogue: "While the concept of the mutually, confirming dialogue unquestionably enriches our understanding of relationships, in general our position is that family relationships have their own specific existential, historic structuring" (Nagy IL:7).

Even when one search for remarks on familial and intergenerational dynamics, through autobiographic fragments in Buber's legacy (Schilpp & Friedman 1967:3-39), references to, for example, his contact with his mother, are not convincing enough to founding a theory for familial and intergenerational contextual therapy (Nagy IL:7). The examples in Buber's dialogical encounters, only describe instantaneous and momentary situations. They refer to encounters within the spur of the moment without any long-term implications for responsible behaviour.

It was already pointed out that the subject for Buber does not have an independent status. That was Levinas' critique on Buber (Levinas NP:37). If the subject does not have an independent responsibility wherein ethics can

---

26 For Nagy, intergenerational relationships are linked with familial dynamics, and not so much with the dynamics of communities of faith. However, these two fields are intertwined, especially in Jewish communities.

take root and be manifested, it becomes virtually impossible to accentuate the ethical dimension within relational encounters.

The research is based on two important critical aspects in Buber's approach:
(a) According to Levinas, Buber neglected the separation of subjects.
(b) Buber did not give special attention to the relationship between generations.

In order to research and assess the contribution of Nagy to the concept of intergenerational relationships, the researchers pose the following thesis:

Because intergenerational relationships are the special focus and paradigmatic background in Nagy's theory concerning familial care and healing (within the framework of the relational dynamics and the concrete setting of social realities and contexts), he views the subject as accountable for the other human being. Thus, the reason why the subject is to be differentiated as a separate entity from other human beings. If that is not the case, the notion of accountability becomes insignificant.

The research will not focus on the question whether Nagy's description of the subject had explicitly any significant impact on Nagy's clinical work. The answer is obviously: No. Nagy was a clinical psychiatrist and psychotherapist. His first concern was the enhancement of the quality of the practice of healing and helping.

With this remark in the background of our mind, it is still important to notify the place of the concept "subject" in Nagy's theory formation. In this regard, attention will be given not only to the concept "subject", but also to other concepts playing a decisive role in the interpretation of ethical entanglements: "Individual", "person", "ego", "self/Self", "object" and "other/Other"[27].

Individual

The notion of "individual" is not a keyword in Nagy's writing. When individual is used as a proper noun, it is not meant to be in opposition to other concepts; especially not in opposition to his theoretic design for a contextual

---

27 Nagy uses alternately small and capital letters in order to underline the importance and weight of the concept.

approach in therapy. The index in the publication: *Intensive Family Therapy* (Boszormenyi-Nagy & Framo 1965), does not refer specifically to "individual" as keyword (Nagy IL:219, 225-226)[28]. Individual as proper noun or auxiliary noun is not used in opposition to context/contextual. It is indeed used in opposition to the notion of a totalitarian system and the powerplay of systemic mechanisms.

Person

With person is meant the individual within relationships. As single entity, the person does not lose his/her identity within the networking dynamics of relationships. Nagy, (in Boszormenyi-Nagy & Framo 1965:75-76), refers indeed to "personality development" and "personality theory" (1965:34). In IL (p 62) there is a reference to "personal identity" and "strength of personality" (IL:373); "What is the objective reality of the person?" (IL:15-17). Person is described as a unique entity, connected to others within the context of relationships (his/her *needs* and his/her *style* of responding) (VR/MK).

Subject

The subject refers to somebody as a single entity; somebody who is indeed a person. This understanding is impossible without a "Thou". The notion of "subject" is used in cases where Nagy (as therapist) wants to describe the psychodynamic or interactional relationship between client and somebody else (with some other): The dynamics of intersubjectivity. In the index of Boszormenyi-Nagy & Framo (1965:51-55, 117, 124-125), there is a reference to "subject role". The following quotation is noteworthy: "Naturally, the self is the experiential center of the individual's world, but the self is always a subjective I, unthinkable without some You" (Nagy IL:9). In the publication there is also reference to "subjective symbolic structuring" (See Nagy F:89). The latter does not mean that the other human being is a symbol in my I-structure (conscious phantasy). It rather describes the position of the self in different dyadic relationships. Both the self, as well as the other, can become subject and object for one another, and vice versa. Relational self-demarcation/delineation takes place not in the "internal dialogue", or within fusion,

---

28 Perhaps, page 256. See individual privacy (Nagy IL:13). In (Nagy F:240-241). There are several references referring to the individual person and the practice of therapeutic treatment (See individual in contextual therapy, Nagy F:240-241; also 334).

but in the authentic dialogue (between subject and subject) wherein both can become subject or object for one another; in other words, context for "self-delineation" of the other (F:94).

Ego

"Ego" is for Nagy (especially in his earlier writings), a concept that profiles psychologically the inner world and motivational drives of the person. It refers more to "the autonomy of the inner world" in Freudian terminology. Ego is part of psychological terminology in Nagy's writings. In Boszormenyi-Nagy & Framo (1965), the index refers to "ego autonomy theory" (40), "ego boundaries" (110), "ego gaps" (94), "ego-mass" (110), "ego psychology" (40), "ego psychology and existential phenomenology" (35-37). In IL there is reference to "ego strength"(IL:109), "ego weakness" (IL:355). F refers to "ego boundary" (F:61-61, 65, 83, 87), "ego-disorganization and reorganization" (F:38).

"self/Self"

The concept "self" refers to the inner, most peculiar existential reality of both "soul" and "body". Within Nagy's dialectics of "giving – receiving", and "receiving – giving", the reference to "self" signifies a kind of "unrest", present in the self. A very extreme mode of "self-centeredness", functions in phrases like: "To give compulsory", and "not to accept something spontaneously" (referring to a kind of martyr-like behaviour). These extreme forms are in fact disruptive forms of self-maintenance and self-justification. However, the point is, these concepts function within the dynamics of relationships determined by ethics.

The index of Boszormenyi-Nagy & Framo (1965:36-84) refers to "self and other". In Nagy (BGT:59), we read that "self-sacrifice" and altruism are normally viewed and interpreted in terms of polarisation (over against egoism). With reference to the notion of deserved trust, Nagy does not think in terms of polarisation, but in terms of a dialectic: Giving by means of receiving, and vice versa. This dialectic is valid even when giving is about outreach to the most vulnerable and helpless people. Their neediness and willingness to receive is in fact a form of giving to the giver. Giving is even not about a strict, formal mode of asymmetry that eventually leads to exhaustion or compulsive giving (leaving the impression of being a martyr). Self-sacrifice is not all about exhaustion, because the most helpless person can also give. In BGT there are also references to "self-assertion", "self-validation", and, in cases of inauthentic modes self-domination (self-maintenance without respect for the other), to self-justification. There are also references to "self-delineation (BGT:75-77, 80, 421) and in F:290; "self-validation" (BGT:77-81, 90, 94, 104-105, 111, 159, 187, 244, 421; F:80, 290, 296, 302-304, 310; "self-actualisation" in F:50; "self/other delineation" in F:44, 60-61, 64, 81, 88-89, 95).

Object

There are many references to object-relation-theory in Nagy's writings. Within therapeutic helping and healing endeavours to schizophrenic patients, Nagy tested the hypothesis of object-relation-theory, but gradually left this paradigm behind when he started to develop his theory for family therapy, and intergenerational dynamics. In Boszormenyi-Nagy & Framo (1965), he uses the term "object loss" (93). With reference to the phenomenon of sensitivity for object-loss, Nagy links it to the collusive character of defence mechanism amongst family members. Boszormenyi-Nagy & Framo (1965) refers to "object role (assignment)" in the discussion of relational modi as well. In the index of IL, there are the following references: "Object constancy" (219); "objective reality in close relationships" (IL:14-15), and "of the person" (IL:15). In BGT, there is only reference to object-relation-theory; in F: "Object relationship" (93), "object relinquishment" (F:44, 48).

"Object" in Nagy's oeuvre can furthermore be linked to the tradition of Fairbairn and other researchers. It is then more applicable to the notion of intrapsychic presentations: "internal objects". With reference to pathological collusions, the differentiation is made between "good object-partners" and "bad object-partners". To be an object for the need of the other human being, implies: to receive from the other (F:94). In this sense, the notion of object is less about need-satisfaction, and more about promoting the well-being of the other/Other.

"other/Other"

In the index of Boszormenyi-Nagy & Framo (1965), there is no separate mentioning of "self" and "other". The index of IL mentions once: "otherness" (IL:21). "Otherness" then means "outgroup" as a different category, and not the otherness of the other person: We may resent them, but we need them (Nagy). "Other" means: different than me, or we. In BGT (73), we read: "Mutual delineation leads to a creative use of otherness." We can conclude and say: "The other" as term, is not exchangeable for the "I" within a therapeutic-theoretical discourse; it indicates merely that all persons/clients (being subjects and therefore objects-to-the-other; to other I's, and others) are in one way or another a kind of "self" (I-identity).

In order to conclude, one can say that the subject-concept as psychic entity in Nagy's vocabulary has not a very high priority. In the glossary of BGT, the concept is not mentioned as key word. Within the chain of concepts (defining the ethical dimension, and mentioned in F:xiv), the reference to "being the object of the other", is the only connection to the previously mentioned concepts. Nagy himself does not bring these concepts in connection with the ethical dimension.

What should be made clear is: *The previously described terminologies are in most of his writings more connected to the dimension of intra-psychic processes than to the ethical dimension as such*; they are intra-psychic categories, not ethical categories.

The meaning of the "ethical dimension" cannot be derived from the way he used these concepts. What Nagy means with "ethical dimension", resides more in the perspective applied by him as therapist. The notion of "ethical dimension" is foundational; it refers to that what Nagy renders as present in the relational networking dynamics of the client, very specifically, in the inter- and trans-generational interaction of relationships.

Albeit, for Nagy it is decisive that the previously described concepts should be interpreted in the light of his paradigmatic approach and attempt to link subjectivity with trustworthy responsibility. Concepts, describing intra-psychic processes, should, thus, derive and render their paradigmatic significance from the paradigm of intergenerationality and its connection to the Other, and not vice versa.

We now return to the scope of this section:
- *What is the status of the subject? Can the comprehension of subject be integrated with the notion of ethics within relational justice?*
- *Is the "I" in Nagy's thinking, merely an entity that eventually becomes absorbed by the "I-Thou relationship" as proposed by Martin Buber?*

As already argued, Nagy's use of Buber does not imply that he reinterprets the realm of the between in the same way it has been applied by Buber. In Nagy's thinking, the "between" is interpreted as an encountering event with juridical and legal implications. This is the reason why the "I" should be a differentiated, separated entity. Only a separated, independent I, can be rendered as "accountable", "responsible", "reliable" for the other.

When the other is not exterior, outside the "I", (the danger that the notions "I-and-the-other/the-other-and-I," become enmeshed in a totality), it becomes virtually impossible to do justice to other people. Collectivity (massification) suppresses the separate interests of the individual. The "I" can only exercise responsibility towards the other, and respond meaningfully to the appeal of the other, when the "I" of the other is indeed a separate entity. Accountability is only possible between two separate entities that are different, and distinct from one another. It is even then possible that the "I" becomes so engaged in an ethical relationship, that responsibility becomes a kind of "obligation".

The fact that Nagy emphasizes that the destiny of the "I" is about being accountable, responsible and reliable to the other, supports the assumption that the question about the status of the subject, is a core issue in Nagy's research and oevre.

In Nagy's thinking, the subject is endowed with a unique identity; it operates within the fundamental dimension of accountability and responsibility. As already argued, the relationship is determined by obligation and is constantly aware of a command that summons the "I" to just behaviour. Thus, the notion of *respondeo ergo sum*: I am responsible and re-*spond*-able; therefore, I am (Heinemann 1954 in F:95, 97). The other is absolutely different, other and completely separate. The subject is therefore also absolutely accountable and responsible due to the factuality of separation, individuation.

The challenge right now is to assess the status of the subject within the paradigmatic framework of inter/trans-generational dynamics. The further question will be: How are the intergenerational, relational conepts connected to intra-psychic concepts?

Gradually Nagy started to interpret the latter (intra-psychic concepts) in terms of the intergenerational dynamics and not vice versa. In order to get clarity on the status of the subject within the networking of intergenerational interaction, the following concepts should further be researched: "mutuality" and "dialogue"; "self-delineation" and "self-validation"; "symmetry" and "asymmetry" in relationships; the "giving child as subject"; "parentification"; an "intrinsic transgenerational tribunal"; the "responsibility of the therapist"; "entitlement". How inter-/transgenerational relationships are represented in these concepts will help to clarify the status of the subject.

Furthermore, in the exposition of these concepts, it will be paramount to come back and reflect on Nagy's conceptualisation of some of the concepts within the paradigmatic framework of Levinas.

Mutuality/reciprocity and dialogue

Without any doubt, justice is a keyword in Nagy's ethical approach to intergenerational dynamics. "We regard justice as a multipersonal homeostatic principle with equitable reciprocity as its ideal goal" (Nagy IL:67).

Sometimes Nagy describes justice in familial relationships more or less in the same way as Buber. However, he does not often refer to the notion of reciprocity. Another reference is in the glossary of BGT: "Justice or balance of fairness" (BGT:417).

With reference to the ethical capacity of the subject, we cannot take reciprocity in Nagy's writings as for granted. The notion of "reciprocity" takes its point of departure in the system of "the totality", and not in the framework of the accountability of the single person, and vice versa. It is indeed possible that accountability can eventually *lead* to reciprocity. In this regard, "balance" and "fairness", two terms from the sphere of accountancy, frame the meaning of reciprocity.

The method, namely, to access the value and meaning of concepts within a judicial paradigm (order of human justice), leads to the following valid question: These accounting terms, do they not presuppose the totality of a ledger, an exterior system that eventually negate the subject and threatens its separate identity?

Often it seems as if Nagy takes his point of departure in a description of a systemic totality. For example, the judicial concept from Roman law: "*suum cuique*" (everyone his/her due; IL:70). It indicates a striving towards "distributive justice". "Distributive justice" is used to identify a kind of general, and collective norm within diversity and differences between people. Nagy renders this general and common measure as a sophisticated application of the *do-ut-des principle* in law: A commutative contract whereby something is given so that something may be received in return as well. Another reference and example are the notion of "retributive justice" ("an eye-for-an eye" and "a tooth-for-a-tooth"). However, Nagy argues that these terms refer in the first place to a collectivity that emerges from the very depth of our being human and existential dynamics: Collectivity is then linked to the contribution of the subject towards the well-being of the other. Due to the principle of mutuality, everyone owes to one another a kind of repayment and reciprocal return. For Nagy, this is also a proper indication of responsibility.

The "ledger of justice" compiles all the accumulative inequalities in reciprocity. They are all ingredients of interactions, revealed to the group in terms of past experiences (IL:56). It is about an accumulation of disparities of reciprocity.[29]

Noteworthy, is that Nagy, despite the impression that he takes his point of departure in a description pointing to reciprocity, eventually argues in a different direction. One can indeed conclude and say that he does not promote an ideal order or system of totality. Justice is not an abstract concept; it is not about a force that promotes a closed system (totality). On the contrary, justice points to just acts; acts of reliability, fairness and truth.

In terms of the research project, the question should be posed if one can identify elements in his writings that proof the following: The relationship from "a to b" (a – b), is not the same as the movement from "b back to a" (b – a)? Is it possible to indicate that despite reciprocity, he reckons with inequalities as a given fact; inequalities that Levinas calls diachronic within asymmetry?

In terms of the research findings one can conclude and say that Nagy follows a very down-to-earth approach: Inequalities are a given fact within the dynamics of relationships.

"Equitability within asymmetry is the key to fair reciprocity, especially in intergenerational relationships" (Nagy BGT:74). Reciprocity is not for Nagy a fixed precondition. Within intergenerational relationships, the dynamics is motivated and informed by "loyalty" and "indebtedness", not by a mechanistic a priori of reciprocity. At stake, is an indebtedness and guilt due to what people (the other) do to one another. The doing good of the other, puts me in a state

---

29 With this concept of accumulation in mind, one can indeed pose the valid question why Nagy still maintains the concept of reciprocity/mutuality.

of indebtedness. However, what the one does to the other and vice versa, is not coming from an outside and normative collectivity. It emerges from the character of the reciprocity, namely "fairness", not from an intentional act from the side of a competent "I". In this kind of reciprocity, nothing is automatic or "natural". Whether the strategies are intentional or unintentional, many disturbances occur. There are indeed many obstacles and unpredictable factors occurring in relational dynamics. For example, one of the disturbing factors is "exploitation"; it interrupts reciprocity and is in fact the opposite of reciprocity. Exploitation is also connected to the power play of sheer dominance.

There are many other forms of exploitation. It is not only the vulnerable that can be exploited. Even the boss, the powerful person, parents and children, all of them can become exploited. A human being can be exploited since there is nobody who is prepared to defend the others' right to be treated in a fair way. Even when somebody is continuously being treated as an object for doing good deeds like in charity projects, the merciful act can be applied as a form of manipulative exploitation. One is forced into a position of always receiving (the guilt feelings of the receiver) without the means to respond accordingly. This is also applicable to children. Most of times, they are merely receiving from the parents and not in a position to repay.

Nagy refers to personal exploitation: The one is abused by the other, covertly or openly, in cases of non-giving or non-reciprocal taking (Nagy IL:57). Another form of exploitation also surfaces: structural exploitation. The latter "… originates from system characteristics which victimize both participants at the same time" (Nagy IL:57). A relationship between people can develop to such an extent that the opportunity to do good, or repay one another, becomes virtually impossible. The account cannot be settled or balanced. Nagy refers to "balanced retribution" (Nagy IL:58). "The meaning of the word retribution includes either reward or punishment given or exacted in recompense" (Nagy IL:57). The point is, that feelings of revenge can develop because one is never in the position to reward.

Structural impediments and the lack of reciprocity become insurmountable obstacles and contribute to acute feelings of guilt. The feeling and experience to be constantly in debt with parents can lead to a connectedness based upon inherent guilt and resistance. In this respect, excessive devotion can be a forced mode of reward with an undertone of guilt or even resistance. The giver can also use the situation to exercise power. Due to the character of sacrifice, the giver can take on the role of a vicarious martyr. In all cases, the fundamental problem is a lack of fairness and merit on both sides.

In a disruptive society wherein injustice and exploitation have become normative, all people involved will eventually become victims. Exploitation is, thus, lurking in all forms of reciprocity. However, exploitation is not the point of departure for Nagy's thinking about subjectivity. It is not injustice, but justice that determines the starting point. The challenge is to do right and to promote fair treatment within all circumstances. Reciprocity is a given fact, even in cases of injustice. Reciprocity must therefore not be confused with "equality".

The subtitle of IL reads: "*Reciprocity in Intergenerational Family Therapy*". In this publication "reciprocity" takes on the form of "due care"; it is an indication of "consideration". At stake, in this consideration, is "merited trust". In IL (80) Nagy poses the question: "How objective can merit accounting be?" This is a difficult question to answer, because the intrinsic justice within a group does not consist merely of a ledger of mutual responsibilities. It is about a complex system, determined also by personal, retributive motivations (Nagy IL:81). Thus, the plea of Nagy for "mutuality" as an "action dialogue" (Nagy IL:82). The latter consists of more than the sum total of subjective experiences of two persons.

For example, in the case of a deceived friend, one is confronted with many layers of entanglements. Underneath could be many suppressed wishes and needs from childhood. Even depression could have played a role. The point is: The relationship has been damaged. The real impact of the damage can only be accessed when the "vantage point" of the friend has also been taken into consideration (Nagy Ll:82). What should be accessed is the unique subjectivity of both.

In a nutshell: With reciprocity Nagy wants to say, that everybody involved contributes to the ethical quality of the interaction according to his/her own sense of responsibility. It is not about the mere exchange of giving and receiving and vice versa. It is fundamentally about the integrity of the partners; about giving and waiting for the other to respond accordingly; about the how of receiving.

Nagy maintains the importance of mutuality and reciprocity. However, the real question is not about the amount of investment by the "I". Nor what the "I" can gain (What advantage is there for me in giving?). The authentic question is about how to create opportunities for responsible obligations. Furthermore, these questions should be motivated by the fact that I owe the other the fairness of responsible responses, not to establish some-*thing* in terms of a reward, but due to the notion of fairness, justice and care.

In BGT the notion of "reciprocity" is not explicitly used that often. There is indeed reference to the relationship between therapist and client. Reciprocity is in this case a core component of what one can call "a contract": Ample but never symmetrical (Nagy BGT:395). Furthermore, in BGT reciprocity is used to indicate dialogue: dialogue as a reciprocity of care.

It becomes clear that when Nagy takes over the concept of reciprocity as applied by Buber in the "I-Thou encounter", he applies it in his own way. It is for him a good model to explain what a relational theory entails within the context of the dynamics of counselling and psychotherapy. It helps to illuminate what is going on psychologically in relationships (Nagy F:54-78). For Nagy, dialogue is not merely the effectivity of a conversation, but the reciprocity and exchange of fairness and the establishment of care.

Dialogue is in the first place about "symmetry versus asymmetry". It is also about "self-delineation" and "self-validation" in processes of polarisation between the selves. In the last instance it is about "inclusive multi-laterality". In the interplay between symmetry and asymmetry, a person's responsible contribution to another is one of the criteria that determines the rules of equitable give-and-take (Nagy BGT:74).

It all seems so obvious. But in the responsible contribution of one person towards another, lurks a magnificent secret! The intriguing question is: How is it possible for a human being to do good to the other? Where does this idea come from? Is it in any case possible that justice can originate from reciprocity?

In fact, doing good, and to exhibit a responsible contribution, do not start with the expectation and guarantee of reward and compensation. In reciprocity, compensation is not at stake, due to the unevenness in reciprocity. For example, there is really no balance between parents and children. For a long period in the developmental process of education there is a disequilibrium. The parents invest more care in the upbringing that the young child can "repay" or respond to in terms of compensation. In fact, instant repayment can be an indication of unthoughtful gratitude (Statement by Gouldner in Nagy IL:59).[30]

Reciprocity cannot be quantified. Thus, the intriguing question: How can we measure the degree of equivalence in the give-and-take mutuality within the realm of daily relational exchange between mother and child (baby) (Nagy IL:59)? It is not about quantification[31], but qualification. Therefore, at stake, is loyalty and trustworthiness. Loyalty and indebtedness form the dynamics of the "interlocking reciprocity" between generations (Nagy IL:353). A "balance of fairness" (relational justice) (Nagy BGT:417), implies in the intergenerational dialogue, a long-term process. It can even stretch after and over the death of parents. Thus, the reason why Nagy introduces the concept of "nonmutual reciprocity". It seems to be a paradox. But in the event of taking without repaying, and receiving with no possibility of giving back, this paradox is most significant (Nagy IL:353).

To talk about reward and repayment between parents and children, is about a unique mode of signifying human encounters. It is about a reciprocity wherein the new generation reflects the care of the previous generation within the mode of caring for future generations! This is indeed a very special and magnificent mode of reciprocity. In terms of Levinas, one can call this reciprocal dynamic a display of operational liturgy; it continues even after death (Levinas HAM:69).

For Nagy, the subject is a separate category, sui generis. It is therefore important to maintain also the exteriority of the other. This is the reason why two categories need further explanation, namely "self-delineation" and "self-validation". He uses them in order to describe the effect of polarisation on the realm between selves.

Nagy introduces dialectics in order to reveal the impact of a polar framework of psychoanalytical theory on the dynamics of relational networking. At stake, in this theory, is inter alia the polarities of "eros-thanatos" and "distance-nearness". According to Nagy, the fundamental ground situation is not established and driven by this polarity, but by justice and hope. The

---

30 In terms of intergenerational relationships, the notions of "ancestors" and "posterity" bring about a temporal dimension which is in opposition with synchronisation.

31 The sociologist Gouldner, differentiates between homoeomorphic reciprocity (tat for tat), and heteromorphic reciprocity (tit for tat) (In Nagy IL).

latter are the driving forces behind the intersubjective dynamics and processes of exchange.

According to Nagy, polarisation can also be described as "the dialectics between Selves" (Nagy BGT:75). In theory for a contextual approach, this dialectics' "the mutual definition of otherness" should be understood not merely as key to interpret the necessity of differentiation over against fusion and the threat of enmeshment. The actual reason should rather be to reckon with the other in his/her self-delineation. This reckoning justifies the challenge to attend to self-validation.

Individuation is established in the earning of entitlement. In *self-validation*, this ethically self-delineating and self-validating processes (Nagy BGT:303), are not about psychological growth, but justice. The desire of somebody to be entitled, is in itself already a driving force. A person can try to entitle him/herself. In this attempt, one can "use" the other. One can even feel to be entitled, but in reality, one is not actually been entitled. In order to reckon with the other in the dialogical process, means: To reckon with, and to care for, the other in the attempt to differentiate him/herself. This process should not be viewed as a complementary event.

The event is not symmetric. Justice within asymmetry is the key for fair reciprocity, especially in intergenerational relationships (Nagy TGN:94). However, "any assumption of an inborn asymmetry between people would contradict the principle of equality proudly proclaimed by the American Constitution and French Revolution" (Nagy BGT:82).

One gets the impression that in some cases where symmetry is mentioned, it is for Nagy more or less the same as equality (*egalité*). Albeit, Nagy operates within the equality concept of the Enlightenment. He is quite sceptic about any kind of inborn asymmetry (which Nagy eventually rejects); he wants to promote a valid asymmetry based on justice and determined by ethics. When Nagy writes about symmetry, it should be understood within the framework of dialectics; it helps to understand better what asymmetry is about. This form of dialectic is necessary in order to prevent equality of becoming merely a vague idealism. Its basic function is to unmask a lack of trustworthiness.

The giving child as subject: The complexity of double-binding

Parent-child relationships are intrinsically asymmetric so that reciprocity is extremely limited. Parents cannot expect to be compensated by their children according to what they had invested in terms of care and education; "… intergenerational giving is not only of a different order of magnitude; it is also of a different quality" (Nagy BGT:82). Children are not born by choice. On the other hand, in principle, (many) parents do have a choice to conceive a child. Being a parent and being a child are not equivalent in magnitude. Thus, the reason why it is not consistent to describe the concept of intergenerational dialogue as an encounter between two selves (Nagy F:242). That should imply a kind of totalising definition and a synchronised statement. In terms of the concept "the-one-for-the-other", the relationship is assymetric and always diachronic. The reason? Because Nagy still wants to protect the independent position of the child. He does not want to see the outcome of parenting as a one-sided achievement. With this statement Nagy wants to outroot the possibility of pathogenic causality (Miller 1979:42).

Nagy's argument boils down to the following: Without bringing the ethical dimension into play, and to recognise the contribution of children, the parent-child dynamic is delivered to the threat of destructive parentification.

For Nagy, the concept "compensation" in intergenerational dynamics is complex. One can even dare to say that explicit expectations regarding compensation by the child is to a certain extent fairer than the parental attitude: I have done everything solely on your behalf, solely for you. In the last instance, the interplay is *double-bind*; there is nothing to be grateful for; there is also nothing for the child to pay back, and that seems to be unfair; it is unbalanced. This is the reason why the legacy of the child's loyalty should be safeguarded and distinguished from the merit of the parent's manifest behaviour towards the child. It would also be unfair to reduce the contribution of the child to merely satisfying the parent's needs and wishes for conceiving a child (manipulative compensation). The compensation from the child's perspective, is much subtler. Without such a wish and intention (from the parent's perspective), it becomes indeed difficult to figure out what the contribution of a child in parenting exactly entails. The child establishes a social relationship with the parents without deliberately and intentionally asking for that. It is a kind of non-intentional contribution; it can be called a "passive ability", passive compensation.

The command to honour the father and mother is in terms of Nagy an attempt to separate the legacy of the child's loyalty from the merit of the manifest behaviour of the parents to the child. The command, thus, breaks the notion of "double-bind".

The parental message, namely that in the upbringing it is an investment solely for the sake of the child (for your concern alone), is according to Nagy a *double-bind* and, thus, unfair. The same is applicable in the case of the following message to a child: You are not responsible for your parents. Both statements are a consequence of brute individualised and fragmented views on the dynamics and significance of life. In the complexity of familial dynamics, the notion that the child cannot make any substantial contribution to the well-being of a family, or that it is inappropriate for a child to make in any case a kind of compensating contribution, leads to what Nagy calls *destructive idealisation*. To put a child on a pedestal and to blame the child for not responding to these extreme expectations, are forms of cruel injustice to the unique developmental state of childhood. In not holding the innocent child accountable for the father's sins, or the parent for their child's transgressions, are complex hidden forces indeed. There lurks always the danger of overseeing the complexity of several hidden forces infiltrating the family system (Nagy IL:78; VR/MK).

Children also give to the parents. However, their giving does not correlate with the input of the parents and cannot be assessed in a reciprocal relationship. The relationship is not symmetrical. "Symmetrical relationships are intrinsically reciprocal [...] By contrast, in the ethical dimension *asymmetrical relationships are intrinsically limited in their reciprocity*. [...] intergenerational giving is not only of a different order of magnitude; it is also a different quality [...] The sequence of the generations itself dictates and justifies the degree of direction of equity. If intrinsic asymmetry in a context is disregarded, the trustworthiness of the relationship is bound to suffer" (Nagy BGT:82). The giving of a parent to the child and vice versa are in principle asymmetric.

The notion of "the giving child" can be connected to the notion of *parentification*. Nagy does not treat this concept psychotherapeutically in the sense of a diagnosis of pathology. It should be assessed and interpreted within the context of the ethical capacity of the subject. No child will opt for being "parentified". However, it does not prevent a child to display in a mature and sophisticated way comforting concern for the parents in situations of crises, loss and despair. In fact, the child is already engaged in a kind of care, even if nobody deliberately has asked for comfort. For this, the child needs acknowledgement. The more the parent gives credit, the less the danger of reducing the child to merely the object of his/her parents' wishes and expectations. This contribution of compensation and care can be described by the very strange and odd terminology of "hostage".

The ledger between parent and child is in the first place a dyadic concept. It entails much more than being a contract based on "quid-pro-quo" (Nagy F:307). The latter is only applicable to interactions in the here and now. However, it does not reckon with the long term, future consequences. On the contrary, the dyadic concept of "ledger" between parent and child implies a unilateral "non-feed-back-like" process of consequences in the parent-child relationship. Despite the unilateral character, there are indeed forward thrusting consequences. The most important consequence flows from the parent to the child, and not vice versa. The ledger implies a dyad. But at the same time the parent is already involved with the ledger of his/her parents, as well as other's ledgers. Even for the child there are other ledgers as well. In this regard, responsibilities entail a whole networking web of intriguing connections. "The ledger of fair give-and-take […] has to extend also into the future" (Nagy F:303). In this way therapy is involved in an ever-expanding context of healing and prevention (Nagy F:xviii from 1986).

The intrinsic transgenerational tribunal: Transgenerational solidarity (the silent partner)

Nagy proposes the term *intrinsic transgenerational tribunal* as an extension of the dyadic parent-child ledger into an inclusive consequential criterion that spans countless generations in the survival of the human species (Nagy F:308). As term, perhaps, an indication of a common mode of truth as pre-text.

Nagy called the norm and measure that is applied for assessing the quality of the tribunal judgement, "solidarity": *Transgenerational solidarity*. This kind of solidarity is for Nagy not merely form and content of this unique judgement. It functions on a much deeper level of interaction: the realm of silence. The solidarity can, thus, be tagged as "*silent partner*" in the relational reality. It functions as an invisible third factor (Nagy F:307). This third factor operates beside the level of current generations, also on the level of past generations and subsequent following generations. This intrinsic tribunal will opt as a court within the ethical quality of intergenerational dynamics.

The implication of the previous outline for the understanding of subjectivity, is that subjectivity is about some intergenerational dynamics wherein the offspring is connected to the deeds of the ancestors. In this context where people do not exist in the same time span, the concept of reciprocity is totally inappropriate to opt as criterion for justice. One cannot detect a pattern of reciprocal influence between different generations remote from one another. "The sequential chain of time is irreversible but not untouchable" (Nagy F:288). The only way to influence the long chain of interconnectedness, and to prevent children of becoming merely objects due to "parentification", is to acknowledge the very valid resource of loyal commitment and trust that the child offers the world of adulthood.

In a very paradoxical way, one can say that the vulnerable trust of a child puts adults in a responsible position. The whole world of mature people is constantly being questioned by vulnerable children. They even question the concerns of coming, future generations. Nagy's notion of a tribunal in a nutshell: The questioning by children puts everybody into responsibility.

When parents are willing to be opened to this trusting by children, they earn and deserve "entitlement". This is then how reciprocal trust comes into play. Nagy refers to this kind of trusting as the golden rule of relational *negentropy*[32]:"Consistent with the good of posterity, reciprocal trustability becomes the "golden rule" of "relational *negentropy*" (Nagy F:304).

At this point, it seems as if Nagy with his notion of transgenerational solidarity, and his uneasiness with future developments, moves into the direction of a kind of pessimism. Contemporary issues like the nuclear threat and climate changes are reasons for concern. In order to survive, humanity needs a new ethics of responsibility, "… to thwart its likely destructive consequences to posterity" (Nagy F:301). But then, ethics should become appropriately effective. He does not mean to alter and to change the basic foundations of ethics. What should take place is that "reliable and trustable human relations"

---

32 *Negentropy* is reverse entropy. It means things becoming more orderly. By "order" is meant organisation, structure and differentiated function: the opposite of randomness or chaos or indifference.

should be rendered as an excellent resource to safeguard a more humane future for all.

With reference to familial dynamics, one dare to say that the traditional "extended family", and to a large extent, even the nuclear family, are disintegrating entities. The implication is that the care and responsibility for children are becoming more and more the responsibility of one parent or in many cases, the responsibility of somebody else (other adults). The parental responsibilities become fairly isolated with not enough appropriate support systems. The implication is that many parents are forced into what one can call "destructive entitlement". This development can be called "a tragic relational ethical dilemma. […] Substitutive retribution is ethically always invalid, even if psychologically understandable" (Nagy F:305).

With less appropriate support systems, it can even happen that parents may force their children to carry depleting amounts of adult responsibility (Nagy F:306). The problem is that the capacity of children is quite limited. This could perhaps become the reason why they start seeking compensation within other more destructive relationships. The victim becomes "unfair victimizer" and results in "destructive overentitlement". A kind of permissive indifferentism is caused that contributes to the escalation of violent behaviour, and the further disintegration of relationships. It impacts on future generations, resulting in the inflation of sensitivity and concern for the other; a kind of permissive right of becoming less sensitive to the rights of others. Eventually, a tragic relational ethical dilemma develops with devastating consequences for intergenerational relationships. "Therefore, the failure of psychotherapists to strive for a precise definition of transgenerational relational consequences amounts to cynical disregard of these consequences" (Nagy F:322).

Personal responsibilities are non-transferrable. Everybody should realise that there is an intrinsic relational tribunal that determines the quality of responsibility and impacts on an accountability that precedes every human choice. One is not sued to appear before the court of reason (Immanuel Kant), but to reckon with an eventual judgement. The latter resides in a conscientious awareness about the "repairing contribution to the hurt human justice". It is in this regard that the concept of solidarity comes into play. A solidarity that encompasses all generations "across the board". It creates hope that does not originate from a Kantian rationality but is founded by fairness and trustworthiness. It is this kind of ethically founded responsibility that children appeal to.

Transference and the guilt of implicit disloyalty

For Nagy, therapy is essentially about action by the client, and not in the first place about empathetic insight. Action precedes insight. It is within action that undergirding perceptions and prejudice could be assessed. Actions reveal the character of deeds and intentionality of motivational behaviour. This is why the responses and level of responsibility of the other must be assessed. This scrutiny brings about insight, especially regarding relational dynamics and the impact of contextuality on human behaviour. To investigate the entitlement of the other and myself, is an important resource for contextual therapy.

The realm of entitlement concerns every person involved in the relational dynamics. In this regard, transference and contra-transference determine the quality of subjectivity. For example, in a family with a handicapped child, and overburdened mother who struggled to cope, the non-handicapped son becomes so committed to the mother and the family's struggle to cope with all the demands, that the son can develop guilt about his transference (towards the therapist). His excessive obligation to his family might contribute to even feeling guiltier due to experiences of implicit disloyalty. To acknowledge his yearning for an own independent existence, and somebody that can promote his need for subjectivity, will be a big concern in therapy. In this case, transference is additionally viewed as an indication of potential disengagement (Nagy BGT:25).

Transference is per definition representation. It can even harm the other (in this case the mother). For Nagy, therapy is about helping the son, or in other cases, the child to limit the unavoidable impact of positive transference. Therapy, thus, probes behind the screen of the transference and its manifestations or representations. When injustice, or even excessive forms of loyalty, are revealed, the whole complex notion of exoneration comes into play.

When injustice, or a lack of respect for entitlement, is discovered and exoneration becomes imperative, the question of a normative and meta-realm surfaces. Thus, the question whether in the relationship of the subject with the other, a meta-component is to be found (a kind of ledger).

Nagy does not derive ethics from a meta-realm (beyond). There is no external norm outside the realm of the intersubjective dynamics, at one's disposal. "The human order is a concept based on a subjective, normative sense of justice or equity" (Nagy IL:68). It does not mean that this order is in itself subjective. In subjectivity the cause at stake is fairness and trustworthiness. It is within this ethical framework (the reason for concern for subjects), that the realm of sound subjectivity is established. The structural context such as "family", and the appeal to be loyal to the subject, create opportunities for ethical actions. This possibility for ethical actions is a given opportunity. Who or what grants this "givenness"? Nagy's answer is: It is the other that comes first due to the facticity of intergenerationality. The other can be "my" daughter, "my" son, or any other that appears within the scope of responsibility. But also vice versa; the other needs me to display care and concern, and to be prevented of becoming a victim of destructive exploitation; of becoming also an "unfair exploiter".

I don't have the power to dispose over the relationship of the other towards me. The "I" cannot determine the obligations towards the other in the sense that the needs of the other precede all forms of projected images. The human order of justice precedes all appearances and projected portrayals. In this sense, the human order is a metaphysical constellation and not a psychological projection. Even not a meta-psychological element. The metaphysical order poses challenges indeed. However, in therapy the question is how to respond to these challenges, and to become engaged in ethical actions. That is the core of Nagy's therapeutic endeavours and engagements.

In conclusion: The ABC of intergenerational contextual caring

The basic point of departure in Nagy's contextual approach is his deep concern and care for the vulnerable context wherein a child is born. He therefore defends the subjectivity of the child and of human beings. Thus, his rejection of any form of causative and external determination, or reduction of subjectivity to a neutral totality and systemic view on our being human (merely to be a member of family X). The "I" is not a term within a relation wherein the self is subordinated to the relational dynamics. The relationship is not "higher" than the self. The subject must also be protected against the idea of complete freedom. The "I" or "Self" (in some cases Nagy writes it with a capital), is also not a sovereign source of a higher kind of knowledge concerning a mystical primordial explanatory principle for personhood as in the case of many metaphysical theories. The "I" is this concrete entity as text and context endowed with accountability and responsibility; it takes actual care for the other; it is about obedience to the higher order of justice.

The subject is for Nagy the person who does justice, and even inflicts injustice to the other and vice versa. The status of the subject resides in the fact that the subject operates within a unique and motivated mode of being; it operates from the ethics of responsibility that is intrinsically intransitive. In this sense, motivations are derived from obligations. The relational concepts, formulated by Nagy, infiltrate psychological terminology and interfere with fixed, static psychotherapeutic theories.

With action is meant something different than merely insight and understanding. To be exposed and to undergo/endure, imply more than feeling and experience. At stake, are concrete activities and a special mode of passivity. The other, whether my parent or child, even a dear one or somebody I care for, cannot be captured by, or incorporated in, personal insights, or feelings as such. Even if I could, my obligation towards the other is not becoming minimised over a period. On the contrary, it becomes even more intense. Responsibility as an ethical obligation cannot become complete; it should then lead to smugness and the negligence of the other. In coexistence our subjectivity is not minimalised or reduced. On the contrary, it makes "… simultaneous coexistence of several individual's rights and motives" possible (Nagy BGT:32). Coexistence is about the individuation of separate persons, and therefore based on differentiated subjectivity.

The quest for humanity within the trace of the Other/ other: Two intersecting perspectives – Nagy-and-Levinas

To deal with the interplay between the thinking of Levinas' more philosophical approach, and Nagy's more therapeutic approach, is indeed a disciplinary challenge. One needs to admit that they are operating from two different paradigmatic and disciplinary positions. Nagy is a psychiatrist and Levinas a philosopher. They operate within two different discourses. Nevertheless, they have one thing in common, namely, both are in search of traces of true humanity. In Nagy's case: The search for the motivational layers of humane intergenerational interactions, determined by an "order of justice" and the establishment of trustworthy responsibility. Levinas' concern is: The quest and source for authentic humanity, founded in the prior of a face-to-face encounter (visage) and directed by the principle of *l'un-pour-l'autre* (one-for-the-other).

Despite different paradigms, it is possible to detect traces of intersection. For example, Nagy often referred to the fact that he is not a philosopher. However, he bases many of his arguments on philosophical resources. Indirectly, philosophy opted as starting point for further reflections in theory formation. For example: Nagy makes an appeal on Martin Buber's "I-Thou" dialogical dynamics. But there are also traces of Hegelian dialectics and existential philosophy when he indirectly deals with Martin Heidegger's ontology of being. Other traces are the judicial philosophy and the use of concepts originating from the judicial sphere of the court. Another important role player is Bateson with his systems theory and focus on the Platonic notion of "mind and nature". There is also Freud's meta-psychological views on the ego, and the implication thereof on Ronald Fairbairn.

It tastes like a fruit salad. It is indeed true that his approach looks like a mixed methodology and is in many cases eclectic. However, there are many turnabouts.

At the beginning Nagy probes in the direction of a "mechanistic cause-effect-schema". From this rigid approach he was freed by the systemic paradigm, in particular, by circularity thinking. He resisted the neutralising reduction of the "person" to a mere functional factor in a system with autonomous characteristics. Thus, his hypothesis that a family should be understood as a quite unique life unit based on the ethical principle of loyalty. With the term "loyalty" it was possible for Nagy to connect the separate persons (being loyal to one another) with the dynamics of interactional mutuality. Mutuality does not operate in terms of mere subjective feelings but is directed by a meta-personal command that makes an appeal on fairness and loyalty. In this way a family could be understood as a functioning whole and intact unit. Loyalty operates along the lines of "guilt" and "obligation". These categories were not viewed as meta-psychological categories within a psychological paradigm. The notions of merit and indebtedness open up the possibility to postulate justice as source for social interaction and relational dynamics. On the one side, justice could, thus, be defined as being distributive (the notion of honest sharing), and on the other side, justice as being retributive (the notion of compensation and repayment). In this way Nagy operationalised the ethical complexity of "fairness".

In BGT (32), Nagy refers to "*useful assumptions*" that can help to transcend both a very strict psychic determinism, as well as "the sheer chaotic power of confrontation" as in the case of Jean-Paul Sartre's existential nihilism. Nagy's concern is to find, and construe, a model wherein the freedom of the person is guaranteed, as well as an approach wherein relations do not operate on the basis of "sheer chaotic power" and "negating nothingness" (*nausea*).

Nagy's presupposition is that a relationship between two or more autonomous and absolute modes of freedom (Sartre), inevitably leads to a chaotic confrontation and demonstration of power. The challenge then is to find a common factor between two or more units of freedom. It is imperative to detect such a factor due to Nagy's concern to rather opt for the notion of taking responsibility for relational consequences, than falling back on an order founded by power. With this presupposition in mind, the relationship between freedom (autonomy) and responsibility comes into play.

According to Nagy, the option to render a place for both "freedom" (autonomy) and "responsibility" in therapy, could be found in the transpersonal dialogical dynamics of Buber's "I-Thou" relationship – a construction from a higher and different order of synchronising unity.

As therapist, Nagy views the social relationship to a large extent as a trans-personal unity. This is necessary because (as therapist) he operates most of times exterior to the client's personal trajectory. He does not maintain this exterior position when he deals with people, belonging intrinsically to the family system. Nothing supersedes personal accountability. In his research and therapy (relying on useful assumptions), Nagy's emphasis is on the relationship as unique entity.

The basic question at stake, is why should two autonomous subjects abdicate from their freedom? The relationship in itself does not explain why two autonomous, free entities (two entities that are psychic determined and being self-sufficient) are willing to be engaged in a dialogue. The relational dynamic does not clarify how a mode of "sheer chaotic power confrontation" could be transformed into a "personalised human order".

From metapsychology to ethics

Nagy's argumentation is quite unique. He does not explain how responsibility is established from the viewpoint of psychology. Furthermore, he does not probe into the probable conditions for the accountability of an "I" toward another human being. Nagy rather postulates an ethical dimension as framework of reference. Since this dimension is an ethical category sui generis, it is impossible to reduce accountability, responsibility and therefore also subjectivity to something else. In fact, there is no abstract explanatory factor for the responsibility of subjectivity. In other words, the ethical dimension concerns a relationship that cannot be derived from a totality and higher trans-synthesis and abstract order of being. Accountability and responsibility are not meta-psychological categories, but subjective-ethical categories. The fact that a subject operates ethically, irrespective of whether the subject is a child or a parent, implies that he/she is touched by an outside factor, by exteriority.

Nagy keeps on looking for a source for responsibility and how to formulate this source. What should be understood is the factuality that human beings take on responsibility and are essentially re-*spond*-able. It seems, even within situations viewed from a psychological or social-psychological perspective, if being is pre-dispositioned to act in an irresponsible way; pre-dispositioned to display egocentric behaviour. The latter could perhaps be called "destructive entitlement". However, every attempt to diagnose exceeds psychological explanations.

The reason why Nagy keeps on looking and searching for the resources of responsibility, could be linked to attempts to link the ethical dimension to other categories like, for example, the notion of "silent partner". Specifically, in the metaphor of the "tribunal" (Nagy F:292-318). This metaphor presupposes an ethical dimension that is original, authentic and foundational; it points to the realm of transcendence. This process of keeping on with his search for a significant factor, could be interpreted as weakness in his theory formation. However, it creates a scientific openness and flexibility.

Accountability and responsibility refer to a relation of the "I" (as subject) to exteriority that is not approachable for, and accessible to, the free act of the knowing subject in an existential epistemology. It refers to a relationship wherein the freedom of knowing and being enabled (theory-and-praxis), are subjected to the critique of some other that renders an *investiture* (meta-*physics* precedes ontology). In this regard, the concept of the "entitlement" of every particular human being (the right to earn a right by means of responsibility), is in essence an anthropological and therapeutic postulate. This postulation can indeed be maintained in terms of the method of falsification (until the opposite is proofed to be true).

Due to the previous outline, the subject should be defined in terms of passivity (Levinas DTA:52).

With this definition in mind, (preliminary to the problem of intersubjective responsibility) it is the secret and puzzle of responsibility itself that must be unravelled (Nagy MG:205). The latter is constitutive for subjectivity; it is not merely added to autonomy. In other words, it is indeed paramount to detect how an autonomous and free subject develops into a responsible subject. But even such an explanation does not shed light on the fact why a subject is indeed a *responsible humane human being*. To import theories, borrowed from Freudian Oedipus-complex-theory, or from general socialisation theories, is for Nagy totally insufficient.

In order to attend to the origin of *humane responsible*, the hunch of the researchers is that Nagy should be reinterpreted in terms of Levinas' ethical model. In this regard, one is challenged to apply some radical assumptions. In order to embark on this route, the focus is on Nagy's reflection on the relationship of the "I" to the "other". To shed more light on the "I-other-dynamics", the further outline will pay attention to Nagy's notion of *multi-directed partiality*. This will be linked to Levinas' notion of *one-for-the-other* (*l'un-pour-lautre*). After this exposition, concluding remarks will be made.

Parallels (l'un-pour-l'autre) *and differences ("visage")*

Within the interplay between Nagy's thinking and the philosophy of Levinas, it is important to reckon simultaneously with parallels, as well as with differences. Dealing with this dual tension gives a very specific profile to Nagy's approach. This is done, in order to deal later with a more confrontational approach to some of Levinas' points of departure. The outline will try to shed more light on what a reinterpretation of Nagy, in the light of Levinas' ethical model, entails.

For Levinas, the ethical responsibility is *an-archic*; that is, it is disorganised, unruly, in turmoil with no controlling rules or principles to give order. Its beginning is difficult to pinpoint because this responsibility is a trace of the other in the self, and, thus, virtually impossible to recall – it is elusive and difficult to grasp. In this sense, it is difficult to describe, to remember or achieve. In fact, it does not reside in one principle (*archè*) that is constituted by the subject. With this very peculiar formulation is meant that the subject is not dominated by the totality of an organising and explanatory principle inherent to the subject. The starting point is with the other. In this sense the other is inassimilable and elusive (*insaisissable*), difficult to find and to comprehend.

In the relationship with the other/Other with whom I am connected from the start, there is always a paradoxical difference in terms of operational levels. It is a difference between two levels: below and above (higher); humility and height. The Other begs me and summons me simultaneously. The relationship between me and the other is therefore qualitative asymmetric. We are never even. The other as other has his/her alterity as content and, thus, can operate as widower, orphan, foreigner and outsider. The other has no status in sameness and is in principle without context.

Nagy also refers to asymmetry. In Nagy's thinking the term refers in the first place to a quantitative difference. The reason for that is that Nagy works with the dialectics of symmetry-asymmetry within the parameters of systems theory and communication thinking. However, Nagy introduces the concept of explicit care. It carries a huge weight so that in this sense, he distances himself from the theoretical framework of systems theory. His emphasis on asymmetry (especially in the relationship between parent and child), thus, attains an ethical quality. The small child that cannot function on his/her own yet, has then a non-status, analogous to the status of the widower, orphan and foreigner. The same is applicable to the victimised person, the family member in his/her misery (the identified patient or dementing parent).

Via Levinas, Buber's dialogical principle (I become myself through Thou) is reinterpreted as the dynamics by which the subject becomes "I" (becoming one-*self*). Levinas' critique on Buber was the untenable proposition that "I" and "Thou" constitute one another. Levinas resisted this kind of reciprocity. Rather, the other renders me to become an "I", so that the "I" can develop into a "me".

Nagy feels quite comfortable with the reciprocal principle in Buber's dialogical paradigm. This becomes clear in the way he uses the notions of "self-delineation" and "self-validation". He operates within the same anomaly as Buber, namely that the "I" and the "other", constitute one another.

In several of his writings, Nagy points out that personal responsibility/re-*spond*-ability and accountability can never be viewed contractually. They are intransitive. It is the same with responsible care/caregiving. The source is neither the contract, nor the reciprocity.

Despite similarities and possible parallels, the following difference can be identified:
- For Levinas, the Other appears before me without any condition. It is about the visitation of the visage: face-to-face. It is about an infinite presence: always there. Even before I start, I am elected to be responsible.
- For Nagy, responsibility is not about a meta-calling. The subject constitutes his/her own responsibility and accountability. But, this act of constituting is in fact about sheer passivity. In the concept of "transgenerational solidarity" and the notion of a tribunal, Nagy detects a mode of passivity outside the control and dominium of the "I": The intergenerational other/others.

According to Levinas, the other is always interconnected to more others (the reality of a plural society). It is now my responsibility to measure and to judge. The obligation of justice becomes a given fact that challenges me. This disposition and the connection with "loyalty" makes it clear that it is not a psychological disposition or the result of a social custom. It is fundamentally about an ontic setting. The commitment to the other, or others, precedes freedom of choice. At the same time, it is about a preferential connection and, thus, shaped by a triadic, relational configuration. Loyalty is linked with indebtedness so that loyalty is in the first instance not the anxiety to be rejected, but about the anxiety to fail the other.

Nagy's understanding of loyalty, is to a large extent parallel to Levinas' preliminary notion of "one-for-the-other" (*l'un-pour-l'autre*), as well as the notion of alliance (*allégeance*) – a kind of knot in mindfulness and not vice versa (Levinas AZ:45).

Because Nagy wants to maintain the dialogical thinking of Buber, responsibility is not shaped by predestination. It has the character of obligation, and, thus, the challenge to reckon with the needs and interests of the other. This obligation is also not based on the mutuality of give-and-take (Nagy BGT:414).

In the case of Levinas, "responsibility for the other", and "responsibility in front of the other", coincide. The one I must answer, is the one to whom my answer is directed. The one "who", and the other "who", coincide[33] (Levinas NP:108).

---

33 *Celui dont j'ai à répondre c'est celui à qui j'ai à répondre. Le "de qui" et le "à qui" coincident.*

The notion of "being-responsible-for" is frequently mentioned by Nagy. "The responsibility in front of the other" is not so clearly indicated. It seems as if there is no other present that makes an appeal to my responsibility. However, that is not the case. The notion of a transgenerational tribunal, operating like a "silent partner" (always existent in the relational reality), points in the direction of "in front of". It is this silent partner that makes an appeal to my responsibility.

Noteworthy in Levinas' approach, is the fact that one's life work and legacy are an investment, stretching over, and even after one's death (Levinas HAM:69). It has an "infinite" effect and a character of disinterest. One can perhaps connect this notion of "infinite effect" with Nagy's notion of "non-mutual reciprocity between parents and children".

Nagy refers to "interlocking reciprocity" between generations (Nagy IL:353). The advantage of this reciprocity is that the new generation "repay" (compensate for) the care of the previous generation. Reciprocity continues within a quite new mode, namely by caring for the future generation. The "balance of fairness" attains in this way a long-term character, and proceeds after the death of the parent. The merit of what the parents have done for the children, becomes a fruitful investment without taking advantage of the fruits for themselves.

We now need to proceed with the sometimes-strange paradoxical mode of interplay between Nagy and Levinas in order to get more clarity on Nagy's contextual approach within the relational dynamics of ethics. We said "strange", because sometimes the formulation is indeed peculiar and complex. The traces are often embedded in philosophical formulations with many layers of significance. Thus, the heading of the next section: Challenging confrontations.

Challenging confrontations: The trace of a peculiar weakness

Human relationships are often exposed to weakness. One can call it the predicament of human vulnerability and failure. On the other side, there is always the courage to be, or what one can call resilience. Weakness without cowardice points in this direction: The ability to always bounce back despite worse conditions of weakness. It presupposes inner strength (fortification) to meet and encounter the challenges of suffering and weakness. In this realm of peculiar weakness, several footprints/traces could be identified that can play a role in the existential confrontation with human vulnerability and the challenge to deal with infringements in a humane way; very specifically the challenge to promote the humane quality of the other – the vulnerable other (The "I" becomes the hostage of the other, but at the same time must also become a hospitable host for the other).

1. A very peculiar vulnerability

"Weakness without cowardice" (faiblesse sans lacheté).

For this first challenging confrontation, we turn to a text from one of Levinas' writings: *Humanism and the Other Human Being* (Levinas HAM:32-36). One can even say that the text of HAM is a concise and very condensed summary of Levinas' other two writings: *Totalité et Infini* (TI) and *Autrement* (AE). In this text the formulation is also less ontological.

The most pregnant mode of describing the eventual significance of responsibility is to describe it in a passive mode: The absolute passivity of the *self*. It refers for Levinas to the fact that the I exchanges places with the Other (*l'Autre*). In this very peculiar exchange, the I becomes the *hostage* of the other (Levinas MG:34). The predicament of hostage creates a very strange weakness (defect) (*une étrange faiblesse*); it is about a weakness that penetrates and strikes the comeliness of being. It strikes like an existential shock (Levinas HAM:32; HAH:11). But and this is the very interesting point, it is a weakness without cowardice (*faiblesse sans lacheté*), because this weakness is the origin of deep compassion and pity (*pitié*). It is about an inability and powerlessness that take on the character of humane humanity by infiltrating and penetrating humanity (*Défaillance de l'étre tombant en humanité*) (Levinas HAM:33; HAH:11).

With "powerlessness of being" (*défaillance*), Levinas describes a primordial feature of being and subjectivity: Being is weak and exposed to failure, faults and vulnerability. And the other is there to remind us that we are fallable and inherently powerless. Subjectivity is a mode of being, wherein the primary focus is not on being itself, not on care for oneself, because the subject has become "obsessed" with the other, touched by the other, who was already there *first*. The powerlessness of being, and its connection with this "peculiar weakness" do not describe a psychological state of being; it does not refer to a psychic or physical condition. It rather indicates the fact that human beings (very specifically) *cannot do* what all other living organisms probably can do, namely, to become automatically and naturally not being obsessed with the being of the other, or something else; the ignorance of just being careless.

The poignant point in Levinas' argument is that if "a sense of vulnerable powerlessness" (*défaillance*) (acknowledgement of failure and faults) is missing, if people carry on with killing and destructive violence, and compassionate pity becomes absent, the false image of "I can cope and manage" becomes in fact an indication of a defect and estrangement (Levinas TI: ix-x). The absence of this very peculiar and strange mode of being weak and powerless, is a serious defect (a kind of existential pathology). Healing could then, perhaps, imply the recovery of this very strange mode of being a subject: Being weak within a vulnerable mode of resilience.

2. The "grace" of powerlessness

A typical feature of existential philosophy is its attempt to unmask the fact that the autonomous subject lives from a kind of gap within the essence of being; nothingness is like a rotten defect in our being; it gnaws into being and unmasks hopelessness (Jean-Paul Sartre). One exists from the vantage point of a defect and, thus, the obsession of to be (courage to be), as well as the desire to overcome the defect. The ontic default developed because the old metaphysical order of a static principle for being disappeared. Adorno calls the Enlightenment a massive deceit (fraud).

Girard in his mimetic theory, argued more or less the same. Girard even spoke of a desire for a mode of metaphysics (*désir métaphysique*). He meant with this new mode of metaphysics, the fact that the one being covets the being of the other. The implication is that the other becomes both model and obstacle. In terms of Hegelian thinking, our being is essentially structured by death and dying; we are becoming *creatures of deficiencies* (*Mangelwesen*) (Arnold Gehlen).

Levinas also refers to desire (*désir*). However, with desire is not meant a need (craving for satisfaction), or merely a functional effect of being. It is about a yearning and longing; a kind of existential unrest, an earnest search and quest. Both are not merely about a deficiency. The desire is about an honourable powerlessness, indicating a sound and soulful resilience. It is about a metaphysical desire for absolute exteriority. Without this exteriority life becomes soulless and void. To be delivered out to oneself (*tout seul*), is to be delivered out to a state of torment and affliction. One finds oneself in a condition of existential imbalance (Levinas: from RA, in MG:41). The other/ *Other* (more or less in a theological sense), from whom I am dependent, is not my enemy, but my "neighbour". The relationship with the other (the other from whom I am radically separated and will always stay separated), is as metaphysical desire constitutive for subjectivity. The existential unrest, the fact that I am addressed by the visage and challenged not to present carelessness, creates a humane condition (*condition humaine*) par excellence. The deficiency of being is about being addressed and directed by the relation with the other. It constitutes the alterity of being (metaphysical relationship); that is, a social relationship that starts irrevocably and always in subjectivity. It represents a longing that does not originate from instinct or psychological needs. It is about an orientation that is evoked by the visage of the other. This is then about an authentic heteronomy: The subject takes (in the mode of responsibility) onto him/herself, the shock of the other. That is exactly what is meant by the freedom of the subject. It does not start with a deficiency in being, but about a powerlessness of being that reflects the grace of being human.

3. About power and disgrace

Nagy is very careful not to make power a constitutive component of therapy. In both his theory formation as in the practice of counselling, he rejects all forms of power language. He is aware of the role of power in society. In many therapeutic "power games" it is about control. But as key to the humane character of human relationships, power is insufficient and inappropriate. To try to exercise power and to maintain control over the other, the attempt to possess the other, force the other into a sameness and equality; eventually one loses the capacity to care. One then fails to create dialogue. On the contrary, one even promotes in fact more loneliness.

Powerful manipulation of the other, destroys the other. To stop this power game, is to realise that the other is seeing me, and, in fact, addressing me. In this kind of encounter, I become aware that I myself become different. The other should not be reduced to the self of the "I". One should rather acknowledge the other so that the other could stay being exterior. The presupposition of all relationships is then that the other enters the self, but in this penetrating event, neither the self nor the other are destroyed.

Human subjectivity is about the brokenness of powerlessness; broken by the primacy of ethics: The a priori of the one-for-the-other principle (*l'un pour l'autre*); powerlessness that degenerates into true, authentic (humane) co-humanity.

4. Patience

Humane humanity is not natural and cannot be taken for granted. It should rather be granted. In the discovery of being tolerant, to endure, one enters into the realm of sound humanity. One then discovers how separated we are from one another. One should postpone the hour of betrayal and "the killing of the other". To endure, is a mode of freedom; one abdicates from one's clinging to the present and one's selfish immediacy. In patience one creates space and time: the miracle of time as future oriented.

The weakness of being in its focus on the other, is a variant for the Hegelian synthesis. It transforms static synthesis into enduring patience (Levinas HAM:32; HAH:11). In this way debating discourses are transformed into the voice of subtle silence (*voix de subtil silence*); weakness without cowardice is stirred as the awakening of compassionate pity; the discharge of a being that gives up his/her possessiveness. "Being weak" is the enigmatic mystery of being responsible for the other; care to the other. Due to the fact that the other is always first, human subjectivity originates from pity and the challenge to instil justice.

In Nagy's thinking, humanity originates from guilt and indebtedness. In this sense, humanity emanates from a deficiency within the inner realm of subjectivity; this deficiency attains the significance of an ethical impulse. It is not an ontological deficit in being itself, but an ethical indebtedness to the other; the first and primordial other. Guilt and obligation are for Nagy not an epi-phenomenon, but constitutive for the human person. Indebtedness and obligation are relational terminologies. Thus, the reason why the notion of reciprocity in Buber's thinking is too limited. These terminologies could only be understood from the internal perspective of the subject that has patience with the unavoidable, existential factuality of being affected by the other.

5. Postponing fear

Nagy views ethical entanglements as indication of our human condition (Nagy F:100-117). The ethical complications and troubles in our lives are in fact playing a key role in the dynamics of being (Nagy F:100). The fact that our life is threatened by death and anxiety, is not the real motivational factor. To be overwhelmed by anxiety and threatened by death are dual experiences. One is fascinated by death, but at the same time resists death, even with violence. This duality is the origin of destructive violence; it is the origin of both inner torment and outer terror.

To obtain sustainable hope and to instil peace in our violent society, require respecting the otherness of the other, becoming aware that the other is demarcated by his/her separateness. In caring coexistence this differentiation does not end in a chaotic confrontation of power-maintenance. Peace is not about the suspension of violence and war. Peace is more fundamental. It is about respect for the otherness of the other.

The real threatening aspect of violence is not actually about destructive behaviour and killing, destroying of the other, but in the disruption of the other's continuity. The violence forces the other into a role wherein people don't anymore recognise themselves. They betray themselves and their engagements. But the worse thing is that eventually violence destructs one's own identity and substance. It forces one to perform actions that destroy all possibilities for significant action (Levinas TO:14; TI:ix).

Instead of destruction, care should be established. For Nagy, the quality of our being human (being a child, adult, husband, wife) is instructed by the other, namely, to take up the challenge of care; it is essentially about a caring commitment. It is not the anxiety for one's own death that dictates being but acts of care and compassion. In receiving this kind of instruction, one should recognise and establish an act of giving to the other (the parent, educator, teacher) (Nagy IL:31, 382-383; *AFTA-Newsletter*:35).

To educate an individual, is in essence an ethical process. Thus, the necessity to abdicate from all forms of violence. Violence is not an authentic expression or component of our being human. The deficiency in being can only be transcended when one poses and accepts the a priori of relationships; the challenge is about a relationship with separate others. It is about a relationship wherein every separate text within context, and every context that frames the text, present otherness, even belongs to the other. Thus, the reason why even a small child can contribute in his/her own right. Everybody exists in his/her own right.

6. The ability of passivity

The Other in Levinas' approach, is about infringement on the self; without any doubt, a very strange weakness in being. It shakes the foundations of sovereignty; it unmasks freedom as arbitrariness. The events that memory cannot recall, mark a trace in the self. The trace of the other is not a genetic trace or marking, but an ethical mark.

The following question should be posed: Is loyalty in Nagy's thinking not perhaps an indication of trace?

For Levinas, the powerlessness of being (as defect) is eventually a sign of humanity, indicating a metaphysical desire. This desire does not originate from need-satisfaction, but from the longing to do something for the other and not to inflict damage; acting and doing, thus, as giving and speaking (voicing). Relationships should never be exploited and abused. For example, when one transfers the relationship into a mere theory, and the I is becoming merely a watching outsider (an objectified position outside the relational dynamics), these modes of externalisation and isolation are already indicators of exploitation and abuse. Even to keep quiet, is a form of denial and withdrawal, a subtle mode of "soft, silent violence".

7. Separation and relating

Distancing and detachment presuppose differentiation and discernment in order to separate from the other. This distinction is the starting point of a relationship, because the other becomes the daughter-of, son-of, brother-of, sister-of, etcetera. The founding of a relationship is also about a process of learning – instruction. Relationships in these cases are totally different than the relationship with death. They precede all our relationships with death, as well as our anxiety for dying. Death and the anxiety for dying could even be rendered as meaningful. The first step to deal with death and dying, is to become involved with the other.

This does not imply a denial of death and dying, anxiety, isolation and hunger. On the contrary. These phenomena are indeed constitutive for human self-development. In fact, they are signs of our human predicament, social disruption, social injustice and inhumanity. Both Levinas and Nagy maintained this viewpoint. The disruption of a society, wherein human beings exist not anymore for one another, but only for themselves, are rendered by both Nagy and Levinas as unacceptable. Such a selfish stance is not authentic and not an original expression of our being human.

On the other hand, one should reckon with the fact that separation cannot avoid a mode of anxiety. That is inevitably the case. From a systemic point of view, the anxiety does have a function. However, the ethical challenge in the exposure to anxiety, resides in the contribution of the one that is willing to care and carry the burden of the other.

Sometimes, parent and adults are afraid of separation and detachment. This is the reason why parents and children are often becoming allies in this web of separating anxieties. They are piling up a lot of unhealthy needs and expectations that in the long run are becoming unjust and destructive. In this respect, Nagy refers to "collusive postponement of mourning". The challenge of working through losses by means of mourning (grief work) (see Mitscherlich 1967), is about facing your sorrow. Not to internalise the loss, is to merely reinforce the loss and separation; it becomes eventually situated in the mind in the form of pathology. Grief work is rather an instruction to the subject. It teaches the subject (as individual) to understand how to give and to receive care in the relationship with the other. *This work is about a transformation process wherein loyalty is transformed into faithfulness. The involvement with connections, is transformed into solidarity.* Merely a geographical or physical separation, cannot accomplish this task; it just minimises the opportunities for giving and receiving.

To establish trust and to promote faithfulness are in particular the tasks and challenges of adults. Nagy refers to the "residual trust" of a child. The latter refers to the fact that the child is dependent on trust, and, should, thus, start to trust the faithfulness and loyalty of the parent and the community of adults. What is unique here, is that the child starts to learn how to give to the parent as well. The undergirding presupposition is that the child can reckon with the fact that the parent will keep in mind the dynamics of trusting. Parents should learn how to deal also with his/her own particularity as person.

The teacher is always the other (my master/mistress). The other is the first framework of reference that renders meaning to reality and things. The significance resides in the acknowledgement of the unique place and value of the other's belongings and possessions. Thus, the reason for my indebtedness to the other. For the process of self-signification, the subject must discover and acknowledge that his/her contribution resides in indebtedness. Awareness of indebtedness sets one free (deliverance) and creates space to sojourn. But then, this contribution, should also be acknowledged and trusted by the other as well.

8. About entitlement and investiture: Heading for "reward"

As for Levinas, it is for Nagy important to realise that power is insufficient to provide a humane perspective on human relationships. The same is valid for family relationships and applicable to relational interaction. Intersubjectivity is also not merely about the coexistence of two or more modes of freedom.

As contextual therapist, it is for Nagy decisive that, in order to operate on a meaningful and professional basis, a different perspective and order should be introduced. Thus, the shift from an ontology of power, to an ethics of justice. "It is […] in the just order of things to earn the rewards that are dynamically linked to offering due care" (Nagy BGT:13). "Due care", the offering of indebted care, has an advantage and spinoff. What? Rewards. Reward consists of the accepted personal freedom that resides in entitlement. And this is already entailed in the "just order of things". Reward should not be confused with "should" or "ought" in terms of sheer moralism (legalism) and abstract idealism. It must also not be confused with priorities, referring to a framework of values, stemming from particular cultural groups. It is anchored in the notion of "universal human reality" (Nagy BGT:13).

Two perspectives are paramount. The one is about "the just order of things", the other is about the notion of "universal human reality".

When one becomes aware of all the sufferings of human beings through the ages and the cruelties done to people, one can indeed start doubting whether there is something like a just human order. Even in therapy, the narratives of people are full of painful loss, violence and deceit. Eventually one can only hope that a just human order will become a safeguarding framework for meaningful caregiving.

In the same way, care cannot be derived from a natural right or law. It is indeed true that Nagy refers to the entitlement of a child. Children do have the right to trustworthy care and appropriate education. Although Nagy does not mention it explicitly, this right and entitlement can even refer to a kind of existential competence or existential calling. Nevertheless, entitlement implies a kind of "reward" due to the offering of "due care" and merit.

It will become dangerous if "due care" becomes a commodity, namely, to earn entitlement and achieve trustworthiness. The implication will be that one is constantly busy to highjack power in order to achieve "manipulative power". The further implication is that one uses (abuses) the other in order to better oneself. But this is merely perverted narcissistic self-concern.

Entitlement is without any doubt an enigmatic mystery. If entitlement is indeed a competence or ability of being, and personal freedom a reward, the question at stake is: Who grants one the competency and freedom? The issue is further complicated by the fact that entitlement is an ethical term; it is about a right that is granted, otherwise it runs the danger of becoming merely an ontological entity (power of being).

Entitlement is a triadic concept. The "I" is rendered a right to do some-*thing*, but this right is given by the other. Entitlement is an act of responsible action. In this sense, it is not static, but dynamic; it keeps on growing and gathers even more responsibility, because care should be understood in a continuum of caring. Entitlement is not usurpation, even not a psychological disposition. Entitlement is dynamically linked to offering "due care"; it is about an investiture (Levinas' terminology).

The peculiarity in Nagy's use of the term "entitlement" points to the following problematic issues:

(a) Entitlement has no subject. A person can be endowed with rights, however there is no subject that grants the person that right. Or is the other that "person"?
(b) Within the realm and phenomenon of "personal freedom", there is no direct object. One can have, and even claim a right, but the right is directed to whom and for what purpose? What is the basis for the claim of personal freedom? The fact that "entitlement" cannot be achieved or earned, makes the term dicey.

Perhaps, the issue is not so complicated. One can indeed gain control over one's environment. And in doing this, one escapes (sidesteps) the absorptive power of things – the threat of becoming merely an object of one's circumstances. However, one should rather become engaged in the situation and start facing the challenge of authentic subjectivity "*by offering due care*". This is precisely what an act of freedom is about. From the start it is geared towards care. It is not in the first place about freedom as such, and then afterwards, about caregiving (*due care*). Both freedom and care come simultaneously into play, within the same act, at the same moment. They are "dynamically linked". The one is not the result of the other, they are co-constituted together.

For Nagy, entitlement is not a kind of ontic givenness; it is not some-*thing* that can be robbed from the other; it is an inspiration evoked by the presence of the other. One is signified by the other by means of the ethical quality of the relationship. If this is indeed the case, entitlement is about humility and servitude. Entitlement is then the powerful force of subjectivity, and not about the self-maintenance of ego-strength. One can even dare to say, that entitlement is a relational quality residing in responsibility. It is, thus, impossible to differentiate between capacity and competence. With "destructive entitlement" is meant a mode of freedom without an investiture; it is then about sheer unbridled freedom and possibly abuse of power.

9. Differentiation and non-indifference (non-carelessness)

Levinas' thinking is steered by the primordial position of ethics. The impetus is an explication of a deep ethical concern and sensitivity. Ethics is the core component in philosophising, in wisdom thinking and human awareness. And in this philosophical constellation, the other and the encounter with visage, are key role players.

Ethics has primacy when it comes to self-consciousness and embeddedness in processes of self-identification. The things at the disposal of the subject; everything that one (as subject) enjoys, work with; the environment wherein one inhabits and live; in fact, the whole of the cosmos is embedded in the realm of social dynamics, and, thus, framed by ethical concerns. Everything attains meaning within relational networking. All forms of being are from the start relational: Being human is in essence relational.

The social realm should not overwhelm subjectivity. What should be promoted in social networking is the humane quality of our being human in this world. Social networking is about relational networking and always exposed to entanglements that are embedded in ethics. For Levinas, the quality of relational networking is determined by loyalty. Even if the therapist in counselling opts as a substitute for somebody else, perhaps an absent father, this (unjust) position should deal with all sorts of ethical entanglements. For example, in family therapy the intriguing question surfaces: How could I become a better substitute parent for you? (Nagy F:99). In order to safeguard the other against emotional or cognitive aberration, therapy should address all forms of entanglements. This is the reason why one should take cognisance of the fact that in ethical networking there is always, at the same time, the threat of emotional smothering (the threat of totality).

Subjectivity is an inner perspective, but at the same time it is objective as well. This duality describes the complexity of subjectivity.

Levinas deliberately maintains subjectivity as primordial due to the trace of Visage/Countenance – an infinite and enigmatic entity. The "I" is never an isolated monad; I am encircled by the other, who is not my enemy but my fellow human being. I am not shaped by developmental psychology, but by the original structure of relational ethics and the otherness of the Other (becoming obsessed by the other). The implication of this discovery implies a total brake with all kinds of narcissistic desires. The discovery of the other as "my neighbour", as well as the abdication from all forms of self-investment, can be described as the shock of being. The impact of this shock on daily occurrences, is the phenomenon of care as exponent of non-indifference.

Nagy's approach is essentially a therapeutic perspective that eventually infiltrates the intersubjective realm of the client. The decisive question is now whether there are kinds of supporting, assisting structures and helping networks available? Are there valid psychotherapeutic discourses and caring spaces at one's disposal wherein it is possible to play back somebody's life story; even back to the traumatic shock-event; that is, the disruptive discovery that I am obsessed by the other as fellow human being?

The researchers are convinced that it is possible, but on condition: The concept of "loyalty" in Nagy's research should not be rendered and interpreted as an ontological systemic givenness (ontic quality). Loyalty as subject matter is an ethical concern connected to justice as a responsibility (indebtedness). The subject should, thus, also be viewed and assessed in terms of his/her original and unique responsibility over against the other; the subject is not a totality, but a re-*spond*-able, humane being (*respondeo ergo sum*).

Applied to therapy, the implication is that the intersubjectivity of the therapist and the client should continuously be corrected and scrutinized from the following perspective: Ethical responsibility is about the grace of a gift; a gift that the client as a total, separate other, "gives" to the therapist (it is rendered). When dealing with the other as "gift", the challenge to the therapist is not to apply his/her paradigm as an abstract theory and legalistic, causative framework of schematic interpretation (explanatory model), but to probe into the basic relational entanglements that harm the dignity of the other (estrangement).

One can indeed pose the critical question: What determines the quality of "giving" and "taking" in Nagy's therapeutic approach?

It is difficult to answer. Is the unarticulated presupposition pointing to a kind of communal measurement anchored in society? But how could one eventually differentiate and distinguish between different measurements (ledgers)? Perhaps, the fact that the therapist opts within the framework of "multidirected partiality", and, is, thus, subjected to critique, as well as the acute awareness of an ethical conceptualisation of "entitlement" (both in its passive and active significance), bring about a critical directive in therapy.

In Levinas' thinking ethics is anchored in subjectivity as a moral conscientiousness. Ethics is not anchored in the "I" of the subject as such, but in subjectivity that, in a philosophical sense, is the knot in the ethical principle, namely the notion of "one-for-the-other" (*l'un-pour-l'autre*). In other words, not the relationship as a volatile entity is the beginning, but the subjectivity as released from totality; that is, subjectivity as the origin for significant differentiation and plurality. The starting point is with "me", but this starting point is given and not an ontic fact; it is differentiated and non-indifferent simultaneously.

Subjectivity starts with a shock; it starts with an alarming uncertainty, and not with an ontological certitude/assertiveness of the subject about him/herself. Neither originates subjectivity from "sound/good conscience". Authentic subjectivity emerges within the wrestling with the question of non-indifference. What have I neglected? Or: What could I have done else, or even more? In the "weakness of being" resides authentic beginning, because my weakness is posed by the vulnerability of the other. To start there is the challenge for all modes of therapy and healing.

10. The significant other: Its meaning

The term "*significant other*" is frequently used by Nagy. The entity that signifies itself, is in terms of Levinas, for the "I" the primum intelligibile, the primary intellectual factor and fundamental reality within an encountering event. Levinas calls it a face-to-face encounter with visage; to be existentially exposed to "Countenance" (the Countenance in encounters). One cannot interpret visage in being categories. Visage appears as speech, command and appeal; it summons responsibility.

Within this framework, one needs to pose the question: Who or what exactly is this "significant other"? Is the significant other, parents for a child because that will be the answer from the perspective of family therapy and education? The problem with such an answer is that it presupposes a kind of ideological sub-structure.

The implication in the case of Nagy is that with such a term (significant other), without any clarification, he would have to start writing in an idealistic and moralistic paradigm. However, there is another option: "The significant other". By applying the term "significant other", Nagy wanted to probe into the basic principles of therapy. Therefore, "significant other" can only make sense if Nagy's presupposition is that, for example, the child discovers the parent as an entity that signifies itself as the other, granting the child meaning and significance. Or that, in the case of a small child, a moment can occur that the parent (mother) has been viewed as a separate person in his/her own capacity and right.

Becoming aware of oneself, would then (in Levinas' terminology) mean: Being aware of the significance that has been granted to him/her by the other. One can take it even further: To discover oneself as the one who is challenged and summoned (Levinas HAM:84). In other words, that the "I" is challenged by the Other towards whom his/her desire and longing are focused. The further implication is, that in the existential yearning for the other, subjectivity becomes immediately being criticized by the Other.

When one translates the previous mentioned fact, namely that the individual is being challenged by the other (Levinas), the concept of *tribunal* springs to mind: One becomes challenged by an "intrinsic, relational and transgenerational tribunal" (Nagy). Being challenged, precedes all forms of being, and simultaneously, this challenge is not self-evident. The preceding occurrence is based on a happenstance that hits me in the core of my self-hood. It puts my self-hood and freedom before a critical forum. Levinas calls this critical summoning: *Assignation* and *interpellation*. The "I-in-the-world" (for Levinas: Intentional consciousness) is assigned and interpellated by the epiphany of the Other's Visage. This is the implication of the phrase: On recognising the visage (*dont je reconnais le visage*) (Levinas EN:2-9). The "I-in-this-world" is a free being; it is not a fabrication; the subject cannot be reduced to a neutral collectivity. Being *is*; it is not caused by the social processes of daily living. It is totally disengaged from totality; it is positional and independent. It is also not merely a particle, but personal; it is not merely about an abstract personage, but about a concrete caring subject. Furthermore, it is a creation, and, thus, not a passive entity that turns up in the pages of a strange bookkeeper (Levinas TO:58). The created and positioned "I", is about subjective freedom, rendered by the other. In its striving, the "I" is totally free from all forms of totality. It represents a mode of atheism (Levinas TO:54). It is constantly being assigned and interpellated by the epiphany of the visage that does not fit into the portrayal of "this world". The visage does not belong to this world; it summons one to "see" and to "face"; it is about a moral challenge that should be acknowledged. This is the reason why Levinas wrote to Buber: An "Other" is my master and my lord (*Autrui, c'est mon Maître et mon Seigneur*).

It is now a question how Nagy's practical and theoretical application of the term "acknowledgement" (coming from the judicial sphere) can be merged with this moral quest for acknowledgement, and the understanding of freedom within the dynamics of relational intersubjectivity. In contextual therapy acknowledgement is not a fixed entity; it is connected to the humane actions of the other that contributes to the original starting of relationships. Thus, the emphasis on: justice as work.

11. Justice as work (*oeuvre de la justice*)

Nagy's anthropology is informed by Buber's anthropological remarks. Later on, these seem to shift to the background of his argumentation and outline. From a more critical perspective, the question surfaces whether in Nagy's theory formation, the notion of subjective action (concrete verbs; modes of subjectivity) becomes eventually transformed into ontological substances; that is, the acts of subjects become converted into ontology, into the form of substantives?

For example, "entitlement", "acknowledgment", "exoneration", "loyalty", eventually become substantives and not anymore viewed as representatives and expressions of the ethical dimension of subjective responsibility. It leaves the impression that the terms refer to conditions of being. But at the same time, Nagy frequently refers to verbs more than to substantive nouns when the terminology should become applicable for contextual therapy. It then refers to the ability of the subject "to acknowledge", "to be entitled", "to exonerate", "to accept/receive", "to be acknowledged", and "to be loyal".

Verbs indicate better than substantives the differentiation between relational entities and fixed totality. The difficulty with substantial terminology is that it often becomes pervaded by ontological undertones. Eventually, it does not present appropriately Nagy's basic theoretical intention, namely, that an individual, as person, does have the ethical "ability" to change the relational dynamics by means of the principle and work of justice (*oeuvre de la justice*): "Justice" is a "work".

12. Levinas within the disciplinary field of psychotherapy

At this stage, it is important to point out that Levinas took on a quite critical stance regarding the disciplinary fields of psychology, psychoanalyses and sociology. His critical assessment should be understood in context, namely his fear that these disciplinary fields tend to dominate the dynamics of relational interaction by means of concepts that reduce the meaning of words to fixed schemata of interpretation and the totality of systems. The framework of reference dictates and precedes significance so that the speaker is reduced to a mechanistic functionary (Levinas MG:31).

Nagy had similar objections. His resistance becomes obvious when Nagy refers to the praxis of care for families. He wanted to maintain his viewpoint, namely that the relationship of the "subject-I" in the encounter with the other (for Levinas: visage), is directly and not mediated. Levinas reflects explicitly critical: The subject-subject-relationship is preliminary; it reflects the intrigue: From one to the other (*de lun pour l'autre*). He disclaims all forms of subject-object-relations wherein the "it" determines the "I" (objectification). The relationship is between my-*self* and the other. Thus, the thesis that ethics precedes ontology (Levinas TO:40).

Between the "I" and the "other" there is no space for formal methodology. Methodology operates in terms of reduced images and theoretical abstractions. Therefore, Levinas is adamant in his critique on the science of psychology and the practice of psychoanalysis. For Levinas, the relationship with the other is asymmetric. The ethical dynamics operates according to the principle of not-knowing and presupposes an attitude of humility and self-renunciation. Furthermore, what irritates Levinas is how clients are delivered out to randomness and the schematisation and classification of people by means of conceptual terminologies (see the notion of an Oedipus-complex). Instead of an Oedipus-complex, Levinas maintains the viewpoint of fatherhood as revealed in Deuteronomy 8:5: Fatherhood is a constitutive category with significance, granting meaning (*sensé*). In principle, it does not instigate estrangement but promote care.

Truth is about respect for the other. It is within this respect for the other that truth happens and occurs (see Aeschlimann in Rouppe Van der Voort 1990:70-71). Truth cannot be captured by the philosophical categories of hypothetical theories making use of classification categories like: libido, sadism or masochism, Oedipus-complex and aggressiveness. The problem is that these terminologies eventually become fixed end-terms for formal and professional classification. Levinas goes even so far as to link these terminologies to the cultural threat of mythological against monotheistic thinking (Levinas MT; TO:50; MG:128).

Not every conversation is about the relationship with an exterior factor. In formal psychoanalysis, the danger is to approach the conversation partner not as "master/mistress", but as object; one out of many. The pedagogical and psychological speech are too rhetorical and run the danger of objectification; the knowing specialist dictates prescriptively the non-knowing receiver (Levinas TO:76).

In terms of the previous outline on Levinas' paradigmatic reflections, it is difficult founding a theory for healing and helping. Albeit, one cannot ignore the field of psychotherapy and professional helping. At stake, in these domains is the phenomenon of intersubjectivity. The problem, however, is that although it is not possible to compare people in terms of totality-generalisations, it is indeed the case that in theories people become classified, and, thus, comparable. Thus, the reason why the tendency to compare the incomparable should be dealt with suspicion and constantly be criticised.

We need to turn now to the question: What is the position of Nagy in this discourse?

Nagy operates from a totally different viewpoint. Within the complexity of relational networking, Nagy's intention is to look for what is helpful and could alleviate the pain of psychic suffering. He wants to attend to the link between suffering and injustice (Van Heusden & Van den Eerenbeemt 1992:17).

Even as in the case of Levinas, Nagy does not validate categories that classify beforehand and estrange people from one another. Nagy is, thus, very careful to apply classification categories like Oedipus-complex to sensitive areas like the relationship between children and their fathers that eventually contribute to further estrangement. Attention should rather be given to caring categories like responsibility, indebtedness towards others within the ethical framework of "ledger" and "justice order". The intention in therapy should not be estrangement, but how to connect people with one another and vice versa. Nagy does not deny the value of psychoanalytical categories. For example, the notion of "transference" that has a specific meaning in therapeutic relationships, can be used. Nagy connects transfer with guilt about disloyalty towards families of origin. However, categories should represent more of an ethical than a (pure) therapeutic perspective.

There are indeed some parallels between Levinas' critique and Nagy's uncomfortableness with categories applied in psychotherapy. However, in terms of the overall intention of the chapter, it is now the time to capture the essence of Nagy's position as therapist.

(a) The therapist does not diminish the fact that the client is connected to others within significant relationships. In these relational connections, the notion of *indebtedness* is paramount. Indebtedness describes the fact that one is related to other/others, and, thus, owes the other/others responsibility and vice versa (the guilt factor; merit). We are indebted towards one another.

(b) Indebtedness operates within the confines of *multidirected partiality*. No therapist can dictate the unique and personal character of indebtedness and has therefore to reckon with the fact that many others could have been involved simultaneously within the complexity of relational issues. It is about the challenge in therapy to side with every particular person involved in the inter-relational networking of systems.

(c) Nagy reckons with the factor of *unpredictability within happenstances* and the dynamics of human encounters. Unpredictability does not imply incalculability. It means literally, that one can by no means forecast the eventual outcome of life events. One must deal with the fact of *surprise in dialogue*.

(d) To reckon with "the third" – the other/others of the client – implies for Nagy that therapeutic interventions and actions should always be qualified and directed by the question: Do I act in a just and humane way? This *justice-question* is valid for both the therapist and the client due to the ethical dimension in dialogue and relationships of responsibility (*ethical dimension*).

The ambiguous connection: Transcendence-in-immanence – the enigmatic factor of disturbance (dérangement)

In the human sciences, immanency has become a buzzword. "Scientific" in many positivistic models means "empirical proof" by means of empirical data and an epistemology of observation. One can understand the importance for Nagy to attend to the interplay between transcendence and immanence. Psychology mainly operates in terms of observation within immanence: The psychic focus is predominantly on individual interiority and personal behaviour. The professional psychotherapist has hardly no other choice because the whole scientific field of psychotherapy is embedded in empirical data. Within the parameters of the human and natural sciences, the notion of evidence is accepted by many as decisive for valid outcomes.

Levinas attends in a very special way to this problem. His emphasis on "metaphysical desire" and the Other (Transcendence) (Levinas MG:192-207) operates on a different level than the intentional analyses of phenomenology. The visible is connected to the invisible, the finite to the infinite. The order of the evidential "receives" even the transcendental; visage penetrates the realm of evidence, without being absolved by this order. Furthermore, Levinas' reflections probe into the realm of subjectivity. The latter is constantly being infiltrated by the mysticism of the Other: Responsibility not as choice but elicited by the approach of the other person (visage). The responsibility of the subject becomes perforated by the Other and enacts the Good – trace of the infinite within daily events.

Furthermore, Levinas wants to defend subjectivity, thus, his focus on certainty (*certitude*). For this certainty he had been influenced and inspired by his understanding of Hebrew wisdom.

Levinas connects certitude to the notion of peace. Specifically, the messianic peace that is much stronger than war (Levinas TI:x). He does not want to promote a duplex order. His interest is mainly in certitude that operates in the mode of unrest. It is about a strange mode of unrest; that is, an unrest that penetrates the order of evidence. Unrest disturbs evidence-based certitude (security). The reason? It is aware of the unique source of disturbance, namely the encounter with the Other, face-to-face. Due to this encounter, the order of evidence receives "the sovereign significance of the Visage" without being absorbed by the Other, or by just following in a docile way (Levinas MG:194). Visage is in fact a significant disturbance of order (*dérangement*). The significance of this disturbing encounter cannot be derived from an order of being. It does not originate from ontology, but, in its focus on the infinite, is directed by a metaphysical desire. Disturbance, thus, links with an infinite order. This infinite order supersedes the epistemological realm of the intentional subject and the intentionality of sheer empirical observation.

In the argumentation of Levinas, one becomes aware of a most significant paradigm switch. This paradigm switch is from evidence to infinity. In this sense, Levinas' approach is quite unique (Keij 1992:116). The interesting point is that, despite the notion of disturbance (*dérangement*), Levinas links ambiguously, even paradoxically, the Other (*meta*-realm) to the realm of evidence. Within disturbance there is still the need for care and recovery. By means of compassionate caring (pity), transcendence is invited into the realm of evidence without reducing this connection to immanence. Transcendence should be prevented of becoming merely an empirical phenomenon. The realm of phenomenology is hereby intruded by transcendence without any form of artificial synthesis.

The connection and disturbance have the character of ambiguity. Levinas calls this ambiguous connection the "*Enigma*". With this *Enigma*, one is wrestling for the rest of one's life. Perhaps, this "*Enigma*" has to do with the meaning of our being human; it is about an *Enigma* to which the human being him/herself is the answer.

The question can be posed whether Nagy has this "disturbed interiority" in mind when he opted for the ethical dimension of our human existence; an ethical perspective that transcends all "facts", "feelings" and "interactions"? (Nagy BGT:32).

Nagy mentions the concept of "dimension" and refers to Buber's "realm of between" and "justice of the human order". However, when one probes into the meaning of all these categories and puts them together, one must conclude and say that ethics and the ethical dimension can never become a big umbrella to cover facts, feelings, and transactions (Nagy F:329). It is because of this threatening tendency towards totality, that the researchers have to be careful not to transfer Levinas' model too fast to the realm of therapy.

For Nagy, facts, feelings and systemic transactions belong to the world of immanence. Awareness of all these categories takes place within the inner realm of phenomena. They are rendered significance and receive their assessment from an ethical perspective. In principle, the "ethical dimension" is a disturbance in the realm of facts, feelings and interactions. These three are in themselves ethically neutral, and, thus, enjoyable entities "*joyeuse force qui va*". The differentiation between the experiential level and the ethical realm is for Nagy fundamental in terms of what contextual therapy has in mind. There must be a clear distinction between these three categories (facts, feelings, interactions), and the fourth dimension, namely the ethical perspective. This distinction is important in order to avoid power-manipulation in therapy. Applied to psychotherapy, one needs to remember that the subject does not "have" an ethical dimension. When the "ethical dimension" comes into play, one must realise that it is still a construction of the psychotherapist according to his/her discipline and subject. It is this construct that eventually becomes applied to immanence.

The motivational layers for hoping

It seems as if Nagy positions himself outside the psychotherapeutic discourse. Keeping in mind possible objections, Nagy wrote "… that is more important to explore the motivational layer in which hope resides for repairing the human hurt justice" (Nagy IL:53).

In Nagy's approach the following issues are at stake:
- Nagy works specifically with the perspective of motivational layers. This is a focal point in order to be engaged in repairing.
- Probing into the realm of motivational layers is essentially about the instilment of hope.
- Hope is focused on the healing (reparation) of disturbed "human justice".

"Motivational layers" and "hope" function in terms of duality. They are indeed intertwined, but due to ambiguity and duality they should not become confused and be merged into one total whole: The two becoming merged into one totality.

There are indeed many driving forces that play a role in human behaviour, actions and engagement with others. Amid all these motivational layers, hope is continuously operating. However, this hope has a unique quality. With hope is not meant a psychological or natural category. It does not originate from needs. It is about an inspiration that renews the zest for life; it bypasses resignation and rancorous behaviour.[34] One can even say, it conquers resignation and rancour.

The following question surfaces: Is "human justice" about a cosmic balance?

Here one needs to take into consideration that Nagy refers to "hurt human beings" due to injustice. It is therefore not about a cosmic balance and reflection; neither about a cosmic reflection on/over justice and ethics, but about a fundamental and ontic understanding of "justice" and "ethics"; that is, it is about ethical thinking concerning the humanisation of the "cosmos".

It is quite interesting, that although Nagy developed a "conceptual framework" and "clinical guideline", he does not refer in these guidelines to the category of hope. Hoping in therapy operates on a different level. The hope of the therapist postulates the hope of the "client": It is about a hope that supports the courage of taking risks. For this endeavour there is no other guarantee than the fiduciary of the one who takes the risk. This is what therapy is about. Success cannot be guaranteed.

Levinas takes a different route than Nagy. For Levinas, the trace of the other is simultaneously the trace of "the Eternal One": HE (God in Third person) (*Ille*) (HE-hood) is never present for the subject, but engraved in culture, especially the Jewish culture.

Unique in Nagy's therapy is that he attends to the complaints of patients. He takes them back to the quest for justice, as well as to hope for recovery from injustice; back to contexts wherein justice has been violated.

The priority of the quest for justice and the recovery of justice, presuppose a subjectivity that is already involved in the intrigue of "one for the other" (*l'un-pour-l'autre*); a subjectivity exposed to the proximity of an already

---

34 See in this regard Hebrew 11:1. Faith (*pistis*) is the hupostasis (*substantia*) of the things we hope for (*elpizomena*). To give up hoping is one of the fundamental existential sins before God (Levinas VTL:34).

differentiated fellow human being with an authentic distinctive sense of being-there, and being named properly; a subjectivity with a non-indifferent sense of care. Hope is anchored in the presence of the frail other; it is directed by the caring principle of "one for the other" (*l'un-pour-l'autre*).

Justice within social dynamics: The quest for loyalty and the establishment of a "balance of justice"

The whole constellation in Nagy's theory formation revolves around the dynamics between "loyalty" and "justice as social dynamics". This dynamic interplay takes place in immanence. Loyalty, social dynamics and balance are, despite the dynamics, in fact closed systems. Thus, the danger that "closed systems" eventually can fall prey to "totality thinking" and "ideological schematisation". This is especially true of a family system. However, the difference resides in the fact that Nagy describes the familial dynamics in terms of loyalty and entitlement. He poses that a child, as human being, is essentially loyal and entitled. It is a kind of primary and foundational givenness and not an achievement. The child, as other, challenges one to maintain justice; to create balance within the dynamics of asymmetry (the child as caregiver).

Nagy refers to balance as being transformed into justice; balance as an ethical principle (balance of justice). The background for this "balance of justice", resides primarily in the dynamics between *justice* (*tsedeka*) and *pity*[35]; it should be established by the person as subject. The balance is not about a judicial order of justice wherein things (guilt, obligation, merit) being weighed on a scale in order to be balanced out. In the centre is not a scale or a court (with a judge) in order to bring about equilibrium. In the centre operates the subject in terms of his/her competence to care within a network of interacting relationships. The centre is about fairness, loyalty and indebtedness.

One can indeed merge "indebtedness towards the other" (Nagy IL; BGT) with the notion of connectedness. Indebtedness can also serve as trace of an original pattern of transcendence (Levinas MG:199). The order of transcendence passes into the order of immanence. One order can indeed enter

---

35 In Hebrew: *Rachamim* = labour pain as metaphor for painful pity and compassion; contraction of entrails in The New Testament (*ta splanchna*).

another order like an osmotic interaction. They interpenetrate one another. Nevertheless, every order stays intact. The second order does not become the first interpenetrating order. The interplay between orders is enigmatic.

The way in which the other competes for acknowledgement by the subject, without giving up his/her incognito, is, in terms of Levinas, an *"enigma"*. The implication is that the human subjectivity is as such engaged in enigmas. The extraordinary has already made itself, in its appearance, invisible in the mode of an enigma. This invisible enigma could indeed be connected to Levinas' idea of trace.

In Nagy's model, existence is from the beginning, about being challenged: "Guilt" and "indebtedness" should serve as links to loyalty. The question is whether loyalty is an appropriate category to describe this ground situation.

Group loyalty can become enclosed indeed. On the other hand, the human possibility of guilt and indebtedness are incorporated in loyalty. This possibility can lead to conflict between different modes of loyalty (loyalty-conflict); it can even develop into ethical entanglements. Due to ethical entanglements people eventually need therapy.

One can start toying with the idea that there could be a link between "ethical entanglement" and the unrest and disturbance in human encounters. Does it perhaps point to the enigma of encounter: Face-to-face with visage? Perhaps to the "prophetic enigma"?

The shock of visage (face of the other in its weakness) creates an existential unrest and disturbance in relational networking; it disturbs the realm of phenomenality. The disturbance becomes a reality that cannot be managed by phenomenological intentionality. This is where the notion of the Other becomes insightful. The Other makes the quest for justice relevant and urgent; it disturbs the realm of phenomenologically based security.

Being challenged means that one becomes aware of the significance rendered to the "I" by the other. It is significant because he or she is indeed an "other". When the "I" is challenged by the "relational tribunal", the child can even become the other that poses the question of justice. But it could also be a different other than the child (somebody else). It could be the parent or any other "other".

The notion of the "significant other" plays an important role in transgenerational dynamics. It should even be linked to the notion of solidarity.

The "transgenerational solidarity" requires "(a) priority of consideration of the welfare of posterity, and (b) multilateral fairness in the relationships of contemporaries" (Nagy F:309). In this complex network of responsibility, it is imperative that the "I" starts to prioritise. In the case of "*hurt* human justice", it becomes extremely important. The tribunal of the justice order represents the proceedings of *social distributive* and *retributive justice*. The challenge is also applicable to the responsibility of the person with regards to the next generation.

The goal is to establish a just order for the social community. In order to achieve this goal, the subject takes on responsibility for many others. For this responsibility it is imperative to prioritise. Thus, the reason why the subject needs support and should not be left in the lurch.

Justice within social dynamics should contribute to a just ordering of society and fair community interaction. This is about a society wherein the subject is supported in his/her responsibility for the vulnerable other/others. It is a society wherein attempts to prioritise, occur according to basic responsibilities; it is about establishing social justice, distributive and redistributive justice, civil-societal justice. All kinds of justice should be promoted by society and not by merely one "I". However, it starts with this responsibility: the one-for-the other.

On challenging the loyalty of the single individual

According to the researchers it is possible to reinterpret loyalty. This reinterpretation should be done within a different paradigmatic framework. The intention is to interpret loyalty as an outreach to the other (Keij 1992:116). It is in this mode of reaching out towards the other, that the single human person is challenged to exhibit loyalty in the public of civil society; to establish a mode of loyalty that operates as a kind of "guide" how to reach out to the other. In this way, the self-evidence of phenomenality could be penetrated. Loyalty as connectedness is, in this sense, not a fate, but a challenge to become humane within justice; to even overcome violence (on becoming human by means of justice). In order to establish this kind of civil societal justice, more than psychodynamic and social-psychological theories are needed.

The paradigm switch, namely loyalty as guide for fair and trustworthy modes of outreach to the other, touches parenthood, as well as the intergenerational dynamics. Loyalty can become a guide how to support children and how to reach out to parents (the parent as other). The further challenge for loyalty to opt as "social guide" (public trace), is about the question how to impact on the chain of generations because the future-other is not-yet, not present in the presence. In this sence, loyalty becomes linked to time extrapolated from the future.

The child is indeed the other. The father procreates the daughter and the son. They are conceived, delivered and nurtured by the mother. Eventually, the father merely becomes a father via the daughter and his son. In the same way the mother becomes mother. This whole interactive chain should be guided by justice as a social dynamic.

The fact that the child uses the other (parents) first, and is dependent on their care, points in the direction of narcissism. Levinas argues in ZZ (1988) along the same lines when he refers to the following intriguing hypothesis: The bodily emergence of a human being, its arising, is a kind of infringement within the realm of "nameless being". It also brings about separation. Embodiment becomes a position; it enters consciousness, the private domain; it receives a name and becomes dependent on the other; it partakes in the elements of being and flourishes. It also discovers that being was always exposed to visage; it annexes its being as its own existence within the sign of allegiance (faithfulness and loyalty). In intersubjective encounters, human embodiment starts to claim its separation and subjectivity. In this sense, the birth of a child disturbs the balance of parenthood and becomes an enigma in the crossroad between "nature" and the "command" (Levinas SaS:128). In the same way the self-hood of subjectivity (individuation) is challenged by a "disturbing loyalty".

Nagy calls loyalty an ontic or ontological entity, being as a "kind of givenness". From the viewpoint of therapy, this assumption can be valued. However, when the subject is at stake, and it is about loyalty as a relational entity (connectedness as a commitment), loyalty is not ontically anchored, but ethically challenged. Every subject makes his/her own unique contribution. The fact that a human being contributes, making an outreach, is not an ontological issue per se, but rather points into the direction of metaphysics (one is summoned), and ethics (one is indebted). In this way, loyalty challenges individuality and even demarcates subjective identity as a separate mode of responsibility (the starting point is the interiority of the subject).

When this loyalty is about a humane condition, (as postulated by Nagy), it is also the induction of ethics in the unavoidable realm of subjectivity. Morality is kindled in interiority and precedes all choices.

It is noteworthy that ethics takes root in the subject. Perhaps the source for the weakness in being. But in the predicament of our vulnerability, lurks already the enigmatic seed of compassionate concern for the predicament of the other, even for the "dying of the other".

Furthermore, the fact that a human being can experience the predicament of vulnerability, is an indication that he/she can reveal a deeper sense of care for "the death of the other"; a concern that even supersedes one's own despair for death. Indeed, a strange kind of substitution. From a psychological perspective the "more-for-the-other-than-for-my-self" could perhaps be rendered in psychoanalytical terminology as pathology – an unhealthy identification and transfer. But from the viewpoint of loyalty, it contributes to social healing and helping.

The abyss of chaotic feelings (confusion due to an acute awareness of the predicament of our human condition) can be sorted out by a skilled therapist. It could even be redefined and tagged with the aid of ethic-relational terminology, like "guilt" and "indebtedness". One can even say that ethical terminology guarantees and establishes the individuality of the subject. The principle of "one-for-the-other" (*l'un-pour-l'autre*) proofs the authenticity of this ethical and loyal establishment. This establishment becomes existent and real, when, for example, a child is intimately connected to a family, or a nation (Levinas TI:255; TO:340).

Albeit, more is at stake. At stake, is loyalty founded by ethics and directed by justice.

The paradigm switch that Nagy intends, implies that loyalty is an outreach, emerging from the other, even the vulnerable other. The child functions as subject, representing the factuality of "one-for-the-other" (*l'un-pour-lautre*); the child as new creation; the subject as *creatio ex nihilo*. In this regard, the principle of multi-directed partiality can do justice to the situation and promote social justice.

The ethical principle of "one-for-the-other" (*l'un-pour-l'autre*), disturbs all forms of superficial certitudes (securities). It even disturbs the continuity of time as causative, linear sequence of temporality.

Time as discontinuity

Connectedness should be about an ethical concern. In order to be ethical, connectedness should be preceded by a breach. This breach or disruption is about discontinuity. For example, between mother/daughter, father/son (etcetera), there is an interval in time: The relationship is in fact diachronic. The diachronic factor refers to difference and non-indifference.

This interval (discontinuity) is ambiguous because it is so easy just to forget about this disruption and breach in time. It can just become forgotten or be neglected. Eventually all forms of sociological or psychological pathology can set in (over-parentification, incest, and many others forms of violent manipulation). The diachronic becomes destroyed, while the other becomes synchronised to the self. The impression is then that differences between persons and generations are based on an original synchronic fusion, on a primary non-difference. However, here the opposite is at stake: Synchronic time is derived from the difference, the diachronic.

It seems to be incorrect to postulate like Nagy and Krasner in BGT: The moment of "healing" resides in "connectedness itself". The following could perhaps be more appropriate: The moment of healing resides much more in the acknowledgement of "*dis*connectedness". A family, as social structure, is exactly about the paradoxical situation of diachronic time; time as discontinuity; time extrapolated from the future.

The remark by Nagy and Krasner about "connected in itself", is to a large extent superficial. In fact, it is even artificial because it does not reckon with this moment of discontinuity; the breach between persons and generations. On the other hand, Nagy and Krasner postulate that healing, and outreach are about a kind of exodus to the other; healing evoked by "due concern" (Nagy BGT:20). This perspective of Nagy's work could indeed be rendered as a contribution to the dimension of healing in therapy. Exactly within this moment of discontinuity, the interval (sterile, deadly time) (Levinas TO:62; TI:29) could pass sound psychotherapeutic interventions. Therapeutic listening to discontinuities in personal narratives, reveals authentic experiences in time. The possibility of "listening backwards", is listening to the ethical agitation as authentic experience of the other. It is, therefore, not an indication of reductionism. One then starts to hear the pain and woundedness in the speaking and silence of the other. As differentiated other and subject, the client bears this painful experience, being wounded, without any guarantee of reciprocity. The only unintentional "reward" for continuous concern or care is "entitlement" (Nagy & Krasner BGT:13, 416) as irrevocable investiture. Via this "entitlement", one is empowered to excercise "personal freedom". One gains a kind of existential competence. It is also then that woundedness is voiced, and the "I" starts to pick up vibrations of the other's pain.

Nagy does not describe this turning point; that is, the moment wherein the eventual destructive entitled person turns to the other who was in fact always and already there (Levinas). Precensing as an ontic givenness. Thus, the reason why Nagy does not want to organise it therapeutically. It is perhaps an advantage not to try to describe this turning point and moment of conversion in order to move in confidence from "destructive entitlement" to "constructive entitlement". However, noteworthy is the fact that the turning point is essentially an ethical moment of "conversion" and change. It does not envelop in terms of casuality; the turning point brings about something new; it is essentially a radical renewal, a mode of *re*-creation.

The vulnerability of the other is a disturbing factor, an original starting point. It functions as challenging factor and creates space for the establishment and enfleshment of affective concern and due care in interpersonal significant relating and in pastoral caregiving.

Multidirected partiality as condition for therapy and pastoral care

We now proceed with the endeavour to reinterpret the thinking of Nagy. The special focus will be on the relationship between the I and the other in psychotherapy. It will be argued, that in this respect, the thinking of Levinas, especially the dynamics of the I-other-interaction can make a substantial contribution to the dynamics of intersubjectivity and healing in caregiving.

The outline will be structured in terms of four modalities: I and the Other; intersubjectivity; subject-object split, and fusion.

A. I and the Other

Nagy: The relationship between the I as therapist and the client, is asymmetric. "Multi-directed partiality" includes the other, and all others interconnected. At stake, in this therapeutic relationship, is the approach and attitude of the therapist. Therapy starts with the question about the "relation" between the therapist and him/herself. This approach is about asymmetry. It implies a total break with the notion of dual symmetry wherein the entanglement is about a dysfunction within the needs of the client. This could indeed be addressed by means of a process of empathetic transference. As argued, Nagy does take another road.

Levinas: The other dictates from a higher position (above), and at the same time from a lower position: being humiliated, without force (*sans force*). The challenge to the "I" is the following: The demand to be obedient is a demand only to oneself. It is about differentiation as an ethical action.

B. Intersubjective

Nagy: Intersubjectivity is an a priori of our being human (human existence). In contextual helping and caring, the "multi-partiality of the therapist performs a multilateral exploration of all possible relationships within the networking context of the client. The latter constitutes a therapeutic platform for dialogue, with the client as subject, encircled by his/her others. "Self-delineation" and "self-validation" describe the separate subjectivity of the I, as well as the separate subjectivity of each of the others. The dialogue is about what counts within the between of "give-and-take". It is exactly here that the general measure of justice, with its distributive and retributive aspects, can be detected.

Intersubjectivity is triadic at least. The family is a social group. The relational networks of a family are indeed complex. There are so many dimensions in family dynamics operating simultaneously, thus, the imperative to deal with them all. This inclusive approach is important so that people can be exposed to the experience that they are been taken seriously and not ignored. It often happens that people are just negated, although they are still alive. It is the same with the memory of people who already passed away.

This networking dynamic of multidirected partiality does have consequences for professional articulation of life problems, very specifically for the language the therapist is going to use. One consequence is "connective speaking"; connective language as an attempt to verbalise what (or whom) is difficult for the client to articulate (Meulink-Korf & Van Rhijn 1991:15).

Levinas: It is indeed possible that the community (the state, caregiving endeavours) could imply a non-comparative stance. But at the same time lurks the temptation to compare as well. This paradoxical stance is necessary due to the attempt to safeguard justice, and to enflesh concern and pity. This possibility presupposes a general kind of measurement, a criteria and scale. However, it is only a derivative. Fundamental is "my" responsibility. The reciprocity is about a structure that is based on an original inequality (Levinas MG:47).

C. Subject-object

Nagy: "Multi-partiality" is in cases of a subject-object-split, virtually absent. This is already the case when one acts as if the therapeutic relationship is strictly a dyadic relationship. The problem is that the client becomes isolated and objectified. From the perspective of the client as subject, a subject-object relationship is about the threat that I start to view the other in his/her participation as object (a collusion). Due to a desire for significance, objectification sets in. This desire can become acute in the other ("evidence of their worth", Nagy F:93). It could even be instigated by concern (care) and the need to cooperate (a child due to a need of a parent/parents). But this cooperation does not minimise the injustice. Injustice disturbs the relationship and makes an appeal on entitlement. The point is, the ability (passive) of the other could become exploited. Unfortunately, this is a very subtle expression of sheer affective violence.

Sometimes objectification is necessary and unavoidable. For example, in cases of medical procedures. However, it does not exonerate one from the responsibility to act in all circumstances with respect for the integrity of the other, including the maintenance of "relational integrity".

Levinas: When one degrades the other to an object of lust, investigation, the gaining of significance etcetera, all the attempts are expressions of violence.

D. Fusion

Nagy: To see, or experience, the other as not being separated from me, is a form of decay; it is about neglecting the ethical perspective. To ignore differentiation implies chaos in the relationship and confusion to persons involved. Several times, the therapist will identify in the client inadequate attempts regarding "self-delineation", as well as signs of inappropriate "self-validation". The problem with non-differentiated modes of being (the totality of "a one-we-subject") (Nagy F:92), established inter alia within all social forms of relationships (also between generations), is that relating itself becomes chaotic; it becomes easily confused with processes of psychological identification.

Without clear differentiation, responsibility becomes problematic and misplaced. When a person is not prepared to take responsibility for his/her own behaviour, relationships become entangled. In the therapeutic relation, fusion is about improper transference. It is about transference that has not been corrected. This will be confirmed by inappropriate modes of contra-transference. The real danger lurks that the therapist takes control over the being of the other. In this respect, the therapist fails and commits a kind of subtle therapeutic violence to the patient. The effect on the patient is most of times an upheaval of guilt due to apparent disloyalty towards the real others in his/her environment (parents, partners, children). The therapist inflicts in these cases further violence to others as related to the client's social networking environment. Every form of "partiality" is then lacking and absent.

Levinas: Fusion implies a falling back to a sterile position even before the hypostasis[36]; it is about a reduction before ethical individuation; back to merely a void "*there is*" (*il-y-a*): Total *in*-difference within the void space of nothingness.

Concluding remarks

Within the interplay between Nagy and Levinas, it becomes clear that Nagy's position in psychotherapy is unique and even extraordinary. Very surprisingly, facts, psychic processes and systemic interaction do not feature so much in his therapeutic approach. The core of his model can be captured by the following therapeutic slogan: *Relational ethics contributes to relational healing and change, while debouncing the fatality and determinating character of "facts"*. In relational networking, there is something that precedes all forms of conversational dynamic; something that penetrates facts, feelings, and transactions. This "something-factor" Nagy calls "ethics" and its link to "justice".

Ethics is rendered as the option for accountability and responsibility. Ethics defuses the fatality of facts, the dominating and determining role of psychic processes, as well as the closed circularity of trans-actions and inter-action.

---

36 The underlying state or underlying substance. It refers to a very fundamental reality that supports all others.

Ethics presupposes that one is not merely free from, but in fact free-for, free-for responsibility. The other side is also true. One should also become *responsible-for*, for being-free. Responsibility is not about a top-down approach. It is rather about servitude, caregiving and diaconic acts of outreach. Nagy refers to "due care" and "earned entitlement". This kind of care should be displayed in all spheres of society, specifically in families. But then this care should not be about self-concern, worry and uneasiness about human vulnerability and our being exposed to the threat of death. It should be about solicitous care wherein the focus is the other, his/her vulnerable predicament and anxiety for death.

The focus is always on other human beings within society; it features within the paradigm of "offering due care", and the notion of "earning entitlement" (Nagy BGT:13). Responsibility does not shrink. On the contrary, it grows and becomes bigger. What is most costly in life, is when one starts with the other first (always prior); when one realises the other is always rendered as prior to me: the other as "*intelligible primmum*". One cannot even capture this moment in terms of rational clarification, because it is about the unarticulated rhythm of humane coexistence.

Care is always about sharing and distributing, because it is based on the demand of distributive and retributive justice. This is necessary to prevent that *one* person in society takes all the burden of care on him/herself, and eventually becomes burnout, with loss of sound distance (over involvement).

The order of justice in society is necessary in order to make the burden less and not more. This order inflicts a consciousness of justice. This consciousness sets in when it helps people to realise that the vulnerable, the weak and the outsider in society need more attention than coping with the demands of the insiders. In this respect, Nagy also reveals a deep concern for coming, future generations and displaced, homeless people in society (Nagy F:xviii)[37].

The spiritual seriousness of Nagy's premise, is aptly captured by Psalm 78:3-4 (NIV):

"Things we have heard and known,
Things our ancestors have told us.

---

37 See the current global migrant crisis.

> We will not hide them from their descendants;
> We will tell the next generation
> the praiseworthy deeds of the LORD,
> his power, and the wonders he has done."

Every generation links anew to the knowledge and education of the previous generation. It is not about a meaningless repetition of past and outdated zombie categories, but about the surplus and overflow from truth and wisdom as displayed in loyalty; a truth that supersedes the limitations of being. Levinas (TO:354) refers to this surplus by using the metaphor "*curvature of the intersubjective space*". In essence it is a spiritual metaphor, capturing the divine intention of all kinds of wisdom-truth. One can even go so far as to pose that "curvature of space" as maybe a sign (Karl Jaspers: *chiffre*) of the presence of God (Levinas TO:354). This is probably what Levinas calls forgiveness: There is a continuous course that inspires women and men in next generations to be prepared to further invest in intersubjectivity. This investment is a sign of loyalty and integrity and not a mirage, or a disturbing phantom of intersubjectivity produced by sheer mechanistic repetition.

According to the researchers, this ethical investment in intersubjectivity is perfectly illustrated by the spirituality of intercession (justice in the place of; on behalf of the other) as told in the Genesis 18 narrative.

Towards a meta-perspective on intersubjectivity: Hospitality as inclusive intercession

In the previous outline it becomes clear that in Nagy's model for contextual therapy, and Levinas' philosophy of metaphysical desire, both are searching for a kind of measurement, ledger or normative criterion in order to safeguard and to establish a humane approach to our being human. Besides subjectivity and intersubjectivity, there are references to the Other and transcendence. Nagy is very careful not to found the ethical dimension in an epistemology of ontological phenomenology. Levinas' metaphysical desire points into the direction of a "meta-perspective" (transcendence).

In an article on Kierkegaard, Levinas links the quest for justice and how responsibility operates in a public space to the very famous story of Abraham's intercession for Sodom and Gomorrah (Gen 18, with special reference to vv 22-23) (Levinas NP:109.113). Levinas connects the narrative to the quest for the "subjectivity of the subject" within threatening social circumstances.

Kierkegaard emphasises the meta-ethical character of faith. Faith is about a leap, an attempt to overcome the obstacle of doubt. It operates on the level of religion. He defends this religious niveau over against the speculative character of systematic philosophy. Thus, the attempt to link the irrevocable and unique character of subjectivity to a religious dimension. Within this context, Levinas poses the question why Kierkegaard subjected ethics to religion. Why does Kierkegaard define the relationship between man and God in terms of a meta-ethical perspective?

Levinas does not want to question Kierkegaard's exegesis of Genesis 22. However, he is quite surprised, even shocked, that Kierkegaard overlooked Genesis 18. The narrative portrays Abraham's intercession as an act of absolute responsibility within the presence of the Other for the other, towards the Other. Levinas formulates as follows: The one I must answer is the one to whom I have to answer. The one "who" and the other "who" coincide. *Celui don t j'ai à répondre c'est celui à qui j'ai à répondre. Le "de qui" et le "à qui" coincident* (Levinas NP:108). The "for whom of responsibility" and the "over against whom of responsibility" coincide. The concretising of this coincidence is portrayed in Abraham's intercession on behalf of Sodom. It is an intercession for the sake of the righteous (*tsaddikim*) that perhaps still dwell in the city. This unique character of subjectivity resides in the unique character of responsibility. It is unique because nobody can replace my responsibility. The knowing about Sodom, becomes also a responsibility for the righteous of Sodom, and at the same time, for the preservation of the city. The responsibility is a kind of election (predestination).

For Levinas, the narrative is proof of the fact that ethics does not originate from a general, abstract collectivity, or prescriptive totality. It resides predominantly in the unique character of subjectivity, namely subjectivity as the priority of responsibility. The unique single person is summoned to perform this subjectivity. The fact that subjectivity resides in responsibility, implies that authentic subjectivity discovers a kind of strange passivity. This peculiar passivity is about a total excessive commitment to the other (burn-up); it is about a sacrificing devotion to the other (burn-out). According to Levinas, the I can never be "too passive". Abraham's burning-up for Sodom, the spirituality of intercession in the presence of the Other, on behalf of the other, helped Abraham to discover the spiritual art of absolute passivity: to wait for the Other.

The text of Genesis 18 is indeed relevant in terms of the research project on contextual therapy. In reading the biblical text, one becomes aware of three outstanding topics:

The plea for justice: Bargaining with the Other on behalf of others

In the Genesis 18 narrative, the other can be differentiated into two categories: "the righteous" and "the Sodomites". Despite this basic differentiation (classification) the petition overcomes the schism between the two categories. Instead of differentiation, the plea makes place for outreach and care, irrespective of right or wrong. Justice becomes "due care" enacted as *diakonia*.

The diachronic factor: Disturbing the causative chain

All forms of unjust classifications fall away due to the driving force in the petition (the conative factor). The Other towards whom the petition is directed (the merciful God), and the other who is bargaining (Abraham), coincide. The mutual dialogue between Abraham and God becomes an illustration of the seriousness of the command: Love your neighbour. This command of neighbourly/fellow love is put into practice (ethics becomes praxis). It becomes operative due to the instigating factor: pity. Pity drives justice and breaks the cultural order of judgement. Judgement entails more than punishment; it can become a gesture of care. In this sense, the diachronic factor is indeed what it means to be: Relating to, and dealing with phenomena (language, culture). Diachronic endeavours and events occur over a period. Diachronic assessment interpenetrates time (the events in Sodom) by disturbing fatal necessities (sheer judgement and punishment). Critical analyses based on pity and mercy (Abraham's intercessory-plea) disturb the chain of causative interpretations. In this sense, diachronic is not supplementary to a synchronic perspective, but paradoxically, in opposition to.

The pre-test of hospitality: Inviting the stranger – on becoming a host/guest for the other on behalf of the other

The test for the integrity of Abraham's plea resides in the event that precedes Abraham's petition in Genesis 18. He invited three strangers, totally foreign messengers (nameless beings from nowhere) and treated them as insiders in terms of the order of unconditional hospitality (Levinas).

One should read the Genesis 18 text in context. The Hebrew name for the biblical text, especially for the five books of Moses, is *Miqra*. It means: to read aloud. The reading of the text demonstrates invitation and devotion. The text illustrates a kind of calling, summoning, worshipping, naming. It even signifies the meaning of fellowship and the art of sharing. Within the language of the bible, *Miqra* means "convocation": to convene and to be called together. It is an exclamation mark and invitation to celebrate (the festivity of celebrating together – having a party).

Furthermore, in the reading of the text aloud (*Miqra*), the intention is not to probe into the word behind the text, but the wording, dialoguing after the reading: The word that emerges from the text, as the significant kerygma and exposition of the text. It reveals the driving factor that sets the text into dynamic movement. In fact, the reading discloses the vibrant meaning of the text that springs from the dull closed network of syllables and written letters. In this sense, the reading "produces", "evokes" meaning. The reading is not merely a simple repetition; it is in fact a mode of transformation, even of creation (Banon 1987:35).

The further importance for reading the text is the context of the Midrash: To investigate, to probe, to research. Probing the Midrash text is directed towards the ethical meaning of the text within the context of the community (convocation) wherein the text should be read and heard. *Miqra* is the place from which one is summoned to question the world. It is the place of interpellation and the forum from where an appeal is made on the convocation. One is called to order, to act responsibly and to obey the law. *Miqra* is also the place from where one makes an appeal to wisdom and significance (Banon 1987:38).

In the narrative there are some basic issues that reveal the intention of Genesis 18. One can call them "spiritual indicators for the establishment of a humane and just society".

- *The text is not about a prophecy, but on "seeing"*. Seeing is doing. The text is in fact an appeal for practising trustworthiness and justice – trace of JHWH in the tent of Abraham and the city of Sodom. The narrative is therefore more than a vision; it is about the operationalisation of morality: Ethics is an optic (Levinas TO:17; TI:xi). The

appearance of JHWH (making Himself visible and becoming visible) corresponds in the Hebrew text with the seeing of Abraham. The fact that Abraham "sees", is the undergirding significance of the chapter.
- *Seeing becomes doing by exercising hospitality.* The seeing enfleshes what encounter, and invitation represent. The three messengers are not tourists, they do not travel in cognito, they present the Holy Other. This is what Levinas calls "the epiphany of visage". The seeing of Abraham represents encounter; requesting grace by becoming hosts; sharing possessions by giving (water, shadow, drinking, eating).
- *Being is not causality.* In the second part of the narrative the focus is on Sarah. The promise of a son to a barren human being infiltrates the fate of causality: Fertility is not a principle of causality. A child is in fact already an inviting and summoning other. Time is diachronic so that discontinuity establishes the reality of continuity.
- *Inviting establishes election and not vice versa.* The third part of the narrative describes an interior dialogue: of the Other. The internal dialoguing of JHWH reveals the significance of Abraham's future – the significance of his sojourn, his offspring and the universal implication of obedience. Invitation becomes election: a blessing to all nations and the whole of the earth.
- *The outsiders become insiders.* Sodom is not the victim of fate. In terms of an ancient rabbinic interpretation, the silence in the city is the screaming of foreigners, widowers and orphans in their quest for justice. Albeit, by means of Abraham's inclusive plea for the city, the whole of the city becomes saved (saving justice).
- *History as happenstance (spaces for care), not as historicity (historic facts).* The narrative could be read as an interpretation; an interpretation of the history of happenstances (the relational dynamics of events) – its significance within the JHWH-human encounter, and not as the theoretical description of facts. It is about the significant meaning of being. In the words of Paul Ricoeur, the encounter is about *a proposition of meaning (proposition de sens)* (Ricoeur 1985); an invitation to care and to exhibit pity.
- *Grace as subjectivity and not as maintenance of a static social order.* In terms of a reading of Genesis 18 from the perspective of the Midrash, the narrative reveals that one should not assess the city merely in

terms of its exclusiveness (the totality of abandoning those who do not adhere to the close order of the city of Sodom). The Midrash interprets the meaning of the text in terms of a critique on the injustice of the city (Midrash 1951, 49.6). It is a critique on totalitarianism: The cruelty of a closed system to sacrifice one in order to maintain the system and establish unity. Girard (1972; 1982) refers to "the emissary victim" (*la victime émissaire*).

- *Trustworthiness as trace of being called (election).* The knowing of Abraham by JHWH is not about the gathering of empirical data for a research project. Knowing is about the intimate knowledge (inside information); an epistemology of close fellowship and communion. It is about starting to love the other due to the trustworthiness of the other. It is about a pre-knowledge that does not analyse but elects, and is in fact, preceding all factual knowledge of Abraham.
- *Petition: From silence (the sacred space) to presencing (responsible differentiation) and to humility (the profane space).* Genesis 18:19-27 describes a decisive turning point. It depicts the mutual dynamics of a spiritual encounter: The mutuality between divine visage (realm of the sacred) and humane humility (the realm of the vulnerable profane); between the speaking of JHWH and the silence of Abraham. The between is breeched in the petition by an appeal on mercy/pity (as portrayed by the faithfulness and trustworthiness of JHWH) and justice (exceeding the human differentiation between the righteous and the evil). The silence is broken when Abraham opt on the basis of an ethical responsibility (accountability): On behalf of the other, for the sake of the other. The ethical differentiation between justice and evil is not done by Abraham. If that was the case, the difference between sacred and profane becomes a void, dualistic schism. According to Genesis 18:25, the Other is the Judge, but, at the same time the Carer. And it is due to this ledger that Abraham's silence becomes a boldness of speech. Verse 27: "Now that I have ventured to speak to the Lord – though I am but dust and ashes – will you destroy the whole city for the lack of five?" (NIV). Abraham's humility resides in the "nihilism of dust and ashes". Levinas connects this remark with Job 26:7 9(b): "He spreads out the northern skies over empty space; he suspends the earth over nothing". This nothingness is not *das Nichts* of Heidegger, but a

hook for the fate of this world; it is a persecuted truth (Kierkegaard), a fragility (Levinas) (see De Boer 1976:55-56). Abraham's "boldness of speech" destroys all forms of totality: The totality is reduced to sheer randomness: "The maybe of perhaps" (Neher 1970:186). "Being" (to be) (être) becomes "perhaps" (*peut-être*).

One can conclude and say: Bridging the gap between sacred and profane resides in the ethical responsibility of subjectivity (accountability) and the ethos of trustworthy humility. Levinas calls it: "*diakonia*"; a kind of humility wherein the "*responsibility for – on behalf of*" and the "*responsibility towards – in the face of*", embrace and meet. *Diakonia* becomes *paraclesis* and vice versa.

CHAPTER 5

Retribution, forgiveness and release[1]

It was argued that ethics is a primary and original event. In this sense, ethics is a kind of avatar of subjectivity – enfleshment (incarnation). Accountability and responsibility are therefore not to be derived from psychology, metapsychology or any kind of theory formation. It is based upon ethics and determined by the human order of justice.

In this chapter, the challenge will be to concretise an ethical approach within the reality of many existential entanglements. Especially in very painful settings of hurt due to injustice. Settings that make an appeal on "exoneration" and "forgiveness". For Levinas, concretising is not to set merely an example in terms of an idea. Concretising is about precision; to be to the point and exact. Because concretising refers to the concrete situation wherein significance is portrayed and subjective meaning becomes evident (De Boer in Duyndam 1984, Preface).

In the previous outline the notions of injustice, wrongdoing and guilt were mentioned. There were references to failure to instil trustworthiness, to unfairness and indifference to care. The lack of responsibilty and accountability, harms and destroys the principle of justice. It leads in many cases to violation, hurt and exploitation of the other.

How should one deal with these issues in therapy and caregiving?

The challenge in this chapter will be to describe accurately the notions of "revenge" and "forgiveness". The argument will be that both the thinking of Nagy and Levinas could contribute to the discourse on exoneration and the praxis of caregiving.

[1] One can also translate with exempt and exonerate. Exonerate is very dubious because in some cases it can refer to the attempt to excuse oneself by means of self-justification. Release is in fact a *form of deliverance.*

One of the overall goals of this study is to get more clarity on the parameters of pastoral care within the dynamics of contextuality. The notion of "forgiveness of sins" is in any case part of the faith tradition of the church. In the light of the tension between the thinking of Nagy (often he refers to exoneration) and Levinas' meta-perspective (frequently the notion of transcendence arises), a more exact description and outline are becoming imperative.

The complexity of forgiveness, revenge and retribution

Revenge is often used by Nagy, but with different nuances. Revenge can refer to a kind of repayment in cases of indebtedness. It can even refer to retribution and retaliation.

In *Invisible Loyalties* (IL:69-73), there is a section on *"Justice as social dynamics"*. Nagy describes the phenomenon of retribution within the history of humankind and its role in judiciary. This description is important to him in order to place familial justice in the context of a more universal social dynamics (Nagy IL:69). The right to revenge (*ius talionis*), could be rendered as one of the most basic forms of "early [...] man's struggle for a sane social order" (Nagy IL:69). The criteria of "reciprocity" and "equity" have their roots in this social basis.

Due to the Enlightenment, the traditional order of justice disappeared; "... a vacuum was created, and modern man has not been able to fill that vacuum" (Nagy IL:72). Nagy specifically refers to the disintegration of retributive justice. "To the extent that strict religious regulation of conduct diminishes in society, the question arises: What takes the place of belief in divine justice?" (Nagy IL:72). Divine justice is for him in this context retributive justice; that is, both revenging as rewarding justice.

Nagy does not refer to a general theodicy. At stake for him, is the quest for an eventual authority of punishment and reward. Without this judicial framework, life will perish. Thus, the question: When God is absent and does not exist, what is normative? Should one proceed with life without a kind of measurement (ledger) within the confines of the following directive: Everything goes and is fine? (The general notion of I am OK and You are OK).

"Modern man's *illusion* of replacing rather than mitigating retributive justice with humanity might constitute one of the greatest hypocrisies, and a threat to the dynamic fibre of society itself" (Nagy IL:69; ital VR/MK).

CHAPTER 5

Within postmodernity, we act as if we need no form of retributive justice at all. It could be an indication of hypocrisy in the public of society. Because there is no social system possible without an order of justice that could provide a clear indication of right and wrong, "… we have to examine the possible effects of a complete elimination of the principles of retaliatory justice and reparation" (Nagy IL: 72). That people are rendered a second change, whether juridical or in informal groups, could be rendered as an advantage. However, what could become an alarming development is the so-called ignorance of the natural sciences regarding the decisive role of justice in society and our human environment. "Attempts to replace the criteria of justice with scientific ones are non-scientific" (Nagy IL:73).

The question at stake, is the relationship between retributive justice and the order of society. What role can retributive justice play in processes of social disintegration? Nagy's argument is that it brings about a kind of equilibrium. Society tends to become a kind of totality system. Retributive justice should be maintained in order to prevent social disintegration. It brings about fairness and balance so that the group can survive (Nagy IL:77).

With this background in mind, Nagy turns to Buber's concept of "justice of the human order". Within secularisation "the order of a just God" (a just and revenging God that is the guarantee for the maintenance of a fair order for our being human) has been replaced by the "justice of a human order". During the time of the Enlightenment, this guarantor is replaced by the rationality of analytical liberalism. Instead of the "divine order", the "justice of the human order" becomes the regulative social mechanism that should take responsibility for the maintenance of balance. Due to this scenario, the implication is that the "manager" is not the "order" as such, but fairness as qualified by retributive justice.

Nagy refers to a "vacuum" in humanistic liberalism after the turn of the Enlightenment. "Our age may go down in history as practicing the greatest apparent consideration, even toward coldly calculating murders" (Nagy IL:74). There is indeed a correlation between a softening of the attitude to destructive behaviour and a more lenient approach to mischief and violent crime, as well as the increasing focus on the individual dimension of accountability. Nagy resists all forms of artificial generosity based on compromise: "To understand everything is to forgive everything" (*tout comprendre c'est tout pardonner*).

The following question arises: But is this vacuum not creating a situation wherein the accountability of the subject becomes tested anew? Is is perhaps now the time to reintroduce (even more than "the principle of reciprocal equity") this intransitive personal accountability of the subject as the point of convergence for ethics and justice? (see Nagy IL:70). In this respect, his plea is not for a mechanistic collective accountability (totality) that opens the door to destructive modes of threatening scapegoating, prejudice and eventual genocide (Nagy IL:78). At stake, is rather the challenge to restore the "justice of a human order" and to revisit the generalisation of concepts like "forgiveness" and "exoneration".

Reservation on forgiveness

The intriguing question why forgiveness does not play a central role in Nagy's ethical approach should be posed here. "The act of forgiveness usually retains the assumption of guilt and extends the forgiver's generosity to the person who has injured her or him" (Nagy BGT:416).

Nagy is careful to introduce the perspectives of forgiveness because it immediately evokes the notion of "guilt". The problem is when guilt is present, the so called "forgiver" can take advantage on the other to constantly remind him/her of his/her guilt by using terminology that reminds the other of guilt. If this is the case, forgiveness becomes sterile. Due to manipulative expressions of forgiveness, the guilt becomes even bigger and excessive. It can easily degenerate into a power game from the side of the forgiver. Without any doubt, within the dynamics of merit and obligation, forgiveness can eventually set free a dialectics of guilt expansion. Within Nagy's concept of ledger, it could indeed be the case that forgiveness even enhances guilt, rather than addressing it appropriately. It can also fortify the "better-than-thou attitude". Perhaps the reason why Buber (SuSg 1962a:227) reasons that there is no place for forgiveness in the counselling room of the therapist.

Another reason for Nagy's scepticism is the practice of ritual absolution (a private, isolated and individual act). His concern is rather to restore "hurt human justice". The focus should then become smaller units like the family. The real challenge is "to place familial justice in the context of its universal social dynamics" (Nagy IL:69). Albeit, what should be restored and addressed is the "hurt human justice". In order to do this, the therapist should reckon with the relevant facts that contributed to the violation of the order.

It could be questioned that when it is about concrete cases of the violation and hurt of a specific human person by other persons, Nagy's terminology runs the danger of becoming too abstract. For example, the notion of "justice of human order" and the concrete challenge to "repair the hurt human justice" can become merely formal ethical principles; general attempts to restore the order. However, the challenge is not to repair the order, but to renew time: To disclose the present for the future generation. Recovery is about an event in time. Something must change in the life of the hurt human being. Deadly time must be transformed into the renewal of time. Albeit, in the centre is always the wounded human being in his/her vulnerability (my own as well as the other's). This should be the eventual criterion in repairing the hurt human justice.

The problem with forgiveness is that it can become blindfolded; running into the danger of overseeing the concrete suffering and real torment of people. Evil is not a mystical principle that can be extinguished by means of an instant ritual of forgiveness.

The judicial context of "exoneration"

For Nagy, the alternative for forgiveness is "exoneration". "Exoneration" does not refer to an order of balance and equilibrium, but to persons and their concrete rights.

Nagy and Krasner (BGT:416) describe exoneration as follows: "Exoneration is a process of lifting the load of culpability off the shoulders of a given person to whom heretofore we may have blamed. In our experience clinical improvement often coincides with the renewed capacity of parents to exonerate their own seemingly failing parents. Exoneration differs from forgiveness. The act of forgiving usually *retains* the assumption of guilt and extends the forgiver's generosity to the person who has injured her or him. Offering forgiveness, a person now retains from holding the culprit accountable and from demanding punishment. In contrast, exoneration typically results from an adult reassessment of the failing parent's own past childhood victimization. It replaces a framework of blame with mature appreciation of a given person's (or situation's) past options, efforts and limits."

Exoneration is for Nagy a judicial term. But what is meant by exoneration interpreted from a judicial point of view? In the idiom of the Dutch judicial system, the term is used in the contractual sphere. In this context, accountability for damage plays a role, as well as the principle of possible exemption. However, exemption is not unlimited. All modes of justice are always subjected to the general principles of reasonableness and fairness.

The importance of the previous explanation of the judicial context, brings to the fore that exoneration is not unlimited. However, the possibility of exemption does not safeguard anybody from accountability. The critical factor and question are always about the criteria of reasonableness and fairness. This is more or less the same in the case of the terminology used in the American judicial system.

With this term (exoneration), Nagy deliberately made a choice for a judicial hermeneutic. Within the German context exoneration refers to "reliable release" (*Enthaftung*). Nagy also mentions the concept of "liability" (*Haftbarkeit*) (*Interview* 1992).

"Exoneration" is a very specific form of "re-assessment". This re-assessment can bring about new insight, change and personal acknowledgement.

In a nutshell: In the context of legal language and judicial terminology, exoneration has a dual value. It can point into the direction of possible limitations of accountability; even to the exemption of accountability[2]. Exoneration can also be connected to many other terms like "balance", "debit", credit", "slate" and "repayment". These terms are all related to judicial and accountancy language and paradigms. For all these terms, especially for exoneration, it is imperative not to understand exoneration from the realm of the affective, but from the realm of the judicial.

Exoneration within the realm of contextual therapy (Nagy)

Exoneration could be rendered as a key factor within the dynamics of relational ethics. It is quite powerful because it unmasks the root areas of destructive behaviour. In fact, it pervades the precariousness of feelings and probes into the motivational and moral layers of human behaviour. Furthermore, it infiltrates the essence of subjectivity. In therapy, this penetrating effect can contribute to human well-being. "Even when parents are palpably destructive, children benefit from efforts to exonerate them" (Nagy BGT:84).

---

2   For the meaning of taking away the burden from the other, see Baakman 1990:43.

The application of "exoneration" to the therapeutic field of language and terminology (Nagy & Spark IL:48, 63), is not to be marked as a new finding by Nagy and Spark. Exoneration could indeed be connected to healing and human well-being. Already in the chapter on "loyalty", and the section on *"Transgenerational accounting of obligations and merit"* (Nagy & Spark IL:46-48), exoneration has been mentioned. In terms of the dialectical character of loyalty, children are positioned and ethically connected to their parents in terms of "repayment". The strange thing is, that despite the fact that repayment has already taken place (the notion of the "giving child"), it often happens that parents are unaware of it. Repayment is quite special because it can stretch over a period of time. It is embedded in a network of relational commitments toward other/others. It can, for example, take place later in life (spouse, children). However, sometimes it can happen that I am so closely connected to my parents due to invisible loyal commitments, that there is no more space for new relational connections (the danger of smothering and collective totality).

It seems to Nagy and Spark, that in more traditional communities, young people are less exposed to the phenomenon of "guilt of disloyalty" than in modern urbanised communities. Perhaps, the reason resides in the fact that in these cases the parents contributed to the new relationship. The implication is then that children of these parents feel free to even project responsibility for their marital frictions upon the choice initiated by their parents (Nagy & Spark IL:49). Due to this difference between rural and urban communities, the link between loyalty, disloyalty and guilt became more complex. Nagy and Spark, thus, focus more on the situation of people who took personal responsibility for their choice of partner. For them the obligation to repay their parents in cases of relational guilt, is more problematic.

The notions of guilt and repayment are always existent between parent and child. But when the child becomes a parent, the inherent right of a baby for care, becomes enough reason to be rendered as justifiable reason for detachment from the guilt of repayment. The adult child feels free to distance him/herself more and more from the obligation toward the parent. The authors go even so far as to speak of the "inherent right *and merit* of a helpless infant" (Nagy & Spark IL:48; italics VR/MK). "Thus, the rewards of parenthood include [...] *the exoneration* of guilt of disloyalty through fulfilment of an obligation" (Nagy & Spark IL:48; italics VR/MK). Parenthood becomes the unique opportunity to pay reparation for guilt about imputed disloyalty. It becomes, thus, clear that it is far easier to develop a deeply loyal devotion to one's child than to one's spouse (Nagy & Spark IL:48).

It could indeed be questioned in postmodern communities with the emphasis on autonomy, whether the notions of repayment and obligation are still applicable in cases where couples make choices on their own without the impact or interference of the parent. Albeit, the interesting fact is that within the judicial framework of right, exoneration is accepted as being obvious. Already the existence of a young child can be an advantage to the parent, because it releases/exonerates to a large extent the parent from the obligation to his/her parents. Perhaps, this could be rendered as the merit of a child. In fact, exoneration can become a means to gain subtle modes of autonomy.

In IL (63), Nagy and Spark link indebtedness to exoneration. When one is in a position of indebtedness in a relationship, the obligation to exonerate becomes even bigger. In this case, exoneration does not say in the first place something about the guilt of the person to be exonerated, but more about the indebtedness of the exonerator. However, exoneration is in this dialectic not automatic and obvious. On the contrary, exoneration can be rendered as the merit of the one who exonerates.

Exoneration and the revolving slate

In IL (68), Nagy wrote, "According to the Scriptures, seven generations may balance out one major sin of an ancestor". The text Nagy refers to, is not clear. However, the point is, the generational account becomes heavy and the person overburdened, even be blamed for issues that one is not responsible for. Nagy calls it the *revolving slate*; that is, a new victim is established because a person with an unpaid debt, transfers the "guilt" and hurt to another relation, other than the one where the debt has been caused. The slate causes a kind of "displaced retribution". The further problem with "displaced retribution", is that the less one is aware of it, the more one can become exposed to emotional exploitation and the gamble of manipulation. The very painful situation can develop that grandchildren are becoming accused by grandparents for siding with their parents, specifically for issues the grandparents blame their children for, namely disloyalty towards the traditions and customs of the family. The parents are then portrayed as even becoming disloyal to themselves and family matters, for example in matters of religious or other traditions/customs (Nagy

& Spark IL:68). Being unaware of the predicament, children can become "unguilty allies" in the strategy of exoneration.

Nagy refers to a case where daughters have been brought up by respectable relatives because of their "mother's life of shame". At a later stage the daughters decided to return to their mother. Nagy comments as follows: "Ultimately, the greatest relief these children can find lies in the vindication in their own eyes of their parents" (Nagy & Spark IL:68). "Vindication" means to be released from all forms of blame. When the children eventually discovered themselves that the condition for the "condemnable actions" of their parents was in fact unfair, vindication set in.

The vindication of parents

The phrase "vindication of the parents" could be related to exoneration. However, they are not the same. The reason: Vindication is about the releasement of shame and feelings of shame. It refers to a psychological driving force (predicament) and less about indebtedness and the challenge to restore justice (as driving force). Thus, the reason why vindication is not the same as in the case of exoneration.

Cases of over-dependency and destructive behaviour of adolescents in their endeavour to become free and to function more independently, are in a very peculiar way linked by Nagy and Spark to exoneration. The destructive behaviour is then a very strange mode of exoneration, an "offering of exoneration" with the message to the parent: You are not anymore prior in our behaviour, we are trying to become released. Detachment becomes a mode of deliverance and in this sense an expression of exoneration.

Often the new younger generation reveals several attempts to act independently. For example, their campaign for greening the earth. In all spheres of life, justice should be installed. However, this tendency does not exempt the parents and older generation to be exonerated from the responsibility of solidarity. "Yet we cannot exonerate the parent generation from their leadership and participatory obligations, even though change will primarily benefit the young generation" (Nagy & Spark IL:387).

About "intrinsic" and "premature" exoneration

In therapy it is often the case that the therapist deals with counselling problems of clients but is at the same time aware of own painful memories about suffering during childhood. "To some degree, *each of us* is obliged to find ways to rebalance and exonerate the shortcomings of our families of origin" (Nagy: F:268; italics VR/MK).

According to Nagy, within the empathetic relationship between therapist and client (especially in cases where children are involved) lurks memories of own suffering and shortcomings during childhood. In the attempt to share skills that helped to overcome own sufferings during childhood, there is the temptation to implicitly start blaming the client's family of origin (indirect scapegoating); "… therapists may easily overlook their own hidden psychic benefit, derived from the *intrinsic exoneration* of their own parents at the expense of the patient's family of origin" (Nagy F:149; italics VR/MK).

It is indeed a question whether this kind of exoneration (intrinsic exoneration) is really authentic. One can argue that the "intrinsic" exoneration is from a psychological point of view beneficiary, but from a relational point of view unfair. Especially not to the client's family of origin.

Besides intrinsic exoneration, there is also the phenomenon of *"premature exoneration"*. It refers to the tendency that caregivers, operating from the paradigm of contextual therapy, tend to exonerate too rapidly their own parents. It can even be the case that such a premature exoneration (intrinsic exoneration) becomes a reason for an attitude of admonishment and punitive moralisation in therapeutic interventions.

Albeit, the aim and outcome of exoneration in therapy should be an increased sense of trust and authentic exoneration, rather than premature condemnation and a hateful severance of objectionable family relationships (Nagy F:197). As therapist, one should also be aware, that all forms of exoneration are in fact relative and contextual. Again: "To some degree, *each of us* is obliged to find ways to rebalance and exonerate the shortcomings of our families of origin" (Nagy F:268; italics VR/MK).

Exoneration as restoring the freedom of action: The benefit of "earned entitlement"

In the text of BGT (181-182), Nagy points out the devastating effects of "failure of exoneration". This is, for example, evident in the way the younger generation in Germany struggled to come to terms with their parents' association and sympathy with the politics of Nazi-Germany. Both the so-called perpetrator and victim need help. Even offspring and future generations are involved.

In this regard, Nagy and Krasner write very carefully: The legacy of ancestral shame and guilt requires redress *and* exoneration insofar as they are possible (Nagy & Krasner BGT:182). The courage to deal with shame and guilt of the parent cannot be accommodated by a counselling room. The initiative should come from the relational dynamics, namely from the parents, siblings and roots. The ability and courage to exonerate do not reside solely in the willingness of the parent or the capacity of the victimised child. One needs to probe even deeper than personal ability and capacity. The quality of the exoneration, as well as the courage to exonerate, will eventually be determined by the ethical quality of the relational dynamics within the specific child-parent relationship.

From the parents' side, redress is possible. For example, in the case of a Nazi-affiliated parent and the relationship with his/her child (son or daughter), the parent can start to view the courage and initiative of the child as an attempt to come to terms with the past, even when the parent is aware of signs of detachment and steps to restore justice. These attempts should not be rendered as signs of disloyalty. On the contrary, they could express a very peculiar and special form of loyalty. If this expressed form of loyalty becomes clear to the parent, the desire to be exonerated could be shared. Reappraisal is in fact a mutual endeavour.

The desire to be exonerated must not become confused with the demand for remorse. In his outline on exoneration, Nagy does not refer to penitence, remorse and conversion. Restoration is not merely about the shortcut of a sudden leap from indebtedness by means of rapid reconciliation (reconciliation without thorough self-identification and self-acknowledgement). Exoneration operates on a deeper level. Its concern is to restore the freedom to act for all involved and to partake in processes of exoneration. Exoneration, as in the case of Nazi-Germany, or *apartheid*-South Africa, becomes an intergenerational endeavour, based on the ethical character of dialogue as informed by the "order of justice".

In a nutshell:
- Exoneration restores the freedom of action.
- Exoneration is not about the balance of an equilibrium. Exoneration is asymmetric.

With reference to the previous cases (Germany/South Africa), and the common reception of symmetry in Lady Justice, Nagy and Krasner make the bold statement: "This measure of balance equity [...] cannot be made to apply to the very young or the very old" (Nagy & Krasner BGT:83). Exoneration is definitely not about a tit for tat game. It is more than a fair deal. It is anchored in the trustworthiness of the partners involved; "... the more trustworthy the parental investment in his or her offspring's context, the easier it is for the child to exonerate her parent" (Nagy & Krasner BGT:84). Furthermore, "the person doing the exoneration can relinquish negative behaviour patterns and earn new options for earning entitlement" (Nagy & Krasner BGT:302). When parents display this kind of entitlement toward their children and reveal a kind of "leadership responsibility" with deep concern for the need of their children, another variant of indebtedness arises, namely, to acknowledge this parental leadership in processes of exoneration. Nagy and Krasner call it *"generous consideration"*. With generosity is not meant a top-down approach in cases of forgiveness, namely, to extend the forgiver's generosity to the person who has injured her/him.

In the parent-child relationship fairness is at stake. Even in cases where the parents are in default to exonerate, one cannot exclude, from the side of the child, the possibility of a kind of "readiness and willingness" to exonerate. Even the attempt to forgive is better than to subject the parents to endless condemnation (Nagy & Krasner BGT:103). "*Regardless of outcome*, attempts to *exonerate* a parent earn entitlement – that is, an offspring's efforts to be fair to a resented or even despised parent – can lead to a self-sustaining spiral of motivation that enables positive behaviour in other relationships" (Nagy & Krasner BGT:103).

What one should realise is that exoneration is not a recipe for "success". Not all attempts deliver the expected outcome. Nevertheless, if one embarks on the route of "exoneration" in the healing of conflicting relationships, the question is about trust and fairness, irrespective of the outcome. In any case, one can force nobody into exoneration. Even the therapist cannot "organise" the process of exoneration in terms of managerial skills. The point is: Exoneration is an act of free will; it is about personal responsibility in the light of an "order of justice", and, thus, about the recovery of freedom. It is only feasible due to the ethical, dialectical character of "entitlement". I am fully equipped and entitled, and when I face this challenge, I confirm my "earning of entitlement" in terms of individuation and subjectivity.

Despite the fact that exoneration cannot be managed, "timing" is indeed important. Timing is determined by the desire for justice and dependent on the loyalty of the client. The therapist should, thus, wait for the appropriate moment: At what point in time is the client ready to work on exonerating his/her parents? (Nagy & Krasner BGT:103). Mutuality is at stake indeed. "A therapist helps to diminish *the myth of one-sided accountability* by rejecting the notion that one person can ever be the sole source of a given family's ills" (Nagy & Krasner BGT:103; italics VR/MK). What is most helpful is when the therapist helps the members of a family to detect the truth of "*earning entitlement through giving due consideration*". Helping people to be released from their burden and becoming unburdened, is the core of helping. Absolute exoneration is not always the outcome. Sometimes exoneration is just to help somebody to gain "existential competence" by "earning of entitlement". In this respect, the therapist can assist the client to start redefining fair balance in terms of that person's relational framework of reference.

Earning entitlement in therapeutic terminology means very simply: To expand the freedom of possible action and the capacity of responsibility. This is a more beneficial alternative for existential guilt and blame. It contributes to the prevention of destructive behaviour, and the redistribution of burdens and benefits (Nagy & Krasner BGT:103-104). In fact, what the therapist is doing is to enhance intersubjective connectivity – *rejunction* – by means of multidirected partiality.

Another benefit is that exoneration is also applicable to the unfinished business of past events and deceased parents. In several of his writings, Nagy refers to "*posthumous* exoneration". It is about the situation of people who want to earn entitlement vis-à-vis their deceased parents (Nagy & Krasner BGT:114). One should reckon here with the fact that it is a one-sided task and "unidirectional". It is however a limited endeavour. "Who the parents were to us, to themselves, and, to others can be reconstructed, but dialogue cannot occur. It is a point at which our parents themselves can receive nothing back despite our good intentions" (Nagy & Krasner BGT:114).

Furthermore, one should also realise that the context of *posthumous* exoneration is inexorable. This should be evident because the dynamics is intergenerational and most of the people involved are already dead. It is inexorable due to the fact that time is irreversible. Reconstruction is possible indeed. This can be done by talking to relatives, or to look at pictures, reading through letters and emails in order to refresh memories. "The very attempt to reconstruct a relationship is a measure of this work's success" (Nagy & Krasner BGT:304-305). Just to ignore unfinished business is contra-productive. "Memories of a 'bad' deceased parent are likely to haunt the offspring-in-flight" (Nagy & Krasner BGT:304-305).

The ethics of relational loyalty: Exoneration as transformation rather than the generosity of forgiveness

The core reason why Nagy introduced the concept of exoneration in psychotherapy, was to transform the relational network. It is decisive that between children and their parents, the focus should not be shifted to other persons because of extended, other forms of loyalty. The parent-child relationship is irrevocable, and it is in this realm that exoneration should be exercised. This does not imply a kind of fatalistic connectedness. What indeed can happen, is change; change in terms of perspective and attitude. That implies also change in the dynamics of the relationship.

For many abused children when they become grownups, the question is whether to abandon the parent or not. When the parent is to be blamed, is revenge an option? This question becomes complex when it is his/her own parent operating in terms of the presupposition that the connection is based on the principle of trust and an ethics of loyalty. In such a case, the challenge in therapy is about reappraisal; that is, the option of renewed action within the reality of the relational dynamics.

The following question arises: But what about forgiveness?

Nagy does not work with the term of forgiveness as such. He reacts against malpractices (a caricature). Nagy understands the tradition of forgiveness as an act and disposition that bypass the complex reality of guilt, ignoring the fact of indebtedness. This ignorance is based on the "principle of generosity". The danger is then that forgiveness becomes merely a generous gesture by the forgiver; forgivenes as being "nice" to people and a moderate gesture to accommodate the wrongdoings of the other. It is exactly this possible connection to generosity, that Nagy questions.

Guilt is complex and should be taken seriously due to indebtedness and entitlement. One needs to reckon with the ethical dimension in this regard. This explains why Nagy rather opt for exoneration than forgiveness.

Exoneration means a kind of cleansing/purification by which the other receives a clean slate. In forgiveness one does not purify the other. One is merely generous enough by turning away from the option of revenge in order to satisfy oneself. One is merely prepared to delete one's demands and claims, but in the meantime, one still clings to the basic issues at stake, namely the reasons for being hurt (Nagy in Van der Pas 1982:32). In fact, forgiveness is merely the false mask of smugness: I am better than thou.

Generosity is about sheer power. The intention is to take control over the other. The aberration resides in the fact that the maintenance of power is built on the notion of balance (symmetry) between obligation and merit. From an ethical perspective such a power game becomes immoral. The reason: It can possibly abuse the existential indebtedness within the relationship between children and their parents. Eventually, it is about a person-to-person exploitation; about non-giving or non-reciprocal taking and not about sheer forgiveness.

Forgiveness is very individually focused and does not reckon enough with systemic contexts and wider paradigmatic issues. Due to complexity, there are many other systemic forces that play a role in generosity and the danger of exploitation. For example, political and economic factors, the social media; all of them play a role in the exploitation of human beings. In these systems of exploitation, the real danger lurks that both parents and children become victims. The other danger is that forgiveness of the parents by the children, also become inappropriate (Nagy & Spark IL:57; Friedman 1992b:206).

Nagy's preference for exoneration is the ethical factor of injustice that plays in most problematic issues a decisive role. For instance, an example is cruelties in war and violent oppressions. In all these cases, exoneration is more appropriate than forgiveness. The advantage is that it works with an ethical basis, namely indebtedness.

In many cases of exploitation, for example parental exploitation, children will blame their parents for unjust measurements. Parents can start to blame themselves for lost opportunities, even when the parent her-/him-self was a victim of oppression. Sadness sets in and the exonerator can start to mourn the fact of irreparable loss or unfulfilled expectations. Sadness can also be presented in the response of (grand-)children affected, as well as by disadvantaged others. The mourning is often about the fact that one realises that many of the attempts of helping was in vain; and now all opportunities are gone. So, then there is sadness in even three generations.

In order to come back to the notion of transformation, it is important to remember that the impetus for transformation should be traced back to entitlement and the justice order. Due to destructive entitlement, the victim is in need for an excessive amount of justice. Transformation can set in if the destructive entitled person also realises that, despite failure, I am still accountable.

Transformation is possible when the "destructive entitled person" starts to "earn constructive entitlement". It is not only the destructive entitlement of the parent that is the focal point (which is obvious), but central is the entitlement of the child in his/her process of developing into maturity. This focal point is a precondition for a new start. In some cases, "constructive entitlement" needs a third, independent factor (other than the parent) that appeals to the responsibility of the mature child. This implies the possibility of a new alliance with another person. The new responsibility can transform the previous responsibility (old relationship) into a new one (a transformed transmission).

Sometimes parents have the experience that children did not grasp and internalised the benefits they wanted to transfer. The inability to accept the benefits, Nagy also calls *destructive entitlement*. It is often the case that the destructive entitlement cannot be traced back to a shortcoming on the side of the parent. To always pose the question about a possible cause that explains parental guilt, is most of times in vain. The important issue at stake, is rather how a person who discovers his/her destructive entitlement, responds in order to start earning *constructive entitlement*. In this respect, all others in the family system (brother, sisters, grandparents) can be called upon to help and to support the establishment of transformation and change. This is where "relational sources" come into play. The advantage is that all other helpers benefit from constructive supporting. This insight is most valuable in the realm of therapy and pastoral care.

Exoneration within the dynamics: Guilt – guilt feelings

In contextual therapy, within an ethical paradigm, family relationships are inevitably about guilt and exposed to several forms of guilt feelings.

In the previous outline it became clear that Nagy &Krasner deliberately wanted to opt for exoneration and not for forgiveness. The reason for this is their fear that the concept of forgiveness is so closely associated with exploitation and generosity that subjective responsibility is undermined. The impression is that forgiveness neglects the seriousness of guilt and the importance of holding the guilty one responsible for inflicted injustice. Thus, the reason to replace forgiveness with exoneration. In contrast to forgiveness, exoneration is the result of a mature reappraisal by the accused parent of past experiences, and the realisation that she/he was also victims in their youth (Nagy & Krasner BGT:416).

There is often in guilt and guilt feelings the tendency that people want to excuse themselves and try to escape the seriousness of displaced responsibility and guilt (the phenomenon of *deculpabilisation*) (Burggraeve 1991:234). Nagy's understanding of exoneration is not about *deculpabilisation* or an attempt to excuse yourself. It is the opposite of denial and blame shifting.

Exoneration says nothing about the guilt of the parent, or that the guilt does not exist anymore. It reveals something about the subject that exonerates. For example, it says something about the suffering of the child due to parental shortcomings. Exoneration also helps to make a reappraisal of all the people involved; it provides new possibilities to assess the abilities of the accused and guilty other.

Guilt is always personal (subjective). My guilt toward somebody else, can only be understood by myself when "I" include the feelings and reactions of others (exterior) in the reappraisal. This can be connected to Nagy's dialectical approach. "Our dialectical point of view not only postulates that the individual is embedded in a dynamically balanced, fluctuating, merit context, but that the latter is an indispensable component for the understanding of individual dynamics and motivation" (Nagy & Spark IL:78).

Guilt *feelings* are intrapersonal. Therefore, guilt feelings as indication of intrapersonal dynamics and internal motivational impetus, can become very intense. They can cause a lot of internal turmoil because they are instigated from elsewhere: Within the context of merit and obligation; "… whereas an individual's *guilt feelings* can be understood without consideration of the other member's feelings and reactions, underlying *existential guilt* cannot" (Nagy & Spark IL:78).

In guilt and guilt feelings the core issue at stake is accountability. In the IKON-*Interview*, the interviewer describes how Nagy visited a woman in a prison in Philadelphia. She killed her child. The mother was totally crushed. Caregivers could follow the dialogue between Nagy and this woman from behind a one-way mirror. Her first question was: "Professor, you came to visit me, please tell me, am I guilty of murder?" He responded and said: "Yes, you murdered your child and are guilty". The caregivers were totally taken by surprise. They spent a lot of time to minimise her guilt feelings. They have tried to convince her that she could not have prevented it due to many difficulties she experienced. The surprising fact was that after this bold feedback and honest response, the woman suddenly became a human being again and started to share and to talk (Nagy IKON:9, *Erven van Toekomst*; Schlüter 1990:29).

The woman claimed back her accountability. Accountability presupposes a relationship wherein this woman is accepted as subject. It is the conviction of Nagy, that guilt and guilt feelings can indeed be healthy. The suffering from guilt feelings has the effect that one starts to *"repay"* (indebtedness and taking of responsibility). The further impact is that we become existentially less guilty because we acknowledge the guilt feelings. If the therapist will try to remove the guilt feelings with the aid of psychological manipulation, even though the person is existentially indeed guilty, the burden of guilt can even increase (Nagy IKON:8; Schlüter 1990:28).

The asymmetry and mutuality of existential guilt: The hurt victim

Although Buber wrote about asymmetry and refered to the relationship between teacher and scholar, therapist and client, humans and animals, the impression for Nagy is that: "Overall […] his emphasis fell on the symmetrical" (Nagy & Krasner BGT:33). Nevertheless, when it is about intergenerational interaction and the significance of the parent-child relationship, dialogue is asymmetric. In this respect, the emphasis between Nagy and Buber is different. However, both refer to existential guilt. Existential guilt is so to speak "beyond psychology". Nevertheless, it deserves attention in the thinking of the caregiver. Existential guilt does not reside in mere guilt feelings but is related to the factuality of consequences resulting from real transgressions.

This is the reason why Nagy acknowledges the reality of existential guilt. Existential guilt comes into play when a person in relationship with the other, harms the justice of the human order (Nagy & Krasner BGT:60). Without any doubt, in dialogue, both a *"reciprocity of responsible caring"* (Nagy & Krasner BGT:73) and a *"mutuality of commitment"* (Nagy & Krasner BGT:415) play a role. However, fundamentally the dialogue is asymmetric.

Trust and trustworthiness are decisive for the dialogue between generations. Valid dialoguing is the fruits of indebtedness and care. Appropriate dialogue is also an expression of unique identity: "… the dialogue as the shaper of identity, suggesting also that the behaviour patterns of any individual are not limited by the repertoire of patterns exhibited by elders or other bearers of cultural tradition" (Nagy F:73). Furthermore, familial dialogue is focused on the mutuality of care. Especially, when it is about the asymmetry between parents and their children. Within the exchange of giving and receiving in intergenerational relationships, there must be a form of mutuality in order to adhere to the principle of justice.

Buber's emphasis on existential guilt is for Nagy important. Existential guilt supersedes psychological guilt. Guilt is more complex than psychoanalytical explanations regarding feelings in the affective dimension of our being human. The criterion for "my" existential guilt is not about a personal feeling of guilt. It rather resides in the factuality of the consequences of my violating the order of justice, and the destructive impact on the victimised other; "… *the extent of injury suffered by the victim rather than the extent of the perpetrator's capacity for guilt feeling constitutes the criteria of existential guilt*, therefore of the intrinsic transgenerational tribunal, too" (Nagy F:309; italics VR/MK). Existential guilt is not about "my" intra-makeup, but about the consequence of injust behaviour on the other (the victim). The suffering of the dupe, the victim, constitutes the criterion for the acknowledgement of existential guilt.

The fourth dimension: Existential responsibility and "survivor's guilt"

The appropriate question is not whether guilt is always existential, but: Is there another mode of guilt possible than mere existential guilt? For Nagy, guilt is a complex concept related to the fourth dimension: *The dimension of existential responsibility*. And that is the difference between Buber and Nagy. Nagy switched from the paradigm of ontological guilt to the paradigm of ethical guilt. Ethical guilt does not exclude existential guilt. However, the focus is different. The primary focus is not on *being*, but on *ethical relating* and other-responsibility.

Without this basis of "existential responsibility", and its connectedness to a human order of justice, guilt becomes reduced to the realm of the affective. Such a reduction and isolation from existential responsibility, lead to inauthentic guilt and neurotic feelings. The feelings are unfounded. In the case of neurotic guilt, the founding could come from elsewhere. For example, from conflicting intrapsychic dynamics. One can call this kind of guilt "super-ego guilt" (Nagy & Krasner BGT:60). It is even possible that a person with relational merit can be manipulated into unfounded guilt and neurotic guilt feelings: "… a person who is actually in a high state of earned merit can nevertheless be manipulated into feeling guilty" (Nagy & Krasner BGT:164). This is possible irrespective of the fact that "an entitled, exploited person, is likely to be angry; an indebted, if ethically disengaged person, is likely to feel guilty" (Nagy & Krasner BGT:164). In other words, one can feel guilty due to what others inflict in the subject; a kind of prescribed guilt without any form of existential responsibility. One can feel guilty without any concrete form of irresponsible behaviour, or damage to the integrity of the other. The criterion does not reside in the feelings of the so-called "guilty" culprit. Therefore, in these cases it is indeed difficult to assess whether the feelings are appropriate or inappropriate due the difficulty to assess the intensions of the other. Only the duped can render in such a case clarity.

For example, a mother can devote her whole life to what she believed was a calling from God to her son; that is, that her son must eventually become a minister. She acted in terms of this "predestined calling" and ignored the fact that it was in fact about another human being. She created a condition wherein her son developed resentment, and guilt is evoked (Nagy & Krasner BGT:228).

Nagy and Krasner refer to this case as "destructive delegation". It is indeed about guilt, and not merely about guilt feelings. One can argue and say that the guilty person is the mother and not her son – kind of misplaced guilt. The son can indeed experience shame for not adhering to the expectations of the mother. But besides the fact of misplaced guilt, the factor of indebtedness is still intact, and can cause real feelings of guilt in him. One's indebtedness toward the other is not necessarily extinguished by the eventual guilt of the other (Levinas VTL:49). It is indeed possible that the son will eventually decide himself about his future. However, that does not necessarily take the indebtedness away.

Nagy's presupposition is that, despite displacement of inauthentic feelings, guilt prevails in one form or another. Maybe as an indication of a lack of freedom to act responsibly, a loss of entitlement, or unforeseen consequence for the other. In one way or another, evil will continue, unless intervention takes place. With intervention is meant, the development of a sound ethical perspective. That is also applicable in cases of neurotic guilt feelings, as well as to the phenomenon of neurotic victimhood. In both cases, help should be offered within the realm of trustworthy relationships.

It could be that people who survived a disaster like an earthquake, or economic crisis can be called "the lucky ones" (the so-called legacy of survivors). The attempt to exempt them from all forms of indebtedness could eventually be totally inappropriate. Nagy and Krasner write: "… a survivor is indebted to the victims who weren't able to escape" (Nagy & Krasner BGT:185). In trying to convince the victims (the survivors) they are not guilty, is in fact an inappropriate response. In the subjectivity of indebtedness lurks perhaps new avenues for the victim to be explored. "The key to ameliorating 'survivor guilt' lies in the survivor's options for appropriate action that will ultimately benefit posterity" (Nagy & Krasner BGT:185). In this case, the appropriate question will be: Can the survivor contribute to creating a safer environment and humane society for the next coming generation?[3] This question is in a very special way applicable to the current global immigrant crisis, and the phenomenon of human displacement.

---

3   Even refusing to use a form of theodicy for the injustice done by others, can be a contribution of a victim to posterity (Van der Leeuw 1991; Epstein 1988:19). Nevertheless, in our theological studies one cannot avoid the complex notion of theodicy.

Forgive as fore-give: The opportunity of compensation and the re-establishment of trust (Hargrave)

After the outline of exoneration, and Nagy's attempt to distinguish between "the judicial realm of exoneration", and the possible misleading application of "the generosity of forgiveness", it is indeed necessary to revisit the question whether exoneration is possible without detecting traces or features of forgiveness, even within the concept of exoneration. Can one maintain such a clear cut and absolute distinction between exoneration and forgiveness? It is in this regard, that we now turn to the research of the American therapist Hargrave.

"We differ from most contextual therapists in that we believe that exoneration is a step toward forgiveness and that forgiveness is a necessary part of healing relational hurts" (Hargrave & Anderson 1992:151). This viewpoint becomes the cornerstone for his reflection in another publication: *Families and Forgiveness – Healing Wounds in the Intergenerational Family* (Hargrave 1994).

It seems that Hargrave is one of the few researchers that connected himself to Nagy's concept of "exoneration" and tried to interpret its applicability for intergenerational dynamics. Hargrave also wants to elaborate further on the topic of exoneration and makes it relevant for theory formation. His reinterpretation is therefore indeed valuable for contextual therapy. For the researchers of this book, it could be an exciting endeavour to compare his reinterpretation with their convictions on healing and forgiveness.

Hargrave was involved in a kind of home-care project in Texas where they tried to combine a "frail-care home" for elderly with facilities for parents with children. This experience helped him to gain more insight into psychotherapeutic engagements with elderly people. It is forecasted that in a global society, intergenerational dynamics will become even more important. More families in future will consist of four or even five generations. Caregiving will have to take cognisance of these new developments.

Hargrave gives preference to the use of the metaphor of the "human body" for the understanding of family dynamics, very specifically when he refers to the possibility of "self-care" and the well-being of one's own life. "As a species, human beings are enormously blessed with the ability to heal physically" (Hargrave 1994:3). This is indeed true regarding the healing capacity of family systems. "Healing in the intergenerational family is much the same" (Hargrave & Anderson 1992:145).

In staying together over a period, it is quite normal that interpersonal and intergenerational wounds will develop. Some are not so serious, and people learn to cope. In some cases, the hurt is serious: "They challenge relational existence" (Hargrave & Anderson 1992:145-146). During serious illness the body struggles to survive. It is the same with "relational hurts". At stake, is then "relational survival". The challenge to the family is about their preparedness and capacity to become involved in a very complex process of helping and healing. Decisive in the process of familial healing are the notions of "exoneration" and "forgiveness".

Hargrave do have some reservations on Nagy's interpretation of "exoneration". "Exoneration is the effort of the child who has experienced injustice or hurt from a parent to lift the load of culpability off the parent" (Hargrave & Anderson 1992:151). Hargrave and Nagy share this vision with one another. The difference resides in Hargrave's argument that guilt, that has been originated from familial relational injustice, cannot be merely exonerated. It can only be done on condition that accountability has been *accepted* for the guilt. In other words, the wrongdoer acknowledges that he/she was responsible for the injustice that inflicted hurt and the pain of woundedness. It is only in the light of such an acknowledgement that the wrongdoer can claim that, if the situation comes up again, he/she will not inflict the hurt again. If one can start to trust the wrongdoer, one could claim that a trustworthy relationship has been restored and restablished. "No longer does the wronged person have to hold the wrongdoer responsible; the wrongdoer holds him- or herself responsible" (Hargrave & Anderson 1992:151-152)[4].

According to Halgrave, without this acknowledgement, exoneration is not applicable. This remark does not mean that one cannot merge forgiveness with exoneration in cases of wrongdoings. "Still, we feel that exoneration and forgiveness are on the same road. Both are acts of giving in the family that earn entitlement" (Hargrave & Anderson 1992:152).

Hargrave (1994) maintains that forgiving differs from exonerating in that forgiveness requires some specific action regarding the responsibility for the injustice which caused the hurt. In a contextual framework, relational justice in a family demands that the person who is victimised and hurt, is

---

4   It is noteworthy to reckon with the fact that Hargrave does not use the concept of "existential guilt" as related to indebtedness. For Nagy existential guilt does not reside in the affective but in the ethical dimension of indebtedness.

reasonable in holding the wrongdoer accountable for the hurt. Trust in the relationship has been damaged. In forgiving, the victimized person is given reason to believe that the wrongdoer accepts responsibility for the injustice he or she caused and promises to act in a trustworthy manner in the future. The relationship is re-established because trust has been restored.

When individuals are violated, they are likely to feel (a) rage as they experience uncontrolled anger toward their victimizer, or (b) shame as they accuse themselves of being unlovable and not deserving a trustworthy relationship. Similarly, violated individuals are likely to act in future relationships in ways that are over-controlling as they try to minimize their risk of hurt, or chaotic since they assume that little can be done to form trusting relationships. They will therefore, in any case, eventually be hurt despite any effort to restore. Some individuals who are victims of family pain experience a wide range of feelings and reactions as they alternate regarding shame/rage, control/chaotic cycles.

In Hargrave's framework, forgiving is accomplished by giving the opportunity for compensation. This could be exercised through an overt act of forgiving. In sum, this framework for forgiveness includes *two broad divisions of exonerating and forgiving*. Exonerating comprises of two stations, namely insight and understanding; forgiving comprises also of two stations, namely giving the opportunity for compensation, and the overt act of forgiving. Hargrave believes that both exonerating and forgiving are appropriate in different relationships at different times. He further points out that the four stations should not be interpreted as stages. People oscillate between stations many times in the attempt to forgive and re-establish relational trust.

Station 1: Insight, and Station 2: Understanding

Insight and understanding are two separate stages during the first part of the process, namely the exoneration part.
- *Insight* refers to the ability of a person to objectify the mechanisms of family pain that caused relational damage. As the individual identifies these mechanisms and transactions which caused pain, he or she has an increased ability to block the transaction and stop relational damage from occurring again in the future. Insight in how the hurt started, can help the duped person to detect the mechanisms that caused the

hurt. For example, unjust action of an old father that manipulated his daughter into the role of a caretaker, evoked feelings and actions of revenge in the adolescent person. Insight in the origin of these reactions helped to prevent a repetition of these reactions and the victimisation of a possible third.
- *Understanding* detects why the hurt happened. The duped person starts to understand via a process of identification and differentiation, how the wrongdoer was exposed to victimisation during his/her childhood (see Nagy & Krasner BGT:416). Understanding involves identifying with the victimiser's position, limitations, development, efforts, and intent. This understanding results in the victim acknowledging the fallibility of the victimiser, although it does not remove the victimiser's responsibility for the destructive action. As understanding takes place, an individual feels a reduction in condemnation and blame toward his or her victimiser.

Station 3: Giving the opportunity for compensation, and Station 4: The act of forgiveness

- *Opportunity for compensation.* In order to give an opportunity for compensation, contempt and blame must be left behind. Wrongdoing implies damage. A deposit in this regard, can be an indication of the wrongdoer's intention: "Forgive" as "fore-give". In giving the opportunity for compensation, the victim allows the victimiser to rebuild the status of trust in the relationship. This is established in a progressive manner by acting in ways that are trustworthy.
- *The overt act of forgiving.* In an overt act of forgiving, victim and victimiser discuss the relational violation openly and come to an agreement that they will seek a new trustworthy relationship in the future. The work of forgiveness, as outlined by Hargrave is defined as an effort in restoring love and trustworthiness to relationships, so that victims and victimisers can put an end to destructive entitlement. In forgiving, the victimised person is given reason to believe that the wrongdoer accepts responsibility for the injustice he or she caused and promises to act trustworthy in the future. The relationship is re-established because trust has been restored. The overt act of forgiving

is not instant and should be assisted in a therapeutic setting. Forgiving is about giving for … In this act of giving, one abandons one's powerful position. This gesture renders space for the re-establishment of trust.

Healing is established by visiting the several stations. The specific station appropriate for the process of forgiving, will differ from family to family. It would be one of the challenges in therapy to direct the family through the four different stations; "… in helping an aging family down this road of exoneration and forgiveness" (Hargrave & Anderson 1992:165).

Within the stations, Hargrave identifies the following elements: Confrontation with the possible instigators of the pain; acknowledgement of responsibility by the wrongdoer; the quest for forgiveness (asking for forgiveness), and the granting of forgiveness (giving forgiveness). Within the whole process, the establishment of a family ritual to "bury the hatchet" as symbolic representation of the violation and pain suffered, could foster familial healing indeed. Perhaps, another ritual: Asking forgiveness "on a bended knee" (Hargrave & Anderson 1992:162); "… it is extremely difficult to ask for forgiveness on a bended knee and not to reckon with the reality of the hurt" (Hargrave & Anderson 1992:159-163).

In assessing the model of Hargrave, it becomes evident that the therapist plays a more active role in the process of directing overt forgiveness as in Nagy's model. Visiting the different stations should take place in the counselling room (Hargrave 1994:186).

Another feature of Hargrave's model is that he views the family as a total unit. The structure and family system determine the different relational parts. This tendency is evident in the way he applies terminology like "intergenerational hurts", "interpersonal hurts" and "family pain". Using this kind of language is in fact concealing issues of partiality so that particularities tend to disappear. It could thus happen that personal suffering and personal accountability are rendered as secondary. The impression is that Hargrave thinks about human relationships in the first place in terms of schematised regularities. It is as if the family operates like a clockwork and functions like an organism. The danger is that the overt act of forgiving becomes eventually a managerial skill, regulated by the therapist.

Hardgrave warns against condemnation and blame that become obstacles in the process of exoneration and forgiveness. For Nagy the factor that needs to be addressed and abolished, is cheap generosity as a superficial trait in forgiveness. The further impression is that Hargrave renders at some places responsibility as "guilt" (*culpa*); a kind of pathology. There is a tendency that the emphasis is so strong on "being a victim", that the victim responds with a kind of passivity and is not really challenged to take active accountability. The victim can become so victimised that responsibility is reduced, and humanity is underplayed. The victim should instead, under all conditions, opt as subject.

One can conclude and say that Hargrave's notions of exoneration and forgiveness become a kind of "idealistic schema". It seems as if his "work of forgiveness" will be difficult to operationalise in a psychotherapeutic setting[5].

Complexity of exoneration and forgiveness: A kaleidoscope of aspects and perspectives

It has been said that both exoneration and forgiveness are complex categories. It is difficult to articulate all aspects simultaneously. It is now time to highlight some of them separately:

- The aspect of "more-than-two (generations)".
- The interplay: Guilt and shame.
- On remaining silent: Therapeutic muteness.
- Exoneration within the framework of death and dying: Post mortem legacy.
- Exoneration as extraordinary: Superseding prescriptive regularities.
- Exoneration: The judicial process.

The following outline will detect the meaning of different aspects. They describe different perspectives of the complex whole during processes of exoneration. They can help to shed more light on the fact that exoneration and forgiveness are complex categories with many facets; forgiveness is a dynamic process and not an instant and final event.

---

5 See in this regard, the biblical text on peace: Isaiah 57:19. This kind of peace is from a different spiritual order than the juridical concept of exoneration. The fact that Nagy (as therapist) does not work with the concept of forgiveness, cannot be ascribed to a shortcoming in his thinking; it is more a case of modesty: Forgiveness as a gift of mercy and grace.

The aspect of "more-than-two (generations)"

Nagy mentions in *Between Give and Take* (BGT:416), that improvement in intergenerational dynamics can be related to the enhancement of the capacity of parents to exonerate their own parents. At stake, are three generations. The person who is summoned to exonerate is addressed as parent (parent of a child).

In settings of destructive behaviour and indebtedness, exoneration can indeed be an alternative route in order to deflect "destructive entitlement"; it opens options for becoming engaged in "constructive entitlement".

We have often referred to the notion of "*the third*" (third factor). In this instance, differentiation is imperative. There is "the third" to whom injustice has been inflicted, and, as consequence to this wrongdoing, responded in an inappropriate (unjust) way. Then there is the third as the one I have treated in an unjust way (my child, spouse, partner). Because I (myself) have been treated unfair by "the second" (my parent) (rotating bill, "revolving slate"), my response becomes destructive as well.

In contextual therapy, the therapist concentrates on "the third" (even the fourth etcetera) due to the perspective of multidirected partiality. Any form of violation towards "the third" cannot be justified. No explanation is acceptable, irrespective of whether one refers to technical terms like "system", "balance", "destructive right" or "rotating bill"[6]. Therapy should therefore pay special attention to the predicament that the victim will indeed have difficulties how to deal with other victims and to forgive.

The interplay: Guilt and shame

Exoneration brings about releasement of shame. "It replaces a framework of blame ..." (Nagy & Krasner BGT:416). Exoneration in this respect is almost "vindication of the parents" (Nagy & Spark IL:68); to purify them from blame.

---

6   A few times, the pastoral theologian, John Patton, mentions in his book *Is Human Forgiveness Possible?* (1985), the name of Nagy. Patton's interpretation of Nagy is predominantly based on *Invisible Loyalties*. In a personal encounter with Nagy, Patton responded as follows: "I once said to Ivan Nagy, after hearing one of his presentations on family therapy, that I felt a little like I had been in an Old Testament class. He seemed a bit disturbed by this and insisted that what he meant by ethics and ethical balance were not based on any religion. I was in no position to argue about the basis of his theory – although I had still my suspicions – but Nagy's views give powerful support to the importance accorded the family by the Judeo-Christian tradition" (Patton 1985:29). Patton makes shame a key concept and concentrates on the act of granting the other forgiveness – the role of the subject is emphasised, without attention to "the third".

Blame can be linked to "shame" and "shamefulness". However, Nagy does not give much attention to shame in his writings. The reason: Shame is for Nagy a psychological term and, thus, not a real relational and ethical notion. Shame refers much more to a loss of personal prestige than concern for the other. Shame also differs from guilt feelings. To suffer from guilt feelings, you pay existentially for your guilt. With shame it is different, because it does not take the situation of the duped enough into consideration. Nevertheless, shame can be a porch to an awareness of guilt. Parental shame can be an indication of personal remorse and become most helpful to children in their attempt to exonerate.

Not really giving attention to shame, is indeed a limitation in Nagy's approach. This is applicable to cases where the other inflicts injustice for which I am ashamed of. Many offspring struggle with the legacy of ancestral shame and guilt (Nagy & Krasner BGT:182). It is also possible that the "I" can become ashamed in the place of the other (vicarious shame) (Havel 1991:255-256).

In BGT, Nagy and Krasner give attention to the issue of "family shame". At stake, is the question whether shame could be rendered as porch for a dialogue about the balance of merit and obligation or not. Shame in family affairs is a very complex phenomenon. It could become a huge obstacle in therapy to detect the truth in relational reality. Often the people affected do not want to be disloyal to other family members.

It is obvious that shame and loyalty are intertwined. Shame refers more to bodily issues, and, is most of times, visible which is not the case with loyalty. Shame often presents as a mode of self-protection. It should be addressed in therapy in order to safeguard the authenticity of processes of exoneration and forgiveness. Help is not in the first place to demask the shame, but to support the person to take own guilt and indebtedness seriously. A person can also be empowered to enter a dialogue with the other with exoneration as eventual outcome. Albeit, what needs to become visible, is loyalty as an ethical entanglement. The fact that one can shame oneself on behalf of the other, should not be viewed as pathology and without any significance. In terms of relational dynamics, it is a sign of existential connectedness.

Another aspect of shame is that one can shame oneself for what others find ridiculous, insignificant or fine. The effect of this kind of shame is that one starts to be ashamed about his/her shame for the conduct of a significant other. It becomes clear that shame is a complex category with many layers. Thus, the reason for multidirected partiality in therapy. One needs to be extremely sensitive not to put the trust of the other to shame; that is, the endeavour to detect in "the vicarious shame of the other", a sound interconnectedness and indebtedness that are not pathological or ridiculous in origin.

On remaining silent: Therapeutic muteness

Exoneration is for Nagy a process. The intention is that somebody is rendered the opportunity to make a new beginning in his/her relational reality. The appeal is on personal accountability within a desire for restoration of relational integrity. The focus is to start with a new beginning in the restoration of the "justice of the human order". In therapy, the challenge is to trace back the fundamental truth of the other. This endeavour means to trace back the track of how the original responsibility and accountability of the other have been violated and contributed to destructive and irresponsible behaviour. In order to do that, more than generosity is needed. One option is to probe into the possibility of remorse; another is to go back to the past situation of being victimised by the other (parent).

It could be that despite all the attempts, no trace of remorse can be detected in the response of the wrongdoer. The impression could then be that the other is merely a monster. However, Nagy maintained that no human being is essentially a monster. To label the parent as "bad" does not contribute to healing and change.

If even exoneration does not deliver a possible outcome, the implication is not that the caring endeavour has been in vain. If the direct goal is not achieved, one should rather keep silent. Silence from the side of the therapist is not an indication of resignation. For Nagy, it is an indication of the therapist's respect for the client, and the acknowledgement of limitations that should be respected. Limitations should be accepted and not be transformed into a mode of artificial "positive labelling". The failure of exoneration should be accepted as a subjective limitation.

Therapeutic silence is about a time of waiting, a constructive pause. In silence the therapist must take time to evaluate the impact of the failure on the client or any other person(s) related to the wrongdoing. Silence is a kind of temporary bracketing with the message: One should merely accept the fact that the incompetent parent was merely a vulnerable human being. All human beings fail and make mistakes. The hunch is that silence is for Nagy not a sign of desperate resignation, but a kind of respect for the client who needs time to deal with possible consequences, especially when it seems that the process of exoneration did not deliver the possible foreseen outcomes. It is inevitably a fact, that sometimes things in life are irreversible. If exoneration has failed, it does not imply that all options have been explored. One should always be open to the surprise of the unpredictability of happenstances in life.

Exoneration within the framework of death and dying: Post mortem legacy

In order to establish exoneration, intrapersonal reflection does not suffice. For exoneration it is not per se a condition that the other (parent) should start to ask exoneration first. Sometimes people are becoming just too old, or too blind, for remorse. The hesitation to opt for exoneration could even refer to possible experiences of victimisation during childhood (destructive entitlement). Postponed exoneration or absence of remorse could be because the other has no courage to take initiative. It could also be that people involved are already dead.

Nagy interprets loss due to death, as "broken dialogue" (Nagy & Krasner BGT:326). When the relationship between parent and child was a caring and empathetic one, the impact will resonate even after death. "For death itself is not the ultimate arbiter of dialogue. Instead, it is a stage which seals out the chance for another intergenerational try at care" (Nagy & Krasner BGT:326). The value of love relationships can be powerful even after death (Maurice Friedman 1992a:194): A post mortem effect. Although it seems as if the balance of obligation is completed with death, the question could still be posed: But is time irreversible indeed?

In *On Meaning Between Generations*, David Krasner describes his father as a person who chronically felt cheated. When one wanted to approach him in this regard, he just sent everybody in a very rude manner away. After the death of his father, Krasner wrestled with his father's legacy, and called the experience: "the ultimate cheat": How will his grandchildren remember him? (Krasner in BGT:409-411; TGN 1994:467-469).

Exoneration as extraordinary: Superseding prescriptive regularities

Exoneration is not something you can achieve. However, this does not rule out the option and competence to exonerate. Acknowledgement of this competence can bring about a kind of freedom. This option is important because it can influence the relationship with the other, specifically in intergenerational interaction it can play a decisive role in the eventual future children and coming generations. The spontaneous effort of a parent to exonerate his/her parent, can become a turning point in therapy with the family (Nagy & Krasner TGN:127; BGT:103). This kind of spontaneity reflects a client's active and genuine commitment to his/her own life-goals (Nagy & Krasner BGT:421). In this regard, a therapist can motivate a client to earn entitlement, namely, to take efforts to exonerate guilty parents seriously, and to reveal these intentions to his/her children or others involved.

The point is: Exoneration cannot be prescribed like a recipe. It cannot be regulated in a systematic way. Exoneration is indeed extraordinary and supersedes the normal rhythm of life.

Exoneration: The judicial process

Nagy and Krasner emphasise the fact that exoneration is a process. However, it is indeed a question if the concept of process is appropriate. Exoneration cannot be a process as in developmental psychology. One cannot split it into stages to be eventually managed. However, what one should realise is that the criterion for valid and true exoneration is the principle of justice. Justice must be done, and one should take care that people are not exposed to injustice.

There are no specific steps to keep in mind. One can merely identify two aspects.

1. Justice must be done: The re-establishment of justice to the victim

This aspect refers to the parent as object of forgiveness: His/her life story in terms of wrongdoings or woundedness should be taken into consideration as well. Exoneration requires patience. It implies that one should often be prepared to take time to dwell and ponder on issues that are irreversible with long term, disastrous effects on a person's lifespan. For example, a person feels uncomfortable with his/her career because the parent prevents him/her to achieve specific life goals and targets regarding a different career. One feels unfulfilled in life; resentment becomes an obstacle in the relationship with the specific parent. The disappointment with the father/mother is about missed opportunities. Just to overlook this irreversible lost opportunity, is not about exoneration; it is in fact a mode of pseudo-exoneration.

The child's freedom has been violated. The challenging question will be how to restore violated freedom so that personal freedom can be reclaimed and even increase again. This is how a sense of personal justice can be re-established.

2. Doing justice to the other (the parent)

To become victimised is about the violation of one's subjectivity and personal sense of dignity (truth). Being victimised can affect one's significance in life. To detect this original pre-truth (the status before the victimisation took place) is virtually impossible. However, exoneration implies to even go back to the childhood condition of the indebted parent (own past victimisation during childhood). It is in fact a challenge to hear the other side of the story as well. The therapist has to probe into past relational networking like sibling relationships, neighbourhood issues, social structures and economic conditions. Probing into destructive entitlement will be challenged by many unanswered questions. The advantage, however, is that it is about trying to restore the dignity of the other (parent), and, in this respect, to take care of the other's legacy. To restore the legacy, is taking care of the middle-generation, as well as taking responsibility for the future third generation. In this sense, exoneration is linked to a judicial process that can stretch over more than one generation.

Irrevocable time and the impossibility of indifference within the triadic obligation of forgiveness: Human being – neighbour – God

Against the background of the persecution of the Jews, and when Hitler was one year in charge, Levinas wrote an article on how "the Hitler-regime" was busy to rob Europe from freedom by destroying time and blocking history. Time became a condition of the irreparable (see Levinas 1994). Since the wrongdoing, the past – in the mode of an accomplished fact (*faits accomplis*) – weighs heavily on the destination of humankind.

The challenge is now the message of the impossibility of the possible: To assemble freedom and time within the now. Levinas sees in Judaism a message of this possibility.

Freedom is to wrestle with the wrongdoings of the past. The torment is an appeal on authentic remorse; it announces a kind of repentance that can serve as generator for forgiveness; a repentance that can heal and repay, restore authentic freedom (*Le remords [...] annonce le repentir générateur du pardon qui répare*) (Levinas 1994:29).

The present, thus, becomes the opportunity for change. Wiping out (deleting) the past, creates new possibilities in the now without repeating the wrongdoing of the past. Freedom, equality, equity, are not established by abstract theories that try to explain individual differences in terms of psychological constitutions. Equality is due to the capacity of the human spirit (soulfulness) to free him/herself from the past.

Remorse and repentance, as well as the receiving of forgiveness, originates from freedom and confirms freedom. As such they co-constitute the present (*un présent*). Although the text cited refers to Levinas' more early reflections, it sets the parameters for his thinking on the notion of authentic change in the present, namely the contours of remorse, repentance and forgiveness that have the capacity to *change* something. This change is not about the restoration of an *archè* (first, unmoveable principle), but about remorse, repentance and forgiveness that establish a new mode of time: *Now* (*presencing the presence*).

This moment of establishing a new present, refers to an autonomy of freedom that should be defined as "created freedom": a freedom founded by heteronomy (Levinas TO:339; TI:255).

From Levinas' perspective, forgiveness is an event that is situated within the following triadic dynamics: *Human being – fellow human being – God*. This is an indication that Levinas thinks in terms of the Jewish tradition. In this wisdom tradition it is not possible to separate any of these entities from one another. This triangle is in Jewish religiosity constitutive for the reality of our being human. This triadic framework is also important for a spiritual assessment of forgiveness. Even the sequence in the triadic interconnectedness is for Levinas not arbitrary[7].

Forgiveness starts with the subject, the "I" of the human being. For Levinas, this subjective starting point is the ABC for understanding the process of forgiveness.

It has been mentioned that Levinas thinks within the contours of the Jewish-religious tradition (Poorthuis 1994:9). When one transfers theological concepts, one should always reckon with the concrete social and historical relational networking that constituted and contributed to its meaning (Levinas QLT). The triadic dynamics of *human being – fellow human being – God*, represents the thinking and doing of a traditional Jewish Biblical and Talmudic perspective. This order opens an ethical perspective on social dynamics –the dynamics of intersubjectivity. How Levinas interprets and operationalises the concepts "revenge" and "forgiveness" should be understood hermeneutically from this ethical perspective.

Due to Levinas' philosophical writings the question should be posed: Who is the speaker that encounters me? In this encounter it is about a subject-object-structure; it is about the relationships between "me" and what has been said (*le dit*) – the content of the dialogue (*quidditas*). The significance of what has been said, resides in the subjective quality of the speaker. The saying is dependent from the semantic structure of the "what"; it is dependent from some-*thing*. Even before one can detect the content of the saying; before one hears the topic of the saying, the I has already responded to a saying wherein the other is presented: The other as an authentic subject. Even if it is a voice of silence (*une voix d'un fin silence*), the "I" is still as subject, the speaker.

In an article on *God and Philosophy* (DQVI), Levinas refers to a kind of responsibility that precedes freedom. It is about a total condition of

---

7   One needs to reckon with the fact that the concept of forgiveness is many layered. In Christian theology there are many views. The triadic interconnectedness can be interpreted differently. Very specifically, in the more reformed tradition, the first factor in the triad will not be the "I" as in the case of Levinas. The starting point, and therefore the originator and guarantor of forgiveness, should be God. God forgives human beings unconditionally. It is on this basis that human beings can and should forgive (Thurneysen 1948:281). Smelik (1943:191-195) refers to the enmeshment or entanglement between the forgiveness of God and the forgiveness between human beings. The latter is theologically speaking, a reflection of the first. Forgiveness is to delete the phrase: "I will forgive but never forget". Even when the wrongdoing has been settled, the difficulty to forget, becomes the obstacle for the future of proper forgiveness. From a theological perspective, forgiveness destroys unforgettable issues totally. This annihilation is, according to Lascaris (1993:266-269), in terms of the imitation of Christ, a "gift". The eventual challenge is to forgive unconditionally.

passivity wherein the infinite already has resonated. In fact, it is about a non-condition, a content without any specific content, because it transcends the comprehension of the subject. The Infinite transcends immanence, but at the same time qualifies immanence. We are therefore empirically indebted with an obligation towards the other; as an *impossible indifference* towards the misery and shortcomings of fellow human beings (Levinas DQVI:116). Thus, the reason to take the speaker (the other) as subject serious and to acknowledge one's obligation and responsibility towards the other: the other as trace of the infinite.

The peculiarity of forgiveness in Levinas' writings: The ethical principle of "one-for-the-other" (l'un-pour-l'autre) *in an anthropology of forgiveness*

Forgiveness is complex, and to a certain extent "strange" and "peculiar", because it is related to a responsibility that precedes freedom. One receives freedom in the encounter with visage. Visage demarcates the contours of both this freedom and the competence to forgive. Thus, the reason why freedom and the act of forgiveness should not be dominated by all-powerful categories like "almighty" (*omni-*categories). It is in the light of this background that the following very famous phrase by Levinas should be understood: "*A world wherein forgiveness is all-powerful (almighty), becomes inhumane*" (Levinas RA).

This phrase is coming from a speech delivered in Marokko (1958) before a gathering of Jews, Moslems and Christians. According to a Jewish saying, nobody, even not God, can substitute the place of a wounded and insulted human being. The Talmud points out the value and autonomy of an insulted, violated human being. Evil is not about a mystical principle that can be wiped out and deleted by merely a ritual. Evil is an insult that one human being inflicts on another human being. Nobody, not even God can substitute the place of the wounded victim (Levinas MG:46). After this remark, follows the thesis that a world, wherein forgiveness is presented as all-powerful (almighty), becomes inhumane (Levinas MG:46). Forgiveness is not about cheap grace that ignores the hurt and damage inflicted by injustice.

In order to understand the meaning of the previous phrase, the triadic sequence is important to maintain. The fact that the human being is first, and then follows the fellow human being (second), thereafter the third: God, underlines another fact, namely that the subject (human being) is the acting agent through whom God establishes a kind of forgiveness that is humane. In this kind of forgiveness, the process is not overshadowed by power-categories that leave the impression that forgiveness can be managed by manipulative powers. An all-powerful, all-mighty forgiveness is a display of power that is not mediated, incarnated by human speech. It destroys the original structure and paralyses the vividness of the triadic sequence. It abolishes the intrigue and violates the "impossibility of indifference".

An all-powerful forgiveness robs the victim (the creditor) of her/his autonomy. The autonomy of the creditor, the wounded or insulted person, creates for the debtor an opportunity to repent and to recover; it opens new avenues for freedom and responsibility. Even autonomy is still shaped by the ethical principle of "one-for-the-other" (*l'un-pour-l'autre*).

What needs to be maintained in an anthropology of forgiveness, is the original, triadic anthropological structure and dialogical intrigue: the intrigue of the one-for-the-other. The for-the-other brings about a healthy split and cleavage in the self that becomes an adventure with God, or even an opportunity for God. When God becomes incarnated by words, the outcome is not the traditional confession: "I believe in God"; it is the *me voiçi* ("here me") by which I pronounce peace for my fellow human being and perform my responsibility to the vulnerable other. When I profess peace in terms of Isaiah 57:19[8], when I bless the other with peace, this peace is a creation of the Eternal. Speaking is becoming an expression of responsibility towards the other; it is about the establishment of language, enacted and originated by the Eternal factor (The Infinite).

The notion of "toward the other" plays a key role in the fundamental proposition regarding the "infinite responsibility for peace". This perspective is maintained in the Talmud as well (Levinas QLT). The offences and mishaps of a human being over against God, are all forgiven on the Great Day of Atonement. However, the offences and mishaps of a human being over against the other, are not instantly forgiven on the Great Day of Atonement;

---

8   Isaiah 57:19 (NIV): "I will guide them and restore comfort to Israel's mourners, creating praise on their lips. Peace, peace, to those far and near, says the LORD. And I will heal them."

compensation (compensating the damage of the hurt other) is a condition for authentic forgiveness (VTL:26).

Offences against God

The great Day of Atonement brings about change (repentance). It refers to penance and forgiveness for offences against the Infinite. The offences entail laws about the eating of food, commandments for the Sabbath and different forms of idolatry. Offences against fellow human beings were ipso facto, offences against God. However, due to remorse and rituals of penance, *The Great Day of Atonement* plays a fundamental role in the dealing with transgressions and offences against God. Atonement is about reconciliation and forgiveness. All offences are totally extinguished; they are radically deleted. Atonement sets one free from all guilt. This new attained freedom and deliverance are performed within close fellowship – the objective order of the community. It is within this space that a human being is forgiven: Fellowship as the intimacy of redemption (Levinas VTL:33).

The unique emphasis of Levinas is that forgiveness for my offences against God, is dependent on my awareness of accountability. The instrument of forgiveness is in my hands (Levinas VTL:32). With this formulation Levinas does not want to project the image that in Jewish religiosity, social ethics dominates ritual practices. He wants to emphasise that the one who can perform self-discipline, is the subject him/herself. It is in the hands of the one who can recognise the visage of the other. The implication is that the subject needs to become aware of an internal moral consciousness. The latter is a precondition in order to restore the integrity of the damaged relationship and moral wrongdoing. The challenge in events of forgiveness boils down to the following imperative, namely, to restore a sense of moral integrity.

Compensating (making good) the other

Forgiveness, exoneration and reconciliation are always a personal endeavour. The insulted and offended person must always be approached personally. Comfort and reconciliation are addressed to the offended as subject based on intersubjectivity. It is of vital importance, that restoring of damaged relationships is fundamentally an "I"-issue. Not history, nor God can oversee or replace this challenge.

In the light of a Gemara text[9] that belongs to the Mishna text, Levinas maintains his conviction that the *drama of forgiveness* presupposes three: *The human being, the fellow human being and God*. If God is the judge, the process is a tribunal wherein all three must be involved. In this triadic construction, God stands not above the process, but functions within the connection man-neighbour-God. Thus, the very peculiar, but crucial formulation by Levinas: Perhaps, God is nothing else than the permanent rejection and repudiation of a history that acquiesces in our "private tears" (*larmes privées*). Such a conception of history views and interprets the inexpressible suffering that people were exposed to, as a necessary stage in a process – the good is established by and through the evil (*gubernatio*). This kind of theodicy, the attempt to make good what is in fact bad, with an appeal on a higher noble goal or neutral principle, should be rejected, because it is then about a fatalistic history that envelops automatically in a very mechanistic way. This conception results in a hermeneutic wherein nobody wants to accept responsibility while tears become a negligible quantity (*quantité négligeable*). In this sense, one can conclude and say that "God" becomes merely a "negating, rejecting factor"; God as the rejecting factor of the history of humankind.

It seems as if Levinas is reducing and minimising God. The question arises: But is God not much more than merely a rejecting factor? Again, Levinas formulates very carefully: Perhaps God is, as the rejecter of a "history without responsibility" and "hospitable concern", in this sense, indeed the "supreme Highest of All": The Judge that renounces history and the One who renders those who shed personal tears, as being the righteous. In this sense, God is indeed the almighty one. God makes the miracle possible that such a history of irresponsible ignorance is rejected. He also instigates solidarity with those "personal tears". The Highest of All (almighty), is in fact the Lowest (most humble) of All – present in the tears of the humiliated and the outcasts (divine solidarity).

Forgiveness and solidarity are in fact obligatory and make an appeal to the whole of being as subject; it concerns me personally (*me regarde*). Levinas also speaks about a dialectic of forgiveness; a reverse of forgiveness: The insulted person devotes him/herself to the cause and responsibility of forgiveness, especially in cases wherein the offender acts with ignorance

---

9   A rabbinical commentary on the Mishnah, forming the second part of the Talmud.

(Levinas VTL:42). The offended person should induce the offender to demand forgiveness.

Whether one is the accused or accuser, victim or offender, the reality is one of irrevocable responsibility; it touches conscience. In some cases, it is indeed difficult to forgive because the offender responds with aggression or sheer smugness. The implication therefore is that the process of responsibility proceeds and is perhaps never completed. Even the offended person is always challenged by the fact that the responsibility towards the wrongdoing continues. In fact, it is not about a responsibility towards the event of wrongdoing, but about a true concern for the predicament of the offended other. The offence and the merit always go together, coexist. There is no offense that cancels out the merit. Both demand their own kind of settlement (Levinas VTL:49).

One can conclude and say: Forgiveness within the context of the Talmud is dialectic. The offended should not rest on his/her laurels. According to the law, the concern for forgiveness is an imperative. The offended should not stay in his/her predicament of being a victim. The offender should not dwell in his/her captivity but must take up the challenge of constructive responsibility for what he/she inflicted on the other/others. The offender should continue to campaign for compensation, because the long-term effects will keep on turning up. Initially, they are most of times invisible. However, later they can reappear in the realm of human encounters.

It could indeed happen that the offender persists in his/her denial of responsibility and refuses to repent and to take initiative in the asking of forgiveness. This does not imply that the victim has no responsibility at all. The victim (the disadvantaged person) still has the competence to render forgiveness and not longer to keep on blaming the other. This competence is about the freedom of the offended person. The wrongdoings and offences of the past should never become part of fate.

When one receives forgiveness, the offender is restored in his/her moral integrity; that is, that his/her moral conscience is reinstituted; the conscience is healed. The ignorance about the scope and effect, is in principle negated and ended. In this restoration God has been actively involved.

According to the narrative in 2 Samuel 21:1-14 (*The Gibeonites avenged*), king David rendered the Gibeonites the right to take revenge by killing seven male descendants. With reference to this quite "cruel event", Levinas poses the question: How on earth can the descendants be punished for the wrongdoing of their fathers? (Referring to the wrongdoings of King Saul). Levinas answers as follows: To punish the children is less an offence and cruel than to tolerate impunity when the foreigner has been insulted. At stake, is the respect for the foreigner in terms of owning hospitality to the foreign outsider (Levinas QLT:61; VTL:49-50). Violation of "the sacred right of hospitality", is in a sense unforgiveable. The foreigner is rendered as the prototype for a human being without context. Violation of the right of hospitality should be avenged. The fact that David made one exception, namely that he saved Mephibosheth, the son of Jonathan, seems as if justice became arbitrary. However, Levinas remarks as follows: The acknowledgement of the priority of justice as an objective principle, does not exclude the "heart of the person"; there is no heart without reason, but, at the same time, there is no reason without heart (Levinas VTL:49).

The I and the obstacle of totality: Delayed justice and immature forgiveness

According to Levinas, it is extremely difficult to merge forgiveness with the concept of society. Forgiveness does not fit into the dynamics of society with its emphasis on mass-communication and mass-production. Society thinks in terms of generalisations. The implication for the "I" is that subjectivity tends to become absorbed by the anonymity of totality. When forgiveness is separated from personal responsibility (subjectivity) and the realm of the Third (as a severe witness, Visage), justice in society becomes easily delayed. Then forgiveness even becomes immature because the flight into a generous gesture of exonerating excuses, does not reflect the existential pain of the hurt victim and the seriousness of the obligation to bestow compensation.

Levinas does not reflect on the dynamics of society in terms of generalisations. Society is not merely the sum of individuals, extended into the whole of a group or allcomprehensive concept. Society is about much more than the sum total of entities counted together. They cannot be calculated since the subjectivity of the "I" cannot be quantified and never becomes a numerical entity. Subjectivity exceeds the limitations of quantification; it is rather about qualification. The insight of the group cannot capture the dynamics of the "I". Subjectivity cannot be comprehended and captured by totality. Nobody is identical with his/her position in the group. Our unique human identity cannot be derived from one's characteristics: One is more than one's mode of being. Identity cannot be detected in terms of achievements, work, tradition or heritage. Thus, the reason why functions in a totality are totally inappropriate to assess personal value.

A society is in practise fully plural. The diversity is huge. We act as if the society is one whole totality. We try to hypothesise all the different others into one comprehension theory in order to manage functions in society and to control individuals. However, in the meantime, we cause a lot of damage to one another. We inflict a lot of spiritual and physical injuries by means of hurtful acts and offensive words. The painful reality is that most of times we are not even aware of the impact of offences on the other due to mass communication and global indifference.

Forgiveness cannot be performed in such a mass anonymity. Forgiveness takes place in the intimate space of subjectivity. It presupposes a dual relationship with the mutuality of dialogue. In society, there is little space for duality because one is always exposed to a third factor: The other/others. One can try to forgive the other but is then immediately exposed to the impact on others. Within the networking of life, there are so many others that could become affected by the offense and the impact thereof on my sense of dignity; so many that can become victims as well. Due to this interconnected networking, my freedom to forgive is limited by the subjectivity and autonomy of the other.

Within intersubjectivity, dialogue between two people is always exposed to the third factor, namely the other human being, the so called "third person". The third party disturbs the intimacy of a love dialogue. The dual relationship wherein forgiveness should take place, "together with God", cannot be established because the potential third person is always present and an obstacle for individualised and subjective justice (Levinas MG:114-115). This is what Levinas calls the crisis of our modern awareness, as well as the crisis of religion.

The real authentic dialogue should be detected in another sphere, elsewhere and not merely in exclusive duality. The real, authentic THIRD, the one who is so easily excluded from the duality between "I" and the "other", is in fact the real Other. This Other penetrates the private intimacy and encounter between two people by means of his/her word; this "Other" stands over against me and face me as visage; looks through me and pierces every form of totality. Only this THIRD is a THOU. With this statement, Levinas does not refer in the first place to theology. It refers much more to the mystical desire and the fact that God can only enact as God if this he is recognised as conversational Partner par excellence (Levinas MG:118).

The status of this THIRD/Third abandoned factor (abandoned from the close duality of intimacy) is without any doubt complex in Levinas' thinking. Perhaps, it could be the widower, the orphan or the foreigner (strange outsider). The real authentic dialogue can even supersede the intimacy of love, because the command supersedes the duality of love (Levinas MG:119). The intriguing question (Kalshoven in TO:26) is: How can the "I", within the ocean of many other I's that cannot be captured into one total concept, still be able to detect this injustice and acknowledge it as being indeed a manifestation of injustice? The irony is that the totality is per sé already an indication of a situation of injustice. In this sense the ability of the "I" to differentiate becomes virtually impossible. In order to perform this differentiation, a new situation is required. It will not be established automatically. Justice does not emanate from the normal flow of injustice (Levinas MG:127). What is most needed in order to "control", "manage" the totality, and to make the I aware of what justice is about, somebody or some instance must summon me and make an appeal on my accountability. I should then be encountered by an entity that is not absorbed by the system; an entity that is transcendent, namely Visage.

Only within the presence the visage of the THIRD/Third, conscience can recover and be restored. As argued, compensation for guilt is possible over against that entity that has been offended and damaged. But you (the other), that also has suffered due to the offense, can only be compensated within the acknowledgement of this Third. This is performed not by being subjected to the other. What should be grasped and understood, is the precarious character of this acknowledgement, namely that I am in the position of an "impossibility of denial" (negation of the negation) (Levinas MG:132).

Forgiveness as exoneration of guilt (I am not any more accountable for my guilt), is only possible within intimacy (a strange form of egoism that excludes a third and forces the subject to become an "I" indeed). Within the totality of society, compiled and determined by the diversity of many different I's, the endeavour to forgive is complex. Thus, the necessity for a kind of judiciary process, a kind of ledger, that addresses the "I" directly as the guilty one (indebted one). This is indeed possible. However, the process can never be separated from economical relationships, financial issues and even the money-factor. Eventually, due to judicial procedures, the injustice and offence will become quantified and therefore dealt with in terms of compensation (material repayment). This aspect of quantifying the loss in terms of compensation may indeed seem "*shocking*", namely, to reduce the human predicament to material values and to make this demand for compensation a condition for implementing justice (compensation as quantification) (Levinas TO:57; MG:135). However, material repayment makes some repentance possible.

It is within this judicial context, that the question of "*metaphysical forgiveness*" comes into play. What about forgiveness by God? Levinas is quite clear with the statement that God cannot forgive on behalf of the victim. Also, not in cases where the dignity of the neighbour/fellow human being has been violated. Levinas maintains the viewpoint: Forgiveness does not start with God and is not the task of God. Forgiveness is the responsibility of the subject him/herself. Offences over against God demand a total mobilisation of oneself; indeed, the most difficult challenge due to the unruly stubbornness of the self to resist radical change and transformation.

The forgiveness by God from all offences against God, is a reminder that there exists in fact no reason for any form of human justification to perform any offence or wrongdoing at all. They are in fact, totally unnecessary. Conversion is to turn around, to turn inwards and to return to freedom with the commitment not to transgress and become guilty again. The quest for forgiveness presupposes the total seriousness of turning around (conversion). In this sense, forgiveness is about a new creation; forgiveness is radical; it creates a new time and mode of being.

If forgiveness needs to be connected to the realm of freedom and responsibility, if forgiveness is about turning around, an act of conversion, what about the passive dimension, namely the art to receive forgiveness and to be granted forgiveness?

Endless time and forgiveness as a purified present

In *Totalité et Infini*, the scope is the reality of Transcendence and its connectedness to the anthropological basic structure of our being human. The question is about how the epiphany of visage is concretised. Within this framework, the following topics are discussed: Eros, fertility, fatherhood (paternity), sonship, brotherhood and the infinite dimension of time.

It is indeed a question how to translate *"l'infinition"*. Perhaps, the best option is to make a paraphrased translation: To translate *"l'infinition du temps"* as *"the disengagement of time from its limitation; from its character of termination and completion"*. Time, thus, becomes endless. The reason for this translation is that the core notion at stake in *"l'infinition"*, is *"fin"* that means "end", but "end" not as final termination (finish). Time that is not terminated by an end does not refer to the fact that time is continuous but presents itself as a gift. In and through the other, I am granted new time and future; time is being given to me. In this connection with time as gift, the other is irrevocably linked to me, engaged with me, and vice versa. In this engagement and interconnectedness, the separation between subject and the other is not abolished or discontinued. This perspective should be maintained so that interconnectedness and intersubjectivity not become fused into a totality of massification.

Eros

The connection between time, transcendence and visage, implies that experiences in life cannot be captured by intentionality (sheer observation and quantification); neither by the rationalistic positivistic split between subject and object. Time should rather be perforated by the infinite. It is in this sense that being becomes transparent for a metaphysical desire.

An example is the erotic relationship. Eros is not subjected to the totality of an intentional relationship. Love is as powerful as death. In such a relationship the subject does not control the object of love by means of rationality and the obsession of becoming mine (posessiveness, namely that I can dominate and determine the relationship according to selfish needs). The hand that caresses does not know the object it is looking for.

When one applies general, common terminology to assess the unique value of eros, it seems as if the erotic relationship is doomed to become merely a failure. It will indeed become a failure if erotic desires are fundamentally about taking, grasping, possessing and knowing. But this is not what Eros is about. To possess and to overwhelm are synonymous with "my abilities", *I-can*. Love, however, is about the opposite. The duality of love in the erotic relationship, makes the totality of fusion impossible. Duality within differentiation (being separate) is the essence of love. It is about a relationship with otherness, with mystery. It connects one with future. One even enters a realm that is different from what is always there and existent – a realm where everything is never I (mine). (*Cest la relation avec l'altérité, avec le mystére, c'est-à-dire avec l'avenir, avec ce qui dans un monde où tout est là, n'est jamais là*) (Levinas TA:81).

The interplay: Fertility, fatherhood, sonship, brotherhood

The formulation and terminology that Levinas uses to describe the connectedness with transcendence and the infinite, are complex and mystical. This mystical way of arguing is applicable to the meaning of the relationship between father and son, as well as to the notion of fertility. The relationship of the father to the son, is about a total other. This other has been generated by the father. The implication is that a human being generates another being although one does not possess any capacity to do this. The creature that has been procreated with its own capacity and possibilities, is separate and unique. The time of the father is not the time of the son. Between the two there is an absolute interval. According to Levinas, it is "dead time". The continuity between the father and the son is established in a mode of absolute discontinuity.

Levinas introduces a new paradigm, namely that the chain of generations is not established by a linear, historical development, stretching from the beginning towards a fixed end. It is erected from the future and established by the not-yet. In the same way as how, humanity (the human being with created freedom) is perpendicular to nature; namely, how family relationships like the father-son connection regarding human fertility are related to the natural flow of time; that is, established by the one for the other. The son is not the "product" of the father; between father and son there is no sign of causality. The son is as son of the father a new creation.

The infinite dimension of time (the fertility of fatherhood)

The mysterious and fertile dimension within procreation resides in the fact that the relationship between the father and the son is essentially a relationship directed by transcendence and established by transcendence. Transcendence creates being. This total new mode of being with the ability to contribute to a unique, other being with a wholly different destination than his/her own (due to the factor of transcending), refers to what can be called a *fertile human being*. Fertility is about the fact that a human being procreates another human being without having the inherent capacity or possibility to perform this event of creation. It procreates a being that (on its own merit) also has possibilities. In fatherhood (despite the inevitability of death), time triumphs over our destiny, over old age and fate, by means of discontinuity (Levinas TO:344; TI:258). In other words, the time of the father is finite. In and by means of the son[10], the time of the father becomes endless, infinite, released from its termination (being is transcended by time). It becomes new time and new creation.

Fatherhood is about a radical discontinuity. The fact that "I" am indeed father through and by the son, and the son is son through and by the father, implies that between the two, there is no law of causality possible. The son (child) is not the product or result of an inherent ability/power (*pouvoir*) of the father. The son is in fact "an impossible possibility". Sonship and fatherhood transcend thus the parameters and limitations of the erotic relationship. The unicity between the father and the son is plural. The son operates within the paradox of created responsibility. At the same time, the son renews the time of the father endlessly. The "I" of the father redeems itself from himself by means of fatherhood. This is done without negating its own identity, namely also being an "I". Because the "I" of the father *is* indeed now his son (Levinas TO:339; TI:255). Futhermore, the son as a unique and separate human being, repeats the paradox of a created freedom. In this way, being is about an infinite and discontinued mode of being –historically speaking, a mode of being, without the fate of a deadly causality (Levinas TO:339; TI:255).

The subsistence of a child

Levinas also refers to the infant (child). A child implies a break, but at the same time opts as a resort or recourse (*recours*) (Levinas TI:255; TO: 339). Both break and recourse come together in the child. As a child, the son still exists as being subsistent in the father; but at this stage, the child is not accountable

---

10 Levinas uses gender language that refers to "father" and "son". He refers to fatherhood and not to motherhood. This reduction is because "the male" is his starting point. According to Duyndam (1984), the analyses of Levinas are prototypic and not exclusive. It would, thus, be possible to read "daughter" instead of "son". In fact, at stake, is the unique identity of the child: The parental relationship and the connectedness with transcendence. This relationship exceeds any attempt to control and classify the parent.

for his/her existence, because the burden is transformed to somebody else (the parent as the other). During childhood, the child is merely playing his/her existence. On being a child, thus, refers structurally to a protective existence (*existence protectrice*), namely being and living under the parent's authority (Levinas TO:339; TI: 255). For this protective condition, Levinas uses the term "maternity" (*maternité*) irrespective of the question whether the protector is "father" or "mother".

When the child is connected to his/her past by means of recourse in order to gain protection, this condition does not describe continuity. It is merely about a kind of concretising of his/her history and past as shaped by the phenomena of "mother" and "father". The further consequence is that he/she belongs also to a family and nation. If the connectedness implies even sacrifice of autonomy (surrendering autonomy), then it is not about a loss but "merit": The giving child constantly revolting against totality and thereby constituting self-hood.

In this context, Levinas addresses and explains the notion of forgiveness in a very peculiar and mystical way. The discontinuity between father and son, wherein the time of the father is renewed by the son, creates a forum for a new beginning; a new beginning with the past as well (Levinas TO:344; TI:259). And this is what forgiveness as renewal of time is about.

Furthermore, what is established within this break and recourse is even a renewed devotion to the past. This new start as established by the moment, namely the triumph of the time as the victory of fertility over the transience of limited, perishable, mortal human beings, is essentially a sign and act of forgiveness. Time thus forgives, and as function of time, parenthood is set free (*un pardon*) (Levinas TO:344-345; TI:259).

Forgiveness functions totally as paradox. It is paradoxical in the same way that future, and the time of fertility operate by means of contrasts. It seems as if time is irrevocable. However, forgiveness renews and changes time. The paradox of forgiveness becomes, thus, a constituent factor of time itself. The paradoxical character of forgiveness for offences (offences seem as if time is irrevocable), is not a symbol or analogy for the termination of time (the attempt to negate time); it rather becomes a metaphor for the progression of the human generations and of authentic deliverance (freedom). Forgiveness renders the human generation "new time". It is in this way that the child brings about the renewal of discontinuity; the new generation is rendered time by the fact that they are the sons and daughters of the fathers and mothers from whom they are now released. In a nutshell, this is what forgiveness implies: It constitutes time as a mode of freedom. Forgiveness – in its paradox of continuity and discontinuity – does not only constitute time; it instigates and keeps time going.

Levinas further argues that forgiveness cannot be merged with forgetfulness. Time is in a technical sense irreversible so that one cannot go back to the past. It is the absolute other, an "Other" that holds my past and changes time. One does not belong anymore to this past other than through the grip of the Other. It gives the subject the opportunity to carry on with life as if the offence had never existed (Levinas TO:345; TI:259). Therefore, the attempt to forget is to try to abolish the relationships with the past, and this is impossible. The implication would be to try to return to innocence and that is exactly not what forgiveness grants. What indeed can be detected in forgiveness is, according to Levinas, a "surplus of luck", namely the very strange and peculiar luck of reconciliation. This "lucky reconciliation" is in fact a daily experience. One is not even surprised by luck, because it refers to the whole mystery of time that makes a total renewal within the happenstances of daily living possible.

Offence and wrongdoing in Levinas' mystical desire for transcendence delete all attempts of theodicy, namely the attempt to justify and explain in rational terms the suffering of somebody else, or of one's own suffering. What rather should be done is to turn eventually towards "Good". This mystery of "Good" could perhaps even be the coming of the Messiah, or the eschaton. For Levinas this turning implies a commitment to the Other; conversion is in fact the establishment of a cleansed, purified present.

It is this purified present that Levinas calls forgiveness. Forgiveness then implies that one cannot bypass the injustice done and inflicted to the other. If that is indeed the case, it becomes impossible to ignore past offences against the other. The past must be faced, and justice should be done. It is therefore imperative to deal with the offences of the past. And this endeavour has nothing in common with what sometimes is called "psychic regression".

This is exactly what Joseph did in Genesis 50:17. He dealt with the past in terms of the dynamics of intergenerationality. Joseph's tears were not about tears of forgiveness, because that was the domain of JHWH. It was grief as an expression of concern and commitment to intergenerational connectedness. He becomes "brother", maybe for the first time. And for this act of transformation, he needed insight; insight as an ethical act of trustworthiness. It was as if Joseph was discharged from all burden; he let his burden and control over the past go. The synthesis is transformed into patience, and the discourse into "the voice of a subtle silence" (*voice de "subtil silence"*) (Levinas HAM:32; HAH:11).

Nagy's re-interpretation of exoneration. Towards an anthropology of accountable responsibility within the tension: Levinas (visage) – Nagy (indebtedness)

The challenge right now is to get clarity on the differences between Levinas and Nagy on issues such as revenge, forgiveness and release. An identification of their different positions will help to understand the tension between the two perspectives. That will also help to demarcate the unique character of exoneration. The further advantage is that it can also help to understand the complex character of responsibility in an anthropology of care, helping and healing. Central and common between Nagy and Levinas is the question about the humane character of human re-*spond*-ability in order to establish a human order of justice. Common in both is the quest for a sustainable humane social order, restorative engagements and encounters with the other/Other; human well-being in reaching out to vulnerable human beings.

For both Levinas and Nagy, the central question is about radical renewal of human relationships[11]. That is in a very special sense, represented in Levinas' plea for forgiveness and hospitality. He uses concepts like "pardon" and "discharge" next to expiation and revenge (retribution, appease, repay). Through these concepts reconciliation could be established.

With Nagy the quest for radical renewal is more implicit. That is the case with his understanding of exoneration, and his therapeutic programmes about the healing of violated human rights. Both of them criticize the artificial way in which in some Christian circles, forgiveness had been deployed in the past.

11 One needs to take into consideration that Levinas was a Jew and understood Hebrew spirituality while Nagy did not call himself a Christian. However, even in Christian faith, the renewal of life is central. In the confession of faith, it is professed that one believes in the forgiveness of sins. Forgiveness, reconciliation and redemption are central to the Christian faith. One should be delivered from evil, sin and guilt. Forgiveness is an unconditional gift and sign of total renewal of the relationship with God and others. Central in all these events is the notion of faith.

In terms of Levinas' critical stance, his argument implies the following: In Christianity it seems as if peace is about "cheap grace" – generous gestures. Authentic forgiveness, however, is not a process within a continuum from guilt towards non-guilt, but about a total, radical event of a new creation.

For Nagy, forgiveness is, irrespective whether in a Christian or non-Christian context, an event within intersubjectivity. It is in the first place not about the renewal of people and relationships, but about the change in power play.

The traditional approach was always to deal with forgiveness within the confines of a theological approach. Within the parameters of the research project, the hypothesis is that forgiveness should be assessed within a non-religious, social-historical context. This approach will be in line with Levinas' subjective approach. In this regard, Poorthuis (1992:251; Levinas HS:80) pointed out that moral religious relationships are not established within the horizon of time and against the background of worldly dynamics. The moral religious relationships are concretised as factual forms through which time and space appear and emanate.

The challenge right now is to revisit the notion of exoneration. Thus, the following research question: Is it possible that the reinterpretation of Nagy in the track of Levinas can contribute to a reinterpretation of exoneration and its meaning for human well-being?

On bending the intersubjective space (Levinas)

For Levinas, it is important to emphasize that the subject is separated from totality. Due to this separation, the "unique I" can be defined in terms of his/her place in a system. The subject, the unique I, is an apology. This apology is from the start a position over against the Other (Levinas TO:357; TI:270). The other is the entity that criticises constantly the arbitrariness of my freedom (a result of totality): the other as an investiture. The freedom of the subject is irreducible; it is a created freedom. The implication is that autonomy resides in heteronomy. To the extent that freedom is limited, temporal and finite, finiteness is not defined within the conflicting dynamics of a power play with the other, but from a free kind of subjection; that is, servitude to the other. The different I's do not constitute a social totality. There exists not a privileged forum wherein all the I's could be combined into one synthesized totality. This would lead to sheer anarchy.

The attempt to create a common level or forum for all the multiple I's, will never succeed, because the free play by volitional subjects, is unpredictable. It is impossible to detect the will of the different subjects. Co-existence and living together are never automatically. They cannot be comprehended from a totality. Eventually, within the wavering of uncertainties, a way is pathed when visage is presented, and justice is demanded (Levinas TI:270; TO:357).

Visage is presented in the presentation and giving of a word/saying (*le dire*), and the receiving thereof in rendering an ear to visage. This act precedes hearing. The demand for justice wherein the definition of subject (as "captive", "trauma", "obsession", "I-split", "summon", "addressed") is proclaimed, could indeed be viewed as the start of trustworthiness. The demand of justice leads to freedom, in fact, it could even be viewed as a demand for the exercising of freedom. The demand for justice constitutes opportunities for family dynamics in the establishment of ethical capacities for dealing with inter-subjectivity.

The demand for justice that creates new avenues within wavering uncertainties, is sometimes called by Levinas: "the curvature of intersubjective space" that could be bended (Levinas TO:354; TI:267).

Inducing totality (Nagy)

When a family is approached in therapy as a systemic and networking whole (whole refers to the setting wherein boarders of the one is determined by the power or capacity of another in order to deal with family analyses and treatment), the therapist is in fact inducing a kind of "totality". But this totality does not smother, on the contrary, it shapes the space for the interplay between subjectivity and the other and the introduction of ethical discernments.

This is the reason why Nagy rather works with the concepts of:
1. Multidirected partiality.
2. The quest for fairness and justice.
3. The bid for authentic dialogue.

The therapist operates within wavering uncertainties that inflict suffering to many. Suffering, due to infliction, is for Nagy not merely a private category concerning only an individual but an exponent of ethical entanglements that demarcate the reality of human vulnerability.

In the attempt to deal with the reality of vulnerability within caring and the shaping of trustworthy interaction, multidirected partiality can help families to escape from totalitarian entanglements (de-totalising). It also helps to create space for a healthy "we". The separation between the I's in themselves (detachment), is necessary in order to prevent the formation of an enmeshed totality (inhumane smothering).

It is within this context, that the researchers are convinced that Nagy's conception of the I (based on Buber's interpretation of subjectivity within the paradigm of Friedman) is to some extent naive. The impression is that Nagy does not pay enough attention to the pre-dialogue, "before" the I-Thou dialogue; the wording that precedes the saying, as well as the hearing that precedes what has been heard. The fact that Nagy precedes from connectedness, disempowers the moral freedom of each of the subjects to hear and to speak individually and personally. In terms of an ethical perspective, authentic dialogue does not originate from an already given pre-connectedness, but from the freedom of an I that, ethically speaking, finds it impossible to destroy or smother the other (which often happens in cases of ethical entanglement – even if the other is "father", "mother", "child", "brother" or "sister").

The impossibility is not about a deterministic fate, or due to a genetic predisposition. It is based upon the intrigue of "the-one-for-the-other". The suffering of human beings, when understood as "multi-directed partiality", could lead to the destabilising of totality. The suffering evoked by the suffering of the other, is the only mode of suffering that is essentially not meaningless.

The ethical intrigue does not start with the question: "Where do I belong? It resides in the question: "Who belongs with me?". The most fundamental ethical question is: To whom do I owe justice? (notion of repayment). This question does not originate from a pre-condition of connectedness, applied as a general principle or obligation. It is founded by and through ethics.

Furthermore, the question of the vulnerable child in family dynamics seems to be the following: Where do I belong? (Expression of a sense of belongingness). However, the most mature question to be posed is: Who belongs with me? However, when a child is burdened by the question: "To whom must I be loyal?" or asks within parent-child relationships: "To whom must I express my solidarity?", these questions could perhaps be rendered as being somehow unfair. Especially when the child still lives in a recourse with the parent, and the parent is not yet discharged from his/her responsibility, these questions are quite valid and appropriate.

What is not naive in Nagy's argumentation is his insistence on the notion of "repairing the hurt human justice". The impression is that he precedes from an original consent regarding the "justice of the human order". Thus, the reason why he renders accountability and responsibility as a kind of primordial position. His focus is therefore to investigate how people commit themselves to this fundamental consent.

The myth of the one-sided accountability

When one applies the previous outline regarding a primordial accountability and responsibility to the imperative of exoneration, one must deal with two movements to be performed by the person who exonerates. These movements refer implicitly also to two positions: The position of the disadvantaged person (the person offended), and the position of the critical judge. The offence is basic. But at the same time the following question is still valid: What is the quality of the accountability of the debtor (guilty person) regarding the damage afflicted. Applicable in this test, are the criteria of reasonableness and fairness in order to detect whether the debtor should repay the damage.

The appeal to reasonableness and fairness takes creditor and debtor further than the quarrel regarding the question whether one should grant the other grace or not. Due to reasonableness and fairness, the creditor can decide to abdicate from the position of being the judge. In doing so, a forum is created wherein both are equal and operate on the same level. This hypothetical platform provides an opportunity for dialogue; they can start talking to one another as equals. The fact that this platform is directed by the normative dimension of reasonableness and fairness, implies a general criterion, a kind of "helping construction". Without this framework, the establishment of a humane society becomes virtually impossible.

In many intriguing family matters, or in group conflict, it could happen that a scapegoat is identified and treated as the guilty one or identified patient. How should therapy deal with the so called guilty one?

Nagy and Krasner write as follows: "A therapist helps diminish the myth of the one-sided accountability by rejecting the notion that one person can ever be the sole course of a given family's ills" (Nagy & Krasner BGT:103). This remark is incredibly important. For example, many family entanglements are attempts to point out a "scape goat" in order to shift the blame to one person in the systemic dynamics.

René Girard aptly pointed out that the "scape goat mechanism" is essentially based on a cultural and systemic myth that implies more than merely being a psychosocial aberration. In fact, it resides in real systems of representation (*un veritable systéme de réprésentation*) (Girard 1982:61). This system of representation is on the one hand embedded in the dynamics of a social-cultural order. On the other hand, culture is informed by existing systems of representation. When this system of representation is threatened, the threatening factor must be identified, and all attempts should be to get rid of the disturbing component. In cultural rituals, these attempts could take on the form of exhortation in order to abolish the evil factor (culprit), or emissary victim (*victime émissaire*); that is, the factor that the group believe is the guilty one, the one that threatens the differentiations of the cultural order. Exhortation is then viewed as a magic factor that can help to restore the order.

The mythical accusation is about stereotyping. It has the following features: (a) Excessive forms of power and power abuse; (b) sexual criminality such as incest and rape; (c) violation of religious taboos. These mythical accusations correlate with factors that threaten society/the group from the inside: a tendency of de-differentiation. The myth is about persecutory representation (*representation persécutrice*), or myth of the persecutor (*mythe persécuteur*) (Girard 1978:465-466). Girard refers to an interesting judicial principle in the *Tractate of the Sanhedrin*: "When a jury finds a suspect unanimously guilty, the suspect must be set free immediately ".

This very strange judicial principle means: In the violation of the myth, one recognises immediately the presence of the other. The myth is never the truth. Truth between persecutor and the one persecuted, is established when the one who is being persecuted turns around in order to face the other. When the persecutor then decides to persist with the persecution, the persecutor attains blood-guilt (guilt incurred by the shedding of innocent blood – Hebrew tradition).

To speak of a common measurement, is indeed complex. It does not refer to a "preceding connectedness". It rather reveals the following fact and truth: We are both the same; your I and mine are identical. This acknowledgement brings about true penitence.

"A-theism" as precondition for justice on earth

In Levinas' thinking revenge (repayment) and forgiveness exist side by side. Forgiveness is not normal and automatic. One cannot extinguish evil merely with the aid of a ritual. Even if this ritual is performed in terms of a sacrament.[12]

The argument is that the separation between heaven and earth is total and absolutely. In no way heaven can take responsibility for the earth. What is imperative for an earthly installation of justice, is a kind of divine absence. "A-theism", as trace of God's absence, should be rendered as condition for mundane modes of justice. For these kinds of representations of justice, human beings (in their subjectivity) should be prepared to take responsibility. This division establishes authentic interiority and subjectivity. It also makes inter-subjectivity (rendered as plurality) possible. Plurality guarantees mundane justice[13]. A human being is predestined for subjectivity; that is, a human being is an exponent of freedom, endowed with responsibility. Thus, the reason why a human being is unique (Levinas DQVI: 118).

The reason for an a-theistic approach is to emphasize the importance of human responsibility. A divine forgiveness that overwhelms unique human responsibility, destroys the original structure of the intrigue: The one-for-the-other (*intrigue de l'un pour l'autre*). In fact, it discontinues human responsibility; one can even say: It destroys human accountability. Inter-subjectivity is not established by a "higher order of being". It is not about totality but represents a unity of plurality. The implication is, that human beings, as subjects, are accountable and responsible to one another. They are so to speak, guarantors for one another. When "divine forgiveness" overwhelms this "safety measurement", the affect is that the autonomy of the hurt human being is becoming violated.

The further implication is not that forgiveness is not possible. According to the Talmud, forgiveness is only possible within the triadic sequence: Man – Neighbour – God. Forgiveness is a creative act. In this triad the contribution of a human being is about: Turning around, conversion, charity, remorse,

---

12 See Levinas RA, QLT and MT and his critique on sacramental forgiveness.
13 For the position of man between God (the alpha and omega) see the poetry of Jan Wit, as in *Liedboek voor de kerken*, 1984, Hymn 1.

penitence and good deeds. It is only within the absolute private domain of my interiority that there can be peace and accord with God (Levinas QLT:44; VTL:37).

The meaning of *Yom Kippur* (Day of Atonement in Judaism) is the establishment of true freedom, a true beginning, and true present wherein the ultimate destiny of being human is opened anew. "Turning around" and "penitence" are within historical contexts, "creation". It represents a moment that can be called "present". It implies that past, history and the flow of time, become interrupted; it brings about a moment that discloses future. As prototype, this change is called in TI (Levinas): The birth of a son, or the becoming of a son or a daughter. He or she is a new creation. In this sense we can interpret the gynaecological dilatation as a disclosure of the meaning of atonement.

Towards the significance of dialoguing encounters: Concluding remarks on a reinterpretation of exoneration

From the previous outline on the tension between exoneration and forgiveness and the quest for an ethical approach to an anthropology for helping, caring and healing, one outstanding issue could be identified, namely that human responsibility and freedom entail more than being free from all forms of evil, suffering, hurt, discrimination and injustice. Responsibility is a bearer and carrier of healing and restoration within the networking dynamics of human interactions. Responsibility refers to significance and the quest for humane encounters that transform unjust violating of human dignity. Responsibility is in this sense a sign, a trace, a footprint, a *chiffre* for maintaining a just human order. In this sense, one can conclude and say: Dialoguing encounters are actually signs of restoration, repayment, compensation, exoneration, forgiveness and reconciliation; they are actually meaning-giving or "spiritual endeavours".

It is within this framework, that a re-interpretation of exoneration within the parameters of Levinas' philosophy of primary ethics, becomes significant. The following concepts contribute to such a re-interpretation: Diachronic time; purification of the present; recourse; convergence; destructive entitlement.

1. Diachronic time and the triumph of fertility over the time of death

It seems as if one is far removed from Levinas' commentary on the views of the Talmud on forgiveness. However, if one probes deeper, that is not the case. In a spiritual approach, the most fundamental question is: Can God alone forgive?

Forgiveness is an act of creation. It means: radical new time. It creates time of the other; a radical new time that is simultaneously immediately "my time". This new time is diachronic, thus, the establishment of a diachronic relationship. And no form of synchronisation can extinguish this diachronic relationship. If one indeed tries to do that, such an act will be viewed as an exercise of violence.

For Levinas a sign or trace of new time is the coming of a child; the kairos of "the son", a son. Levinas calls this new establishment of a son (triumph of fertility), forgiveness. The son is "new time" as generated by the father. However, it does not imply that the son is a by-product and caused by the father. Between father and son exists an absolute interval: "deadly time".

2. The purification, cleansing of the present

The imperative of "not to forget", the "impossibility of not-to-remember", penetrates the present by means of remorse and repentance. The child (the son) is a sign of the impossibility to forget. The child is future, and as original subject, searches for recourse within the space of fatherhood and motherhood. The child is also connected to a tribe/group, nation, and family whose permanent revolution (transformation) is constitutive for a child's selfhood. And it is exactly due to the facticity of this child as new creation, that it becomes impossible to forget the past. To try to forget the past, will be to destroy his/her interpersonal being (intersubjectivity). What the presence of this child does, is to forgive the past, and to transfer that what is not forgotten, to a "cleansed or purified present". Due to this cleansing, the mother/father receives in the presence of the daughter/son, a new change. The cleansing belongs to the new order of insight. This new order can perhaps be interpreted as repentance and conversion (turning around, by the son/daughter). This is what Nagy calls re-taxation.

3. Recourse as generational accountability

Re-taxation can inter alia imply that the son/daughter becomes recourse for the father/mother. The surprising discovery is then: I have not realised before how burdened you (my father or mother) was since your childhood. This recourse can also imply that the son and the daughter start to make an appeal on their accountability by posing the question: Father, what exactly have you done; what did you commit? Or: Mother, where have you been? How do you position yourself right now?

This question that makes an appeal on accountability, can lead to penitence and remorse from the side of the parents. The question can even become a kind of guarantee. The child is willing to step in on behalf of the parent by holding them accountable. In this way, parents are saved from guilt and deadly fatalism: Children create together a presence for both parents. It can be compared with Isaac that evoked accountability by Abraham. Abraham heard in the voice of his son, the voice of the Eternal Other.

4. Exoneration as reversal (to turn about) and display of mercy (*chèsèd*)

In terms of Nagy, exoneration can be rendered as a radical turn-about – a kind of reversal (*tesjoewa*) from the side of the one who has been exonerated. What happened is that from the future to the one exonerated, a kind of reaching out has been established by means of loyalty. In principle the parent-child relationship is irreversible. In fact, time is irreversible. The relationship is about the interaction: from subject to subject. It is non-simultaneously. The child that is questioning the parent, is from the perspective of the parent a reaching out from the future that is factually not the time of the parent. The questioning summons the parent to be judged; it can even become an accusation. The child owes the parent a question; the parent owes the child an answer.

This interplay between parent and child, reveals the wonder of being a family. Sexuality and birth carry from start the weight of trustworthiness, trust, accountability and responsibility. The latter does not generate naturally; it is not about genetics. This "abnormality of accountability and responsibility with intergenerational dynamics", have nothing in common with attempts to glorify the nuclear or extended family within cultural contexts. It has nothing to do with artificial sanctification; it is not about the function of the state or the projection of abstract ideology. At stake, is the "respect for intimacy"; the close intimacy of trustworthy relationships that is the opposite of fusion or powerful totality.

The norm for appropriate family dynamics is not about a "good family" as ideal model. Such a model is in most cases an obstacle. The norm is not an ideal, but the doing of mercy and grace (*chèsèd*). Even in settings of divorce, *chèsèd* prevails. It even profiles the practice of all human relationships as ethically structured; intersubjectivity is in fact about ethical relationships (Levinas). This is also the reason why the turning around of the one who has been exonerated towards the one who exonerated can be described as penitence.

5. Destructive entitlement and the making good (pseudo-exoneration) of the unforgiveable

In retributive justice there is often a lot of hypocrisy present in contemporary, global society. Levinas resisted this kind of mischief. He referred to the attempt to justify the violation of the foreigner in 2 Samuel 21:1-14. By no means that should be the case. Although the narrative seems to be harsh and cruel, it is an illustration of the seriousness of violating the right of the foreigner in the Old Testament.

"Destructive entitlement" can be used as a hermeneutical tool to understand the pathological modes of destruction as "grief" about the right on recourse: The right that has never been exercised. The intention is not to justify destruction, but to try to understand the destructive behaviour from the perspective of grief. Far away from the hypocrisy of pseudo-exoneration, far away from a cheap "forgiveness".

The following question should now be posed: But what is the advantage of still referring to "entitlement"?

Entitlement could be interpreted as a kind of capacity and competency of being; as merit, emanating from due care. Entitlement, as connected to destruction, is ethically speaking impossible. One can only refer to destructive entitlement as a tragedy.

As said, entitlement can only be maintained in terms of due care and appropriate caregiving. In cases where due care is linked to revenge, it is not about revenge in terms of what has been done against me, but is revenge about what has been afflicted to somebody with whom I am intimately connected. It is in this context, that "destructive entitlement" makes one sensitive and aware of the grief that forms the basis of the destructive acts. One can even speak of the justification of grief; grief as mode of justice; grief emanating from trustworthiness and is the result of sustainable loyalty to the hurt parents, parents who suffered due to injustice. The parental hurt should be revenged by the children. It is about revenge as obligation.

Directives for practical theology and pastoral caregiving

One should now pose the question: But what is the implication of the previous outline for practical theology, specifically for pastoral caregiving?

According to the researchers in practical theology and pastoral caregiving, the advantage of the previous outline is to backtrack a specific desire for peace in human existence. It is about a yearning to pledge peace; to receive peace and to grant peace. The challenge is: how to live peacefully with fellow human beings. At stake, is the peace granted by forgiveness; peace as a gift. The implication of this peace-giving is a radical transformation in co-existence with the other. In this co-existence and encounter with the other, it is fundamentally about a mode of being, resembling the Trace of the Other. It is about a "strange trace" (an anachronism): a trace of his/her absence. But this trace penetrates the phenomenological realm of being.

Theologically speaking, to detect the trace of the Other, is to start knowing God. It means: It is about the content of knowing, knowledge that can never be reduced to the content of consciousness. The content never becomes an object for the conscious. "Knowing God" implies: To become engaged with his/her trace via the visage of the other. As in the case of irrevocable accountability and responsibility, this knowing is prior; it precedes every choice; it describes a learning curve. The words indicating the personal meaning of this encounter, connection and contact, are describing in fact a continuous, heuristic process.

It is impossible to manage forgiveness in pastoral caregiving. It cannot be structured or organised. Pastoral care and therapy cannot operationalise forgiveness. The endeavour of exoneration is exercised in all sobriety; in fact, it is carried by hope and focused on the renewal of time. This is about a mode of hoping without illusions; it is about tracing the Footprints of the other. These Footprints are copied in the concrete situation of "non-religious time" and "social reality". In terms of a theological articulation of the concrete situation, the modes of prayer and praise are applicable. To speak "about" God (over God), is impossible. Everyone can only hope on God, even when one raises one's voice – only as sign that one should not keep quiet: the voice of a speaking silence. Because it is about the time of incubation – the time of having no words yet (HH Miskotte, personal conversation).

Forgiveness and the quest for sacrifice: The liturgy of the sanctification of life

Mythology contains many stories about murdering of a father, mother, child or brother. They are stories about the sacrificial killings and death rituals. One can say: Literally about a *sacri-ficium*; sanctifying by means of a holy "trick" or ritual. A kind of new life (new possibility) is thereby established for the members of a clan or the offspring. The death of the "identified victim" attains merit with positive affects for the group or nation. It can even render identity to that group over a longer period.

An example is the myth of Oedipus and its role in developmental psychology. In the myth, Oedipus was king of Thebes, the son of Laius and Jocasta. As was prophesied at his birth, he unwittingly killed his father and married his mother. Due to guilt and penance, he blinded himself and went into exile. Sigmund Freud translated the myth into psychological terminology. Oedipus became the prototype of a guilty youth, animated by a murderous rivalry with his father in order to gain possession over his mother. Within the dialectics of hate and guilt, growing into adulthood is displayed as a rivalry with the father (male figure). In this ambiguity, the entanglement between the sacred and destructive violence, a revolving slate, is established.

With this Freudian interpretation in mind, Nagy refers to the fact that the motivational determinative force of merit can be traced back in the history of many nations and religious circles, even in the narratives of families. In this regard, Abraham's offering of Isaac in Genesis 22:1-19 comes into play. "Abraham's willingness to sacrifice his son in obedience to God served as the basis of the covenant which was believed to have pledged God's loyalty to his people. Christ's sacrifice revolutionised the merit of millions of subjected or condemned people for centuries. The self-sacrificing acts of a nation's heroes and the vile acts of their enemies determine the motivations of countless generations of young men who are born into an idiosyncratic merit context" (Nagy F:109). The implication is that the relational structure of loyalty, encompasses the historical network of merit-calculation of a group. The child becomes captured in the struggle of the parents to repair a very ancient injustice. In this process the child becomes the scapegoat for the injustices of the past.

This could indeed be the mechanism of a myth. Myths create indebtedness and open up the possibility of classifying "identified patients".

Surprisingly, Nagy did not realise that in the narrative of Abraham and his son Isaac, it is precisely about the opposite. In this narrative, it is not about the merit of Abraham's willingness to sacrifice his son, namely, a sacrificial murder in obscure obedience to a higher, supreme entity (superhuman being). It is about a demonstration of refraining from any act of murderous killing in order to establish a relationship of non-rivalry. This act of non-rival intervention can become a blessing for the whole of the earth. Of this blessing the offering of Isaac is a vivid illustration and witness. In the Jewish tradition, the story is called the *Aqedat Jitschak* – the bond of Isaac. The point in the narrative is that Isaac is *not* sacrificed, and that is what the merit of Abraham is about.

The narrative is embedded in the ancient tradition of child-offerings in order to safeguard future fertility as granted by the deity. In the Genesis verdict, however, the background is the demand for obedience in order to promote humanity and authentic human relationships. Because in the relationships with the other (*autrui*), the I is immediately related to God – facing the visage. A moral relationship is all-comprehensive. It refers to both self-consciousness and an awareness of God. Ethics is about facing God: Ethics is an optic (Levinas MG:42).

The impression is that the narrative is written as a test for Abraham's faith. The merit then resides in the fact that Abraham illustrated his choice for God over against his son. It was a choice for more holy interests than a concern for his son. In this case, the narrative becomes horrible and an illustration of a perfidious "God"[14].

The narrative is written in the mode of a dialogue between Abraham and his son. It is not about the fusion of a murderous totality, but the plurality of walking together within a gradual ascent of a sacred space (Deurloo in ACEBT 1984:48). The interesting fact in this dialogue is that Isaac took the initiative, and by doing so, he "owns the relationship" (Goedhart, no date). And in the

---

14 See in this regard, the exegesis of Miller 1984. See as corrective, in Isaiah 1949:199 the commentary of Rashi on the meaning of the grammatical imperative in Genesis 22:2 (from the verb "*lqch*").

"yes" of Abraham, he confirmed the relationship, as well as who he is in this relationship. The relationship had then been established ethically. Isaac also responded with the very intimate remark of: "My father", because he had been confirmed as "my son" by his father. Isaac's question about the offering (the lamb) is therefore an indication of the trustworthiness of the relationship.

In Abraham's response to Isaac's question about the lamb, Abraham's answer is that God will provide. This is a quite remarkable response. It is not about an attempt to play down the seriousness of Isaac's question, it is rather an indication of the seriousness of the whole sacrificing predicament: Abraham realised he had to step in on behalf of his son. The question of the son put the father into a position of responsibility. It became impossible for Abraham to give a meaningless, faithless answer.

Within the dialogical dynamics of "my father – my son", Abraham's answer is in fact a promise, a *promissio* as expression of trust and personal not-knowing; a kind of taking a deposit in the now of action. Despite the not-knowing, the answer, the words, bind the speaker. Abraham's words are immediately an expression of action with the further implication of complete commitment, covenantal binding, sacred accountability. In fact, Abraham's binding answer is becoming a substitute, a replacement for the victimisation of his son. His answer is promise and provision as indication of his pledge.

His answer is prophetic and an illustration regarding the absolute priority of trustworthiness of a human relationship that exceeds the narrow confines of mythology. In taking the knife, Abraham's firm gesture is in fact his failure, because the command is not to kill (to slaughter) Isaac, but to raise him up. In terms of Abraham's provisionary and promissiological firmness, steadfastness (an exemplification of substitutionary trustworthiness), the narrative is an explication of the ultimate seriousness of a commitment of one human being over against another human being: *The other*. The whole dialogical event between father and son, becomes a prototype for an existential learning curve and lesson in sacred, covenantal interconnectedness. The answer is about bonding and not about superficial assurance and pacifying comfort. In the saying (the word): "God will provide", the guarantee is confirmed: This is exactly how it is going to be. In fact, both received a lesson in what is meant by the concept: Torah.

The outcome of this lesson is that Abraham called the mountain: *Adonaij Jireh* – the Lord saw. The question could be posed: But why not

Moriah? "Because the place which was most important was not "Moriah" – where Abraham was about to do what God wanted him not to do – but the place *on the way to Moriah* where the encounter with Isaäc occurred" (Goedhart 1978:27; italics VR/MK).

In the *hinnènni* (here am I), Abraham negated his failure (the taking of the knife) and confirmed his "yes" regarding the provision and promise he spoke on behalf of, towards and for his son. That becomes the proof of his pious obedience and God-fearing. Abraham's piety is expressed in the moment when he said "Here am I" to the messenger. It is exactly in that moment that he stopped the murderous killing and exchanged it with a provisional confirmation. The son is not anymore, the guarantee for the father, but is established as a true authentic "other" (*autrei*).

Abraham's obedience becomes an abdication and abolishment of all forms of "ontocracy"[15] (Van Leeuwen 1966:*passim*). Life becomes again "fertile", because it does not revolve anymore around the principle of self-maintenance (Van Riessen 1991:235). In the deposit that Abraham received beforehand, due to God's promise, he did not hold back and robbed his son from JHWH.

And what about Isaac?

He posed questions, but furthermore, in his silence, he put his father back into a position of accountability and responsibility.

And what about the scapegoat?

The price has been paid. There is no need for extra-exoneration anymore. The goat becomes a monument; it commemorates the fact that *the father heard the voice of the son as the voice of the Infinite – the Eternal*. Within the interplay between "hearing" and "speaking", both the father and the son were set free: The narrative and encountering event are indeed about the origin of true, authentic intersubjectivity; it illustrates the true liturgy of servitude – the revival of life.

---

15 The domination of being and the maintenance of a causitive ontology that explains everything in terms of an abstract principle of being: Being for the sake of being alone.

CHAPTER 6

Pastoral care within a contextual paradigm: In defence of "gratuitous subjectivity"

In general, it seems as if care is focused entirely on the interior of our being human. It is not so obvious within many psychoanalytical and psychotherapeutic circles to pose the following question: Is subjectivity predominantly about inner psychic processes within the exclusive realm of personal awareness and ego-consciousness?

The human encounter is about a networking dynamic. To face the other, to approach the space of visage, is to become exposed to an intersubjective context of interacting obligations and ethical frameworks exposing the subject to a kaleidoscope of moral challenges. Levinas (MG:71-72) refers therefore to the fact that the authentic inner life is not about a pious exclusivity and a well-established world. What emerges is the huge challenge to take care of a humane human relational dynamics within the intimate space of consciousness; a consciousness that is like a hut open to all sides and directions. It is as if one dwells in one of the temporary shelters for the *Feast of the Tabernacles* wherein the concrete memory is about life as an exodus. Memory operates like a web of vulnerable consciousness, a precarious, but divine dwelling place for subjectivity.

The challenge is right now to link subjectivity to this humane web of interacting others and interrelated consciousness. The intriguing question in therapy is: What is meant by healing, helping and well-being within a contextual approach to pastoral caregiving?

The objective of the whole research project was to reframe the pastorate within a contextual paradigm and intersubjective perspective. The hypothesis was that "context" is about a paradigm switch from psychic interiority to ethical dynamics of interactional intersubjectivity. The paradigm for healing interventions is not merely personal insight, but the establishment of trustworthy relationships within the scope of the human order of justice. With this paradigm switch, the researchers wanted to explore the term "contextual pastoral care" as indication of a pastoral methodology that can serve as vehicle for channelling the insights of Nagy to the field (discipline) of pastoral care. Traditionally, this field is closely related to the pastoral ministry and the parameters of local congregations. Pastoral care is embedded in the dynamics of the congregation as the networking of ecclesial fellowship (*koinonia*) – bonding in terms of vicarious suffering.

The proprium for pastoral care: The ecclesial space of fellowship

The basic presupposition that can be derived from the previous outline, is that, in terms of the contextual, therapeutic model of Nagy, one can say that human life is portrayed by the prior of a responsibility that precedes all forms of freedom. It does not imply that responsibility enslaves human freedom. It is also not about a freedom that excavates responsibility from within. Responsibility qualifies the networking relationships; the network of sister- and brotherhood, of motherhood and fatherhood; on being a brother and sister within interacting sibling dynamics. However, the opposite is not true. Familial networking does not qualify the responsibility. The responsibility does not emerge from brotherhood/sisterhood. Brotherhood/sisterhood derives their character from the responsibility for the other. With reference to Levinas, it means that even before my freedom of making choices and the challenge of making decicions whether I should act or not, I am "predestined" (called) to act in a responsible way. This pre-status, namely being summoned to act in a responsible way, qualifies the dynamics of sisterhood and brotherhood.

What are the consequences of such a primordial disposition of responsibility for theory formation in pastoral care and contextual-therapeutic insights, specifically for a contextual approach to caregiving?

With pastoral care is meant a very specific mode of care that is embedded in the congregation (fellowship of believers). The question at stake is: What is meant by "congregation"?

The intention is not to describe and formulate a basis theory for ecclesiology. The goal is to detect a few directives that demarcate the basic field of being a church and some ecclesial parameters for reflection on the core character of pastoral care within a congregational context.

(a) On being the church: Congregation in eschatological perspective

The congregation, the church, can be defined as a human, social entity within a messianic perspective. One can even say: The congregation as fellowship (social and inter-humane) within eschatological perspective. With "messianic perspective" and "eschatological perspective" are meant a transcendent infinite; a "more" that supersedes the liminalities of ontology. Translated into moral categories, it means that ethics (morality) is in opposition to politics; it transcends the demands of prudence, even the parameters of aesthetics. Ethics is unconditional and universal. In this respect, the eschatology of the Messianic peace supersedes the ontology of war (Levinas TO:15; Levinas TI:x).

Eschatology does not introduce a teleological system of totality. It is not the task of eschatology to prescribe the direction of historical events. The eschatology (eschatology of the Messianic peace) instigates a relationship with being outside the limitations of totality, or the confines of history. Eschatology explodes in the present without being encapsulated by past and present events (Levinas TO:16; TI:xi). In other words, in eschatology it is not about the question what follows after past and present, but what is eventually at stake in life (the Ultimate Factor): the judgement over totality and history. The infinite passes hereby into the finite as continuous factor: now and forever.

Eschatology has a radical function. It takes the jurisdiction of history and the future away from the limitations of frail subjectivity. The implication is that eschatology summons being (subjectivity) to full responsibility; responsibility, thus, becomes a calling (Levinas TO:16; TI:xi).Peace is about the ability to speak. The eschatological vision penetrates the totality of war (breaking through their exclusive power structures) and imperialistic enterprises wherein nobody dares to speak (Levinas TO:17; TI:xi). Eschatology has a visionary function. It pierces through totality, perforates it, in order to open the eye for the possibility of meaning without context. The moral (ethical) experience does not emanate from the vision, it establishes the vision. In this sense, ethics is an optic (Levinas TO:17; TI:xii). The peace always refers to the realm of eschatology. This kind of objectivity does not imply that it should be embraced by faith alone. It appeals to an epistemology of knowing that is linked to a metaphysical desire.

The previous references to Levinas' view on eschatology, and the possible link to the notion of "congregation", do not mean that the researchers are of opinion that Levinas practises theology instead of philosophy. Concepts like "eschatology", "messianic peace", "vision", "Word of God" within the encounter with "visage" (*Parole de Dieu dans le visage*) do not describe theological practises, but the priority of subjectivity within a spiritual understanding of the meta-horizon of responsibility: The in cognito presence of the divine as incarnated in the vulnerable presence of the other within the now-dynamics.

In a fragment from a conversation with Formet and Gomez, Levinas remarked as follows: In my relationship with the other, I hear God's Word. This is not about a metaphor. This is extremely important. In fact, it is literally true. It is even not about a kind of mediation – it is the mode wherein God's word resonates (Levinas TO:150).

(b) The social realm of being the church in a global world: The plurality of the human society

The congregation is compiled by the human society within a very specific perspective: the messianic perspective. Every part partakes in the whole, every member is a part, representing the whole (*pars pro toto* – a part, taken for the whole). The implication is that every member in the congregation partakes in the whole of fellowship and social interaction in society. Every member is situated within the units and different sections of society; every part is exposed to totality. Believers partaking in the "whole", does not mean that they are absorbed by the social dynamics, nevertheless, every member functions within the relational dynamics of society. This is more or less the situation of all people irrespective of whether they are Christians or not. The difference resides in the fact that the congregation demarcates, signifies the situation (thematises it). The further implication is that the whole of society is exposed to both the "enlightenment" and "critique" of the eschatological perspective with all its possibilities. At the same time, the congregation (the church) lives by the moral (ethical) experience that is established by the eschatological vision. This establishment demarcates a kind of fulfilment in terms of deposits. For example, the deposit of the one-for-the-other principle (servitude and reaching out) as impetus for ethical engagements and caring interventions.

Care and pity are all about traces left by the eschatological Other. It takes place in terms of fragments within contexts that are also exposed to change. It is in this sense, that the congregation focuses on the plurality of society and civil environmental encounters. The congregation is, thus, a compilation not of equals or of people sharing the same values; it is about plurality, the diversity of "others"[1].

The focus on the plurality in society, implies that responsibility does not emanate from brotherhood. On the contrary, responsibility shapes brotherhood.

In this respect, the remark of Zygmunt Bauman in *Life in Fragments – Essays in Postmodern Morality* (1995) that our world is not anymore about my house, city or land (nation), and has become a global entity, is most challenging. Even time encompasses much more than my individual life. However, what is indeed new and unique, is that individualisation, and the fact of global displacement, have become opportunities for personal responsibility. At stake, is the phenomenon of indifference about the predicament of the other (inflation of compassion). Especially when the other does not belong to my family or exclusive circle. In a plural, multi-cultural society, the other has become exposed to the predicament of vulnerability: the "barrenness" of the staring face without context (*contextlessness*). What is indeed questioned in the diverse plurality of contemporary global society, is the authenticity of hospitality and the quality of the care for the other. The facelessness of the masses forces all of us to start "seeing anew". Bauman thus proposed: "… the breaking up of certain hopes and ambitions, and the fading of illusions in which they wrapped social processes and the conduct of individual lives alike, allow us to see the true nature of moral phenomena more clearly than ever. What they enable us to see is, above all, the *"primal" status of morality* …" (Bauman 1995:1; italics VR/MK).

What one should understand is that the plurality of postmodern society is not about an unproblematic synchronising whole. Plurality in postmodernity is complex indeed. However, what is important from a congregational perspective, is how more and more people, from different contexts and cultures, are contributing to the humanising of life. More and more people

---

1 See the interpretation of Strack/Billerbeck (1994:474) on a reference in the Talmud about the concept crowd/multitude (Greek: *ochloi*).

are crossing the borders of national exclusivity in order to contribute to the establishment of a more humane society.

In the complexity of a plural society, the challenge for the congregation is to become "home" for the homeless; the ethical imperative is to provide place for the displaced outcasts in society and local communities. To feel at home is to create space for the homeless; that is, to take responsibility for the other and accountability for the vulnerable.

(c) Fellowship: The dynamics of unity in the congregation/church

The unity of the church refers to a mode of peace as exponent of eschatology. In the dynamics of fellowship, sisterhood and brotherhood lurks a challenge, namely obedience to an absolute command. This command is about a summoning coming from the enigmatic other – the face-tot-face encounter with Visage (De Jong in Boendermaker 1978:128). Fellowship is therefore constantly directed by the presence of the other.

In terms of Levinas, fellowship is to become aware of a metaphysical trace – the peculiar trace of the Other. The challenge is not to try and track the footprints[2], because in themselves they are not signs. One should rather reach out to all the Others that reside in the footprint of "*illeity*"[3] (phenomenology of impersonal being; a sign or trace in the empirical sphere that refers to transcendence: *He is there*) (Levinas HAM:99).

(d) The ethical experience: Execution of the eschatological vision by the koinonia

It is Levinas' contention that the moral (ethical) experience does not emanate from the vision of eschatology, it is rather the execution of this vision (*elle consomme cette vision*) (Levinas TI:xii; TO:17). In this sense, the congregation never possesses as a deposit what has been received from eschatology. However, this vision constitutes the real unity of the church. The congregation/church signifies and thematises the unique human situation

---

2   Although the terms "footprint" and "trace" are more or less the same, "trace" refers more to the general concept of a mark left behind; footprint refers more specifically to the meaningful contour (signification) and character of the mark.

3   *Ille* is the Latin form for the third person. *Ille* is a form of addressing the presence of transcendence by means of traces. Because God is transcendent, already ahead, and only leaves traces. *Illeity* refers to transcendence as presencing: He is there. He is there as trace, is about testifying that the infinite passes through the finite.

from the perspective of the messianic peace. This peace is the vision that keeps the church going; it is established as ethical experience with the vivid awareness of the Highest Other, the Servant of all (Matt 25:31-46; Is 58:6-7) – the footprint/trace of *illeity* that encompasses all the other.

The unity of the church is in terms of the eschatological perspective, always existent in this footprint/trace, namely in its outreach to the other. Fellowship is thus unified around the execution of the eschatological vision. As an ethical concern, the unity of the church is not sacramental because it does not materialise and realise eschatology (realised eschatology); it is ethical and plural.

The ethical dimension in being the church in a postmodern society wherein people become more and more individualised, implies that the Christian congregation should become the open community of brothers and sisters (see Pasveer 1992). This inclusive openness does not mean to ignore particularity because inclusiveness can, thus, become a delusion.

The church is in the first place not a social phenomenon, determined by sociological dynamics. It is essentially established as fellowship – *koinonia*. In fellowship, members partake together in something that is greater and more comprehensive than the sum total of its members and character of its smaller units or particular relationships. In *koinonia* we deal with a community that is not the result of a social contract. It is prior, primordial to all forms of relationships and therefore first. When an outsider enters the *koinonia*, it is of fundamental importance to treat this "foreigner" with dignity and hospitality; to treat the other as guest. The fellowship is not founded by emotional connections. The latter should be negated in order to create space for the other (on becoming a host), sometimes even for anonymity.

(e) The principle/intrigue of the one-for-the-other (*l'un pour l'autre*) in fellowship: Deconstructing the totality of social-ethical entanglements

The challenge in fellowship is to understand the social-ethical entanglements. One should understand them from the perspective of the one-for-the-other (*l'un pour l'autre*) (the diachronic perspective). This perspective is not about the solution of the ethical dilemma, in fact, it is the starting point. It is about the deconstruction of totality in order to boil down to the ethical experience within contexts; that is, experiences that contribute to the disturbance and disorientation of subjects. This is where pastoral care starts.

Acknowledgement (Nagy: crediting) is within fellowship decisive. Acknowledgement entails more than positive "labelling". This mode of tagging is only possible if it is accompanied by acts that deserve acknowledgement; acts that represent deeds of caring, concern and compassion based on the *koinonia* principle of mutual *diakonia*. This approach is not about a top-down model and demonstration of power. In fact, it is a demonstration and enfleshment of the New Testament's principle of mutual empowerment and support (Miskotte 1991:11-12). People encounter one another in terms of trust and confidence. Within mutual confidence and trustworthy relationships, it is possible to support all and articulate (nearly) everything.

(f) Towards a humane society for future generations

Pastoral care cannot be reduced to care for psychic interiority (a psychologised *cura animarum*). Pastoral care is indeed the endeavour to take responsibility for the future of human beings (*transgenerational solidarity*), and the whole of the earth and the creation (*cura terrae*). In other words, pastoral care in contextual perspective is sensitive to the political context and the challenges in civil society (political pastoral care). Thus, the importance of constant critique on totalitarian systems and constellations. Liberalism alone does not suffice. One needs to boil down to justice in the community. What is needed is a sensitive concern for responsibility and accountability in the affairs of familial relationships, care for children and future generations, for excellent education and the preservation of the environment (See Korf 1975).

To be summoned for the healing of people, and to become responsible for the quality of life and conservation of the cosmos, presuppose the sacrifice of stepping down from unbridled materialism (spiritual deliverance). The challenge is to instil justice for all and for all generations. To stockpile money and possessions can indeed be a hampering factor in the challenge to care for the other and to invest in the spiritual well-being of children and coming generations (Hamel 1987:145).

What is most needed in pastoral care within the plurality and diversity of postmodern society, is to revisit its basic point of departure. Paramount for inter-relational healing is a paradigm switch from exclusive psychic interiority to an inclusive and wholistic understanding of care that is focused on the promotion of a humane and just society: The humanisation of caregiving – the fostering of a *humane exteriority*.

Care of human souls as care for justice and ethical networking: Towards an "a-theistic freedom" of subjectivity

Decisive in pastoral care is to maintain care for human beings in their relationship with the holiness of God. This is in the first place, not about an emotionally based connectedness, but to maintain a kind of "*a-theistic freedom*": The enigma of responsibility wherein God cannot do in my place for what I am summoned to perform, namely, to step in on behalf of the weak and vulnerable other.

This freedom is all-comprehensive, including heart, soul and the whole of life. It is very concrete and even material: devotion with body and mammon/money (all inclusive). It is about subjectivity and its link to a "metaphysical desire". God is the total, absolute Other, the Holy One. This relationship cannot be expressed in terms of "being", because the Other is "wholly Other". The focus therefore on the care of human beings in and through ethical relationships; is to maintain justice in ethical relationships, and to support and to empower human beings in their quest for authentic freedom within the complexity of liberation. The intrigue for the other as "nutrition for subjectivity", cannot maintain any form of indifference. In non-indifference, the Infinite is established beyond the subject-object split of a "*noësis-noëma schema*" (intentional-and-intended content of the human mind in epistemological dynamics).

The freedom "incarnated" in the *one-for-the-other* structure (*l'un-pour-l'autre*) is complex and difficult. One cannot hide beyond the masks of totalitarian schemata. Obedience and "re-*spond*-able responsibility" are about huge and difficult challenges indeed. These operationalisations imply the end of sacrificial violence; the deconstruction of self-justification and practice of scapegoating in familial dynamics; they should also result in the abolishment of the "revolving slate". Within the framework of a humane order of justice, the violence and offence toward the other human being (a third), is not to be justified in terms of any explanatory model; not from a systems approach, nor from the notion of "destructive entitlement", or even the threat of the rotating (revolving) slate. In this respect, pastoral care transcends the narrow confinements of exclusive interiority. Its scope is general, universal, teleological and focused on the unique essence of subjectivity within the networking dynamics of intersubjectivity.

Professional pastoral care: Legitimation and social scope (The Word)

Pastoral care is legitimised by the Word. This dialogical dynamic is an appeal to personal re-*spond*-ability – being accountable before the Word.

Pastoral care is embedded in fellowship (*koinonia*); the congregation is the container and carrier of care. Every member is involved and called to helping and healing. Care is not the sole responsibility of the offices in the church (the office of minister and pastoral caregiver). Official clergy are both slave and server. The offices in the church are *essentially* about servitude and unqualified reaching out (*diakonia*).

Even in the profession of healing and helping, the caregiver is "a servant", reaching out to the other with compassion. As representative of the gospel, the pastoral ministry is about the embodiment of religion; it is enfleshed in social and community publics (Josuttis 1988:17). One can understand that members of the congregation often expect from ministers to maintain the existent social order. Their intention is most of times to maintain totality and avoid an encounter with possible distrust and failing belief in the eyes of the other/others.

As said, pastoral care as legitimised by the Word; is a sign of truth and freedom. In a very strange and paradoxical way, pastoral care, in its contextual and social embeddedness, is a strange exponent of "natural religion". It is within all contexts that a human being is summoned to act in a responsible and accountable way.

The traces of humanity: Exteriority and the ethical breach

Nagy's theory is closely connected to notions like "the justice of the human order", "transgenerational tribunal", "the dimension of relational ethics" and the "general, universal scope of therapy". The general component in Nagy's approach is about a responsible recognition of the footprint/trace of humane humanity within intersubjective dynamics. Nagy bases his ethics not in a kind of cultural relativism. He incorporates a metaphysical perspective. The "*humanum* of humanity" is not about a natural phenomenon with its origin in mere empirical experiences. Its origin is exceptional indeed. This strange origin establishes an infinite responsibility. It seems to leave the impression of being natural, however, it is not natural but implies in fact a total breach with what is called "natural". It is about an ethical breach and infringement.

The huge disappointment is that Nagy does not explicate the source for this unique mode of infinite responsibility. In this regard, his silence as therapist is a shortcoming indeed. His restraint can cause huge confusion, because a vague and general comprehension of humanism without any connection to a source, can reduce humanity to a vague value that can be manipulated by the selfish needs and emotional instability of the subject. And this is exactly what Nagy wanted to prevent. He deliberately sets himself off against the totality of an onto-theology that possesses and dominates.

It was Nagy's fear that theology had become too closely associated with totalitarian denominational concerns (imperialistic denominationalism). The real danger lurks that religious groups can try to provide an ideological basis for values justifying the privileges of one group over against another. It is rather Nagy's intention to promote the "ethical dimension", "accountability", "responsibility" and "entitlement" as unique entities transcending the realm of subjective values. These concepts should be anchored in a realm that grants value to subjectivity; subjective signification resides in receiving, not in controlling.

Nagy connects ethics to intersubjectivity. However, the terminology he applied points more to an ethics that is eventually anchored in subjectivity; it is intrinsic and engraved in subjectivity, internalised accountability.

Does responsibility and accountability refer to merely a subjective state of being so that the subject controls the quality of responsibility and accountability (the subjectification of ethics)?

The question should be posed: But what is the difference between ethics anchored and engraved in subjectivity, and ethics as a kind of deposit in subjectivity that can be claimed by the "I", something to be grasped and performed? The answer points in the direction of the following: Anchoring refers to an event that enters from the outside; its origin is exterior so that it disturbs and wounds. Ethics is not the voice of my interior – coming from the inside. It enters from beyond and summons me (Levinas EO:85-86).

When one takes this perspective of "entering from the outside" (exteriority) into consideration, Nagy's approach can indeed be applicable to the practice of pastoral endeavours.

Debriefing: The interplay between subjective encounters (facing the other) and ethical entanglements (indebtedness): A way out?

There is a huge difference between Levinas and Nagy.

Levinas is a philosopher and probes into the paradigmatic frameworks of Western thinking (wisdom). He even formulates in an enigmatic and *meta*-physical way when he wrestles with the interplay between rational analysis and mystical insight. Concepts often bounce back in a paradoxical way with a confusing effect.

Levinas is in search of the original structure of our being human. At the core of his thinking are reflections on the encounter with another person. Meta-physical encounters evince a particular feature: The other impacts on me unlike any worldly object or force. In this encounter the questions pertaining what is good, why does somebody do good, and what are the driving forces behind acts of well-doing, are paramount. These questions are linked to the original structure of subjectivity. This original structure renders access to the absolute other and could, thus, be described as an "objective-structure"; subjectivity provides the key for gaining access to the absolute other (Levinas NP:31).

Nagy is not directly a philosopher although he often wrestles with the philosophical meaning of texts in his attempt to understand the thinking of, for example, Martin Buber. However, he clearly stated: "I am not a philosopher; I am interested in what makes therapy work." He even does not pose the question: What is meant by helping in therapy? He asks instead: What helped really in this case? In this sense, he is a pragmatic in his approach.

Nagy's hypothesis is that there is basically an original intersubjective structure that is ethically constituted. He links with Martin Buber's thinking and the interpretation of Maurice Friedman. He applies their ideas, as congenial with his own thinking, to the field of family care. Familial dynamics and the notion of "family" are the main focus of his practical engagement and concern about the quality of the intergenerational dynamics. It is within this focal point that he discovered that patients are stuck in what can be called "ethical entanglements".

Due to the influence of Buber, Nagy works with the assumption that in all these entanglements, guilt plays a decisive role in human well-being. When patients wrestle with guilt, another third factor arises: Indebtedness towards the other. Immediately, the other person to whom one owes the guilt, becomes a factor in therapy. Since he is a psychiatrist and inspired by systems theories, he developed a "theory regarding relationships" wherein guilt, especially the factor of indebtedness, plays a core role. The relational reality is prior. Thus, the reason why guilt cannot be reduced to the level of mere personal feelings. Guilt is not about a projection of guilt; it is essentially about indebtedness within the ontic dynamics of "being-with" within interactional relationships.

For Nagy, in families, loyalty forms the basis for the appeal of the other, and the intriguing argument that the relational dynamic is qualified by the ethical dimension of justice. This approach helped Nagy with the insight that many forms of irrational guilt that patients believe has their origin in themselves (subjective interior), even irrational behaviour, reside not in the intrapsychic structure of the patient, but in the realm of ethical entanglements and should not be ascribed to delusions. He often uses judicial language to describe the character of these ethical entanglements; "… we have felt, that it is more important to explore the motivational layer in which hope resides for repairing the hurt human justice" (Nagy IL:53).

Loyalty as habitus within the we-structure

Nagy connects justice to the fundamental, irreversible situation of family members in their mutual interaction. This fundamental situation could be portrayed and described by the notion of loyalty. Loyalty is not the result of decision-making and free choices. Loyalty is an ontic feature of mutual interaction; it describes the identity of a person as enfleshed in habitus; the mode of being in familial relationships as indication of personal, self-integration within the "I-we-relational dynamic". The mutual tension between the "I" and "we", has an interpersonal, and, therefore, also an intrapersonal character. The tension is constituted by the fact that individuality and collectivity do not coincide. The further contributing factor is that the "we" is in fact an entity that supersedes the confines of the personal. However, Nagy still deals with this "we" as being the interface of relational dynamics and mutuality. At stake, here, are the notions of "indebtedness" and "obligation". They describe and demarcate the ethical realm of "justice as social dynamic". Due to the influence of Buber, "the between" in mutuality has an ontic status. Thus, the link between justice and the order of being. Nagy calls it the "justice of the human order". The latter is reflected in the quest for fairness within the encounter between parents and their children (the relational resources in family therapy).

Fairness is a decisive factor in the dimension of relational ethics, because it refers to the qualitative character of interactions. Furthermore, relational ethics is important because it deals with what one can call (in Levinas' terminology) "disturbed interiority".

There is a close link between relational ethics and the notion of "context" in therapy.

But what is meant by contextual therapy?

Contextual therapy: A qualitative and ethical approach to interrelationality

Nagy's emphasis on a "contextual approach" to healing, helping and therapy, is most helpful. Psychotherapy could indeed benefit from this more concrete and intersubjective approach.

One can say that *"contextual" is about the dynamics of relational ethics, and the factor of ethical entanglements within the mutuality of human encounters.* As such, "contextual" is merely a concept. In combination with ethics, contextuality can be redefined as *the ethical dynamics of relational interaction, indicating the quality of intersubjectivity*. The advantage of such a definition is that the therapist should not anymore be concerned about a "trick" or "skill" how to manage the situation therapeutically. In the encounter it is rather straightforward and quite simple: Just "plant seeds" that invite the other into the dialogue and summon human beings to responsible and re-*spond*-able responses to difficult life challenges (Nagy & Krasner TGN:321; BGT:277).

In contextual therapy the priority of the third factor is decisive: the other/others and their predicament of being hurt. Context is not in the first place "my" immediate situation, but the setting of the other. Thus, the challenge to redefine contextuality. But by whom? The real redefinition of the relational context can be done by people constituting the relational context.

The people themselves redefine the relational context. This is the prerogative of everybody involved, parents as well as children, grownups as well as youth.

The bottom line in contextual therapy is: to repair the hurt human justice. In this sense, the description of psychic and interactional forces in the mutuality of relational interaction attains the character of ethical opportunities for healing. This is important because the healing of psychic wounds and hurt in therapy, cannot be dealt with appropriately on merely the level of personal awareness. The therapist should probe deeper: in and via an act of interactional humane encounters.[4]

With reference to the critique of Levinas on Buber, it is important to emphasise the prior position of subjectivity. Not the relationship, nor the connectedness is a priori, but the subject, challenged by the intrigue of the-one-for-the-other (*l'un-pour-l'autre*); especially, the ability of the subject to exchange places and to replace him/herself in the position of the other. (Levinas AZ:208; AE:186). The other is already as trace/footprint present in subjectivity. Thus, the notion of responsibility as an *irrevocable* and *irreversible* entity. Furthermore, responsibility represents itself as a relational trauma; that is, the trauma of separation. Responsibility presupposes separation because it does not start with mutuality, but by the summoning of oneself: subjectivity as responsibility.

The attitude of a *multidirected partiality* is, in terms of methodology, important because it opens up different avenues for dealing with intergenerational dynamics, especially, when one has to deal with future generations as well.

The "dialogical model" has to focus on the humanity of the other human being. The objective of "*humane humanity*" is the logos which precedes *dia*-logos. The logos is not about an abstract principle; it is about a face (visage) – the visage of the other. With "logos" is then meant not a "discourse", but the priority of word (a first word) that flows from the visage of the other and presents itself as a trace that infiltrates the field of phenomena. This original "event of wording", is about a foundational plea and command, directed towards "me". In this event, the "me" is summoned, and predestined for an irrevocable responsibility that precedes my choices and decision-making.

---

4   See in this regard, the impact of an introductory article of Buber to Hans Trüb's publication: *Heilung aus der Begegnung* (1971).

Levinas even formulates in a very provocative way: Because the significance of the other precedes my initiative, it has "the appearance of God". This discovery of significance precedes all my initiatives to render meaning (Levinas TI:279; TO:356). This prior wording-event speaks from an absolute exteriority directed towards me. In this event, the me becomes the "I" that can respond with: "Here am I" (*hinnéni*) (1 Sam 3:4; Gen 22:7).

The researchers want to link this first event of "wording", with the LOGOS in John 1:1: "The word planted in you" (James 1:21). Even Levinas refers to the infinite that commands me in my own wording, in and through my mouth (Levinas AZ:210). An irreversible affection (which is to be finished/completed by infinity) is established (*Affection irréversible au fini par l'infini*) (Levinas Trl:26).

Applied to theology, one can even toy with the idea that theology starts with the awesome wonder of "*subjectivity as witness*". In other words, subjectivity is as pure interiority not a secret hiding place in me; it is an embodied witness about what is pure exterior. God draws a straight line with a bended stick (Levinas AZ:210).

It is in fact possible that the subject can reject the calling and unique predestination. For example, one can try to suppress the non-indifference; one can even resist and reject it and, thus, start to practice evil. For example, to start to pretend that one is not the keeper of one's brother/sister. Evil is ignorance regarding the injustice and hurt of the other (my fellow human being).

It is even possible that one can hurt and damage the non-indifference of the other, for example, a child (Matt 18:6). This non-indifference is vital, because it establishes a relationship between unequal entities. It is, therefore, important to have in every society a judicial institution that safeguards the otherness of the other and prevents that the other is moulded into the totality of a mass sameness. Plurality should be maintained at all costs: The social community not as a unity, but as intimate proximity. Proximity then as an ethical category: The presence of the other as neighbour/fellow human being.

Ethics is not like a prepaid deposit inherently part of subjectivity. I do not dispose of ethics, and, thus, envelope an altruistic character. It is the other that summons me to responsible behaviour and non-indifference. In other words, the exteriority establishes the interiority, resulting then in an aptitude and attitude of compassionate outreach to the other. Subjectivity is in this sense, dependent on exteriority and should be tuned in on the other. Unfortunately, it seems that many of the different disciplines like sociology, psychology and physiology are "deaf" for the silent voice of the voiceless; even blind for the faceless visage (Levinas TI:267, 354). Perhaps, that could also be the predicament of theology: The finite is so enchanted by ontology that theology misses the awe of eschatology.

What is most needed is the more of ethical-inspired capacities, namely trustworthy responsibility and fair responses to the appeal of the other. The visage of the latter instills appropriate responses of caring. In other words, the appeal of the other grants possibilities and opportunities. The response (as re-*spond*-ability) realises and materialises the possibility and being options. This realised possibility/opportunity is established as entitlement.

Entitlement and relationality are interconnected. Relationality is a very special gift and opportunity due to its connectedness to entitlement. Therefore, it is exactly at this point that the intriguing question arises: Who is the author of one's entitlement?

The "design" of entitlement: The merit of competence

Entitlement should be reinterpreted as a "being competency" framed by ethics. It means that this unique ontic capacity or competency should be earned. This earning of entitlement is linked to merit; merit not as achievement, but as a gift to being; merit as rendered opportunity to subjectivity. I am, thus, a human being due to granted opportunities.

The problem, however, is that entitlement as opportunity is exposed to indebtedness. One should always reckon with offence, guilt and the revolving slate. What is then most needed, is to be released from the burden. This is where the notion of *exoneration* comes into play. Exoneration is the quest for recovery and healing; the healing of integrity; that is, the reinstitution of freedom – freedom of action; it is about the quest for blessing so that being can become a blessing for others.

In family relationships, exoneration can contribute to releasing the child from fatal transmissions. The one who exonerates (often the adolescent youth) can become free in order to carry on with his/her life. For the parent it offers exciting, graceful opportunities for a new beginning; a re-establishment of trust and new chance to earn entitlement within the setting of harmed relationships. In order to respond to these new opportunities, "conversion" is becoming imperative, namely to" turn around" from destructive to constructive entitlement. This interpretation of exoneration comes very close to what one can call: *the receiving of forgiveness*. To receive forgiveness is about the true character of penitence and remorse.

In terms of the ethical dynamics of forgiveness, it is indeed important to assess the value of the contribution of forgiveness in processes of healing and the restoration of freedom. It has become clear that Nagy's interpretation of forgiveness does not suffice. It is merely focused on the dimension of transaction and interaction (the third dimension). The real danger lurks that forgiveness is reduced to "generosity". The one who grants forgiveness is still the one in control, the director and owner of forgiveness. It is quite interesting that it is exactly this danger that both Nagy and Levinas wanted to prevent. Both had serious critique on the way forgiveness had been exercised and performed in the religious and Christian, liturgical tradition. The impression is that exoneration has been offered as a kind of gain and profit to the younger and coming generations.

For Levinas, evil is not a mystical principle that can be extinguished by performing liturgical rites (Levinas MG:46). His critique touches the area of a top-down duality. To exercise forgiveness in terms of all-powering categories, is to destroy the anthropological and triadic structure of the one-for-the-other.

Nagy's thinking is more or less analogous. The triadic dimension comes into play in Nagy's emphasis on the role of coming future generations, and his attempt to indemnify them from the effects of the revolving slate. Thus, the importance of a judicial approach and interpretation.

Without any doubt, forgiveness is associated with grace. The question is then: What exactly is the implication of grace on the notion of forgiveness?

The "loyal" (gracious) earning of entitlement: The surplus of gratuity

Nagy does not specifically refer to grace in his contextual approach. Entitlement and the connection to loyalty could be rendered as more or less an equivalent. However, entitlement does not safeguard one against judgement, it only grants the opportunity to earn entitlement and to receive it anew. But, as Levinas argued, there exists no absolute, total gratuity. There is only a "surplus" that can be called gratuity (Levinas in Burggraeve 1991:279).

But what is meant by "surplus"?

"Surplus" refers to "amazing grace". It articulates the hope that my resisting stubbornness, my guilt before God, due to the hurt, harm, injustice, wrongdoing, offence against fellow human beings (my neighbour), are wholly forgiven. The only authority in terms of forgiveness is justification by the Infinite (justified by grace alone). In Nagy's terminology: One needs to be entitled in order to earn the entitlement. And this state of being entitled, cannot be achieved. It can only be received. In ethics one needs to deal with the paradox that only irreducible subjectivity can assume responsibility (*La subjectivité est dans cette responsabilité et seule la subjectivité irréductible peut assumer une responsabilité. L'éthique, c'est cela*) (Levinas in NP:107).

The mandate of pastoral care: The diaconic outreach of the fellowship of believers (church) to the other/others

The research data and previous outline should be linked to the discipline of pastoral care. Relevant for the research project is the question: What is the mandate for pastoral care?

In his theory formation, Nagy also wrestles with the question about the mandate in therapy. He identified the transgenerational tribunal as mandate for therapy. In BGT (98) he wrote that the justice of the human order, challenges every human being to partake in the human order. The context of the human order of justice, and the transgenerational solidarity, create together a "silent partner" within the dynamics of intergenerational relationships. For Nagy, the question is not so much about the ontic status of this order, but the fact that it represents the normative factor of justice. In this sense, the transgenerational tribunal, functions as kind of eventual judgement.

Judgement presupposes a mode of personal responsibility that precedes freedom, prior to all choices. This is what is meant by mandate. The *mandate implies a transgenerational solidarity*. The justice of the human order requires that each person contributing to this human order, simultaneously receives his/her share of returns from it (Nagy BGT:98).

"The context of the human order of justice and transgenerational solidarity is a silent partner to intergenerational relationships" (Nagy BGT:98). With this mandate, Nagy wants to make it clear that, in a therapeutic endeavour, it is not about self-maintenance, or to promote a disciplinary theory for the professional field of psychotherapy. It is about an objective criterion (critique of the logos) that expresses concern for the well-being of the other. Thus, the reason Nagy in some conversations referred to the intriguing phrase: "That's my theology".

Contextual caregiving: Guidelines for the practice of pastoral care

The practice of pastoral caregiving should be inferred by two directives in a contextual approach:
(a) To promote the unique contribution of subjectivity within relational entanglements, and to establish the complexity of "the-one-for-the other", "on behalf-of-the-other" (substitution and replacement), within the realm of intersubjectivity.
(b) The imperative of justice within trustworthy ethical dynamics and relational entanglements. The other is always "fellow-human-being" within networking intersubjectivity; interaction with all others as well. One has, thus, to take responsibility for the vulnerability and even the responsibility of the other.

With these two directives in mind, pastoral care is a mode of receiving, namely being taken care of. It expresses and articulates the principle of being *safeguarded by the Word* (Word of God: The need to be comforted and directed by God's care).

Care boils down to ethical concern and triadic responsibility. Therefore, Nagy's noteworthy emphasis on the ethical attitude of responsibility with the focal point: The vulnerable and hurt human being. His emphasis is on the fact that familial relationships are always relationships of care. This is also how it should be: A situation of care and space for learning, nurturing and education. Non-indifference means that human beings should be vulnerable to the hurt and wounds of the other. They should also take caring responsibility for the re-*spond*-ability of the other/others. Without any doubt, vulnerable caregiving is a huge and complex endeavour. For many parents to take care of the vulnerable complexity of their children, can indeed become a painful burden. The earning of entitlement is a continuous process and difficult to establish over a longer period.

Care and the pastoral praxis are framed by the notion of "repairing the hurt human justice". To put this principle into practice, one needs freedom. Freedom to start with repairing the hurt human justice. At the same time, this principle provides free space for practical engagements. This freedom to "repair human justice" can also be interpreted as legacy. Nagy means by legacy, the ethical imperative to the current generation, namely, to discern what in life should contribute to the meaningful survival of the next generation and their offspring (Nagy TGN:476). This discernment is exercised within an acute awareness about the legacy of past generations. In other words, the narrative regarding the freedom of entitlement in the history of a family, is an important resource for providing security for the carer or parent.

One is safeguarded by an active component (I take care and protect), as well as a passive component (there are others who take care of me). Safeguarding is not shielding off or violating independent responsibility. On the contrary, it is a mode of compassionate being-with. When a space of proximity is established, this intimate space is not about smothering, but to safeguard free expression and responsible decision-making. When one steps in on behalf of the other, or acts as role model (a kind of resource and legacy), it can be viewed as a relational resource and act of safeguarding freedom. It is not about robbing the other from freedom and responsibility. In this respect, one can refer to legacy as a meaningful source for constructing appropriate memories. The legacy can also serve as example of how the obligation of the ethical imperative exemplifies what counts in life and what will be meaningful for next, coming generations. It could capture the meaning of substitution and the embodiment of solidarity.

The question can be raised if the ethical imperative and substitutional solidarity are not merely variants of a masochistic morality?

In an IKON-*Interview* (1986), Levinas responded as follows: He is not afraid to apply the concept of masochism when it is about an attempt to heal and not to hurt. When it is about safeguarding and providing security for a vulnerable human being, and to take care of the woundedness of generational interrelatedness, solidarity is not about pathology, but about solicitous care. Safeguarding, and to act as guarantor for the other, should be rendered as a kind of relational resource (legacy[5]) for children and vice versa. It should not be interpreted as a threatening factor. Because, the issue at stake, is to take care of justice, and to establish trustworthy networking in caregiving. In this

---

5 Legacy is not about an obligation to repeat past mistakes. It is about the obligation to free offspring from violating habits, harmful traditions and inappropriate legacies (delegations) inherited from previous generations (Nagy & Krasner TGN:476; BGT:418).

way, a grandparent can opt as guarantor for children and grandchildren. The memory regarding the acts of guarantying, can even function as meaningful resources of what trustworthiness implies. Legacies could be empowering and not dehumanising.

Pastoral care and the diaconic outreach to human beings

Pastoral care has been described as care in order to establish the humanity of our being human, and the challenge to protect and comfort from within the following relational duality: Human being – holiness of God. The care is not so much about promoting the "justice of the order of being", but engagement with disturbed interiority. It describes the infringement of the Other in the self (subjectivity); it is about the character of deep concern; that is, being touched by the other's predicament.

The priority in caregiving is not so much about information and the gathering of data, but about the engagement and acts of involvement. Acting and hearing are not in opposition, but two perspectives emanating from the encounter with the particularity of the other; responsible action and caregiving emanate from a face to face confrontation with Visage. The latter Levinas describes as an epiphany of Visage, established within the longing of a metaphysical desire. In an IKON-*Interview*, Levinas called this event: God's word within the encounter with Visage; Visage addresses and speaks (*La parole de Dieu dans le visage*).

The non-indifference for the other is, in this sense, founded in a unique setting of knowing, namely the otherness of the other. This knowing is not about a free process of decision-making or based on natural necessities; it is about a metaphysical event. In this event, the encounter is not about visibility and seeing of the other. It is not about the intentionality of empirical experiences, the appearances of phenomena or immediate data (thus, not *donnée immédiate*, Bergson 1924). Visage refers to the intervention of a meta-realm within the intersubjective encounter, namely, to be addressed from beyond, and not to be captured by dominating thematising or synchronising totality. Speaking and addressing are about modes of asking for; modes of giving and expressions of hospitality and peace. They refer to the "surplus of truth", beyond the capacity of being. One can even describe them as the bending of the intersubjective space and representations of possible "traces of the presence of God" (Levinas TO:354; TI:267).

Kenotic *diakonia* to the other: Human beings in their quest for justice and helping

In diaconate caring, non-indifference implies vulnerability; it can even be rendered as an empirical exponent of the obligation toward the other (impossible indifference). It exemplifies an indisputable responsibility regarding the misery and mistakes of the other (the neighbour) (Levinas DQVI:116). This ethical vulnerability is therefore a vulnerability regarding the vulnerability of the other; it is about the suffering on behalf of the suffering of the other. Vulnerability is, therefore, in the first place not a pre-psychological category; it is about substitution. This substitutive vulnerability is the basis of care and comfort.

Care presupposes the ability, capacity, jurisdiction, competence, even material competence of subjectivity– the vitality of diaconic servitude. Diaconic outreach is personal; it attains features of the New Testament's concept of *kenosis* – the total emptying of Christ in his becoming human in the flesh (incarnation) (Phil 2:7). *Kenotic diakonia* is about the attitude of servitude and enslavement on behalf of the other, for the sake of the other. This diaconic imperative implies total differentiation and particular subjectivity. Therefore, the call in Matthew 10:35-39 to distance oneself from the family on behalf of the other, is not about disloyalty towards familial ties, but about distancing and breaking (detachment) with every form of totality that suppresses subjectivity. The call sets one free for discipleship (Matt 8:22); one is summoned to act in service of the caller (the Lord). In this diaconic differentiation, lurks the art of transcending all forms of totalitarian limitations; it is about the challenge to move beyond the priority of tradition and family ties – to claim personal freedom and authentic subjectivity. In fact, visage disturbs my personal comfort zone, and I become exposed to the command of the vulnerable face of visage: The command to exemplify diaconic servitude. This coercive imperative is not about bondage, but a caring intervention in order to set one free for the hurt of the other. Not to respond to this command (sheer negligence), in, for example, family dynamics, obstructs the exit to freedom.

Unrewarding servitude

The parable of the workers in the vineyard (Matt 20:1-16) is an illustration of the impact of negligence and disobedience to the call of servitude and diaconic discipleship. It is about fairness and not in the first place about calculation and reward.

In terms of Peter's calculating and quantifying question in Matthew 19:27: "We have left everything to follow you! What then will be for us?", the following parable about the workers in the vineyard is an illustration of the fact that in the entanglement "man-neighbour-God", servitude and commitment in the kingdom of God are never about quantifying calculation in terms of cost-benefit analyses as in the case of bookkeeping.

At stake, are two things: The question about what is meant by a "good act". See in this regard the question of the rich young man: "Teacher, what good thing must I do to get eternal life?" (Matt 19:16). Also, the calculating question of quantified rewarding as return on the investment of service: "What then will there be for us?" (Matt 19:27). The framework of Jesus' response to the good and merit question, is the command and mandate, namely, to exemplify the Torah. That is what good is about. These commandments should, thus, be acted out. The implication then is sacrifice, that is, to go and sell possessions and to give to the poor.

The question in Matthew 19:27-30 assumes that merit and a privileged position are first in a hierarchal order. After the first, could follow a second, a third, etcetera.

In the parable of the workers and their demand for payment and reward, it is not so much about a position, but about timing. The difference between the first and the last is about the time of the hire. The parable reverses time. The good resides in the fact that the last becomes the first. And the deserved place of the first (merit), becomes the obligation towards the last. The difference in time is not made equal by the reward. In fact, the difference has been maintained. The fact that all the workers become interdependent and are in this respect interconnected, is the illustration of "good". This is the will of God. The good is about what is good between unequal entities within non-simultaneous time events. Goodness is not an equaliser.

At stake, in the parable is the exemplification of solidarity between the first and the last. But, where should solidarity start? Perhaps, it should start with the last, because the last benefited from the merit of the first. The parable ends with a total reversal of order: The first will be last, and the last will be first.

The parables put the notion of justice and fairness on the table. It brings us in contact with the challenging realm of ethics. One can even add: the realm of faith. Ethics is not determined merely by the position of the first and the last. The directive is the entanglement "man-neighbour-God" as the contours for clarifying the humane setting of our being human. One can only speak and act within the contours of this triad. It is within this triadic entanglement that the I is summoned to respond in a responsible way. The I is then summoned to become the first, the second, and even the last. This responsibility is characterised by the fact that authentic responsibility is not about reward and repayment, but the privilege of being called and predestined to servitude. It is from this spiritual perspective, that pastoral care can operate in diverse, plural, and social contexts. In this sense, diaconic care can feature as contextual care.

Pastoral care within ethical entanglements and violent aberrations: The challenge of a contextual approach in family care

The fact that pastoral care is involved in the entanglement of others within the networking dynamics of other/others, one must take the ethical dimension seriously as well as its implications for the practice of caregiving. This is where contextual pastoral care comes into play. One is involved with particular subjects within social and community intersubjectivity. This involvement works with the presupposition of a passive ability of accountability and responsibility (Nagy); pre-reflexive non-indifferentism (Levinas).

As pastor, I always operate within the realm of the between (the between of others). The between is not neutral but demarcated by ethical relationships. It implies a relationship with exteriority, determined by justice. Justice is embedded in relational networking and "the other-dynamics". An attitude of multidirected partiality is applicable in the act of caregiving. The pastor should therefore reckon with the ethical interiority of every particular entity involved in this entanglement. Everybody can claim its right for justice and quest for humane freedom in the search for fairness. This becomes a valid claim due to the exposure to vulnerably and hurt: "… a quest for multilateral balances of fairness in relationship" (Nagy & Krasner BGT:399).

The presupposition for the operationalisation of pastoral care engagements, is the following: A human being is vulnerable due to the vulnerability of fellow human beings. Therefore, everyone should promote the responsibility of his/her fellow human beings. The challenge is to probe into the preliminary situation of every particular person separately (inner perspective). Contextual pastoral care is the attempt to probe into that fundamental prior setting of interiority in order to set it straight and to restore justice.

Nagy designed a working model for practical caregiving and helping by means of the principle of multi-directed partiality. In practice it means that family members are invited and elicited to redefine their context ethically.

For example: Joyce was addicted to alcohol and in the process of parenting neglected her two-year-old daughter. In a therapy session, together with her mother, the therapist asked whether he should call her in the presence of her mother, "Joyce" or "mother". In her family, Joyce was always merely Joyce and never "mother". To be called "mother" would immediately imply the connection to her little child. In her response, Joyce indicated that she will prefer "mother". She just wanted to experience, despite the family entanglements, how it feels to be addressed as "mother". To be addressed as "mother", has the implication that the family totality has been penetrated and reversed. The totality has been infringed. Joyce was suddenly challenged by the trustworthiness and fairness of responsibility. She is therefore summoned to act in a re-*spond*-able manner.

The complexity of family entanglements

Familial networking is closely connected to ethical entanglements. It is of paramount importance to deal with family-images, because they can become very idealistic and detrimental in the manipulation of human beings. For example, the family of an unemployed father can become stigmatised in a very specific social and community environment. In many cases, stigmatisation contributes to destructive family entanglements. On the other hand, in a social scientific research project, the identification of unemployment, and its impact on the family dynamics, can attain a different meaning. In fact, it can provide important information regarding effective family interaction and hampering factors in communication.

It is, therefore, important for the pastor, to know how to deal with information. The pastor should take extra care how to reckon with the context wherein the data have been gathered.

A family is not a "holy entity"; it is in the first place an ethical entity. Within a contextual perspective, personal responsibility should be emphasised in order to prevent the formation of totalitarian familial entanglements. The emphasis is therefore on the establishment of personal responsibility and trustworthy relationships with the other. Prior in care is, therefore, not the context of the family but the quality of the encounter.

How should family be defined?

The researchers' preference is to view "family" as an interactional dynamic of intergenerational relationships, structured basically around the ethical principle of accountability within the realm of intersubjectivity. Although socially regulated, family should provide a trustworthy space wherein people could become co-responsible for one another. Due to the factor of differentiation, members are not equal. They should, thus, not become equalised and pressurised into a form of total simultaneity. If it is indeed necessary to refer sometimes to the family as a unit and "holy space", it should be made crystal clear that "holy" is an ethical category, referring to trustworthiness and accountability; family, thus, as dialoguing space wherein people can start talking and conversing freely to one another.

The Lutheran ethicist Trillhaas (In TRE:xi; 1983:1-23), views family as a political regulation that emanated from the marriage of the spouses and their parents' marriages. Family is a very original community already described in biblical times. It can be called an institution of creation (order of creation). However, family should not be moulded into a fixed and static entity. It is rather about a resilient and dynamic space of interaction; family dynamics can adapt and change according to political and economic circumstances.

The child should therefore be under no circumstance be overwhelmed by the possessive power play of parents. The child is a unique creation of God, so that parenthood should be viewed as the continuation of God's creative involvement in the destiny of our being human.

The notion of family as an "order of creation" is also maintained by Emil Brunner. Karl Barth had a different view. For Barth, family is a kind of "emergency precaution/regulation" within the larger paradigm of freedom in society (a community entity). As "emergency precaution", the family still exists under the authority and jurisdiction of God's word. Both Brunner and Barth had in mind the nuclear family unit and not so much the extended family. However, family is not a biological necessity, but more a social functionality (for Barth and Brunner see TRE xi:6).

What one can gather from the previous outline, is that parenthood and the family system are contextual and situated in a social and cultural environment. Within a dynamic approach, discontinuity between parents and their children, opens up a more humane approach in caregiving. It is not the biological factor, or the notion of control and possession, that shape parenthood. One becomes a father and mother in terms of the quality of accountability within discontinuity. Parenthood and being a child, a brother or sister, are determined by ethics. It is determined by the irrevocable status of accountability. This status is not defined and determined by biological procreation, or by the physical condition of being (biologically) fertile or not. Parenthood is not about production and reproduction; children are created not procreated.

As already said, if one still wants to link family with the notion of a "sacred space", one needs to be careful. Sacred must not be interpreted as a "holy and fixed totality – sacred whole". It should be assessed in terms of ethics. It should not be encapsulated by an exclusive approach, disturbing the asymmetry of intersubjective connectedness. In a nutshell, family is contextually determined and embedded in social and cultural dynamics.

This perspective is promoted by David Augsburger in his book on *Pastoral Counselling Across Cultures* (1986). Family reflects the values and customs of cultures. It is culturally shaped and situated.

In their critique on Augsburger's cultural approach, the researchers point out that family is for Augsburger merely culturally situated. The limitation in his theory is that the family system is not ethically shaped. Augsburger thinks more in the line of family systems theory, and the approach of researchers like Murray Bowen. His focus is on the psychic dynamics of need-satisfaction. The most basic need is to be accepted unconditionally (sense of belonging). The therapeutic endeavour is then to address the fear for loss and the anxiety for rejection. For the researchers, it is indeed a shortcoming in pastoral theology to focus predominantly on psychological need-satisfaction without a sound ethical foundation. The further shortcoming is that Bowen's cultural model does not provide space for ethical entanglement, trustworthiness and the unselfish outreach to the need of the others in their quest for justice.

Augsburger thinks in terms of paradoxes: individual versus group; independence versus dependency; love versus justice; horizontal loyalty versus vertical loyalty; biological family versus spiritual connectedness. Dynamics is categorised in paradoxical dialectical units without real ethical embeddedness.

What is indeed to be valued in Augsburger's approach, is that he acknowledges the importance of family interactional patterns that can be expressed in a variety of different formations within different cultures. It is difficult to detect one normative and outstanding pattern relevant to all circumstances and appropriate to all people. In this respect, there is correspondence with the view of Nagy. However, the fact that Augsburger also places family dynamics in a more Christian framework and refers to the sacramental character of marriage, is not convincing enough. The critical point is: He does not found his theory in ethics within the quest for relational justice.

Furthermore, in Nagy's approach, contextual is not in opposition to universal. The actual opposite is totality. The basic perspective should rather be: It is not totality that determines quality and identity, but personal accountability within a relational dynamic that qualifies the whole. In this ethically determined networking, the other signifies him/herself.

Cultural plurality does not safeguard ethics. It does not prevent totality-thinking. It can even contribute to cultural relativism. In order to think in terms of an ethical, diverse paradigm regarding the cultural, plural appearance of family, a different perspective than the cultural and phenomenological approach is needed. Family care should thus appeal to the notion of accountability. And the latter is not the spinoff of culture and society.

Family is constituted by the sustainability of mutual accountability and responsibility. Without doubt, one should reckon with the fact that family is also an economic and social unit. The responsibility is also intergenerational and stretch out towards future generations. Albeit, in the last instance, it is not biology, nor psychology or sociology that determine the significance of family dynamics in pastoral care, but the link between responsibility and the notion of creation by God. The creation paradigm prevents totality and safeguards simultaneously distance and discontinuity between parents and children. Creation safeguards a humane approach to human relationships. The child cannot be possessed and is not the product of procreation. The child is a unique creature and subject. Human beings are accountable and summoned to become keepers for another. Cain is summoned to become a keeper for Abel[6]. This imperative establishes true authentic brotherhood.

---

6   See Cain's response in Genesis 4:9: "Am I my brother's keeper?"

The imperative to care for one another, is basic in pastoral care. It is more basic than several myths that are maintained to describe motherly love. To refer to motherly love as natural is in fact naïve (see Elisabeth Badinter 1989). But to make the opposite assumption can also be part of a myth. Even to accept that small children are predominantly selfish, is an expression of stigmatisation due to the impact of mythological totalities. In his book *An Intimate History of Humanity*, the historian Theodore Zeldin, writes: "… recent observation of the very young (from fourteen months) has revealed that they are capable of many kinds of generosity, not haphazardly, but in ways appropriate to the needs of others. They can recognise people's feelings and perspectives much earlier than was previously thought" (Zeldin 1994:391).

It is a huge misconception to generalise on important concepts like parental love and children's capacity for trustworthy relationships. One should be careful to describe familial dynamics in terms of "natural responses". Familial love is not self-evident and obvious. To a large extent, family is a wonder that does not originate naturally. The wonder and sacredness of the family reside in the irrevocable character of relationships, namely the accountability for that what is always different.

Adjournment of violence

One of the main threatening factors that violate the quality of family entanglements is inflicted injustice. Injustice violates the fairness of familial interaction. Disloyalty robs the other from human dignity. It is therefore paramount that pastoral care should focus on violence as a disturbing factor in the application of the ethical principle of the-one-for-the-other to the reality of significant human interactions. The vulnerability of the other, summons one to exercise solicitous care.

There are many forms of relational violence that can impact on the quality of family interactions. The following forms of violence (violent aberrations) need to be articulated: Authoritative forms of destructing modes of power abuse; education as a totality of manipulation and suppression of freedom; sexual harassment (incest). All these forms of violated subjectivity should be adjourned and therefore be addressed in pastoral care.

Calling in pastoral care

Pastoral care is closely related and connected to the notion of calling. Calling implies, one has the capacity to respond and to answer, not to play hide and seek. Calling implies the following insight: One is predestined for responsibility; one should respond to the command and cannot resist the ethical imperative; one has to respond and act in obedience. In calling one should serve, so that the ethical demand could not be highjacked for unethical purposes, namely, to impose dominating structures of power abuse.

As said, responsibility is a complex phenomenon. It is not merely personal. It is also about taking responsibility for the responsibility of the other. And the responsibility of the other resides in his/her ability to respond with non-indifference. It is my responsibility to reach out to the other and to support and empower the other. Calling is not a psychological phenomenon; it is ethically structured and operates in the confines of predestination (election).

In pastoral care, the responsibility of caring interventions is related to the conviction that God calls and summons. The calling is not related to an abstract principle, or an overpowering dominating force. It is a calling from the true, trustworthy and faithful God. One should, thus, respond in obedience, and start to combat the destructive and violent forces that humiliate human beings; one needs to start caring for the revolving slate.

For solicitous care, natural abilities are totally insufficient to deal with evil. Pastoral competency is not a biological or psychological trait. What is most needed is the exteriority of a divine calling; one is summoned to the endeavour of responsible caring. Care is framed by a passionate concern for the vulnerability of the other (non-indifference). Without this concern, caring is totally inappropriate. Concern is about a sensitivity for all forms of destructive violence. Specifically, the masked forms of violence that lurk in total entanglements that endanger subjectivity.

Education

It has been discussed that Nagy identified two features of family relationships: It evolves around loyalty and the irreversible character of the relationship between generations. Important for the research project is to add the notion of education.

The family as space for nurturing and education implies a pedagogic dynamic; the dynamic is determined by the order of justice as ethical framework for education. The presupposition is that the eventual goal and outcome of the educational process are to enhance the quality of human dignity by promoting human freedom.

Education is a pedagogic endeavour that is focused on a person that is differentiated from "me" and "we" as subject and other. The person is an absolute other. If education is about domination, manipulation and possession, the educator is guilty of an act of violence. In intergenerational relationships, education is sensitive for exploitation. Its objective is to establish peace and success. It focuses on experiences of hurt and wrongdoing; on destructive entanglements in order to promote trustworthiness and justice. Education can be viewed as an opportunity to start with ethics and eventually also to address issues like faith, convictions and questions concerning the link between belief systems and judicial concerns (righteousness).

One needs to reckon with the fact that education, as pedagogic process, is complex. Education is about influencing a free human being. Education does not want to suppress subjectivity, on the contrary, it wants to enhance freedom and to create a significant space for the making of mature, meaningful (informed) choices. In this process, discipline is at stake. At the same time, the challenge is to merge discipline with empathetic concern so that possible forms of violence could be addressed.

It is non-negotiable that all forms of education should respect the freedom of the child. Simultaneously, one needs to take the vulnerable position of the child into consideration. Education is an investment in trust and confidence. It bases the educational process on the ethical foundation of mutual trust and the unique competence of the learner. The learning child is always vulnerable and can be hurt. Due to vulnerability, the "educator" must always take the defencelessness of the small infant into consideration. For this task, the notion of non-indifference is decisive.

In pastoral care it is important to support parents in the upbringing of their children. Therefore, the "for-the-other"-principle, and the responsible contribution of the other, should always direct processes of guidance and learning. Educational guidance is always exposed to possible hurt. It is paramount to always reflect on the notion of vulnerability for the sake of vulnerability. Vulnerability should always be an ethical concern and not merely a precarious affect. Exploitation of vulnerability can contribute to severe forms of anxiety. In fact, it can cause huge damage to processes of individuation and self-identification. Even over-parentification can cause destructive and violent reactions.

The education process should never degenerate into competition and rivalry. Such a conflict creates a win-lose tension and is eventually reduced to sheer power struggle. In education, the danger that the child will always become a looser and exposed to authoritative manipulation, is quite evident.

Sexual harassment: Incest

Incest is a serious form of violence against a child. Nagy and Krasner mention the fact that to ignore fairness in the ledger of parents and children, can lead to severe and destructive consequences. The expectation that the adolescent, or even smaller child, should be sexually available is indeed horrible (Nagy & Krasner TGN:118). Incest is the most severe form of parental "other-violence". In fact, it destroys the important factor of fairness; it is an evil exploitation of the asymmetry in the parent-child relationship. The damage is severe, because trustworthiness is exploited. Trustworthiness becomes a destructive bondage wherein it is difficult for the child to become released. The bondage is so detrimental that all forms of contact with the parent are based on manipulation and inhumane exploitation. In fact, all forms of care and concern become artificial and ineffective. Connections become compulsory and are not anymore based on the sound ethical principle of responsibility and justice. Incest also has long-term implications. The whole realm of trust becomes infected; that is, trust as basis for future relationships such as marriage and eventual parenthood.

The consequence of incest on human sexuality is incalculable. It violates human intimacy and moral values such as respect and trust. It damages the integrity of the other and the establishment of trustworthy relationships. In the pastoral encounter, the caregiver should be extra sensitive for the vulnerability of the other and the fear to trust and to be connected.

Incest also has an impact on the next generations, because they can suffer indirectly from this violated trustworthiness. They can even develop an excessive need for attention and concern. One can understand why the transgenerational transfer of destructive entitlement will indeed play a role in transgenerational structures of loyalty. It affects the notion of "invisible loyalty" and fosters suspicion and disloyal entanglements.

Pastoral care should pay extra attention to the re-establishment of trust in all these cases. One needs to "hear" the quest for trustworthiness. Signs of "invisible loyalty" towards the perpetrator (the father or any other) should be addressed in order to restore trust. Signs of guilt and guilt feelings should be picked up, because incest is an offence, and, therefore, should be made public in order to lead people into sound acknowledgement, healthy remorse and constructive confession. In all cases, forgiveness should not be introduced as an artificial mode of exoneration to just pacify and cover injustice. Forgiveness should only come into play to get closure and establish peace (Imbens & Jonker 1985:202-204; Renes 1994:26) after acknowledgement of authentic responsiblity.

In all these cases, blaming, scapegoating and partiality should be avoided. At stake, is rather fairness, respect, trust and integrity. These values should be restored. It is also paramount to promote dignity when dealing with the victim of incest. A dignified sense of subjectivity should be restored. The person should be addressed as a wholly responsible subject. However, it is not only the victim who should be taken care of, all possible others, also children of the victimised woman, as well as the guilty father or victimiser (Meulink-Korf & Van Rhijn 1995:43)[7].

Towards the adjournment of violence in pastoral caregiving

During the outline of a contextual approach, the core destructive factor in an ethical approach is violence and exploitation. The latter destroys subjectivity. Thus, the importance to give attention to attempts to adjourn all forms of violence. Pastoral care within destructive entanglements cannot avoid dealing with violent behaviour and should meet the challenge to combat violence.

What is most needed in a strategy of adjournment, is *patience*.

With patience is not meant a lenient attitude towards violence. Injustice cannot be tolerated with a mild approach. Pastoral engagements are

---

7   For more literature on incest and a contextual approach, see Cotroneo 1986:413-437; Gelinas 1986:327-358; Nieskens 1995. See also Galle-van Luttikhuizen 1995:36-46. For responses from a feministic perspective, see Van Keulen 1995:8-11; Kosian 1994:45-52; Plantier 1994:52-57. Den Dulk 1995:31-44 also refers to the impact on women although it could have been more nuanced. See also Den Dulk 1996. The researchers are of opinion that more attention could have been given to Nagy's viewpoint on "invisible loyalty". It should also be acknowledged that Nagy's position is more or less in line with most of the feministic critique, especially, on the notion of personal responsibility as postulate for the relational reality. For a more extensive discussion, see Meulink-Korf & Van Rhijn 1995.

preliminary and not about instant solutions. The overall goal is to promote justice in human relationships.

Human vulnerability can indeed become chaotic and cause destruction and injustice. Many family conflicts revolve around accusations pertaining negligence about care for the other/others. If people cannot experience the care, they can easily start to think that nobody really take cognisance of my predicament.

There is an acute need for change and transformation. Conflict needs to be addressed. The change is not promoted merely by identifying psychological aberrations. For change one needs non-indifference, solicitous care for the other, responsibility, vulnerability, the paradox of investing trust in settings of distrust and rejection. When these constructive directors are not present, one can understand why conflict exacerbates and contributes to even more violence in family interaction.

In a postmodern society and the emphasis on wealth and prosperity, adjournment becomes extremely difficult. The social media design many alternatives and options. The complexity of society is indeed an obstacle in the endeavour to adjourn and to limit violence. It becomes indeed a huge challenge for parents to support their children in their endeavour to establish freedom and fairness.

Parenthood and the education of children have become a complex endeavour. The support of the whole community is needed in order to help parents in their effort to establish justice. What should be promoted is social networking and cooperation in order to establish justice in society. It is often the case that one parent must take care of the upbringing of a child. Without efficient support systems, the parent can become dependent on the child for the fulfilment of basic emotional needs for intimacy. Without any doubt, this kind of over-attachment eventually contributes to emotional exploitation and subtle forms of parent manipulation (see Nagy & Krasner BGT:367, Nagy F:289).

The challenge is twofold: (a) Education needs the support of a just society to provide meaningful assistance in the upbringing of children. The society must cooperate with parents to establish intersubjective modes of trustworthy relationships. (b) The adjournment of violence. Anxiety must be addressed, therefore the urgent need for structures to combat fear for loss and rejection. In this regard, an ethical relationship with the Other must be restored.

CHAPTER 6

Towards a reformulation of basic concepts: The measure of familial dynamics (directives and norms)

With measure (normative dimension) is meant: Appreciation (validation) and respect for the integrity/dignity of every person separately to whom care is given and who receives helping and support. The notion of measure is not to design an external principle, but to support family members to start acting in a reliable and trustworthy manner; that is, to exercise mutual care. The notion of measure is introduced to detect and promote the quality of the familial dynamics and the impact thereof on every person involved.

To pay respect for every member and person involved, is a complex process indeed. It includes everyone separately; it should focus on common wellbeing (their common life together) and processes of sharing interaction. This mutuality between every person separately and the social coexistence together, does not imply all the people involved, living together under one roof. They can even live separately (the grandparents, handicapped child etcetera). Not living together, does not necessarily mean a dislocation and disruption in the family. To pressurise family members into one unit is not always beneficiary for all. Thus, the reason that one can question the advantages of "home care". To take care of persons with dementia can become a huge burden for the family system. It is perhaps time to reassess this practice (Pot 1996:141).

The question could be posed how it is possible for a person not living with the family anymore to contribute to the quality of the family dynamics?

For example, a mentally handicapped child has been put in a clinical unit to take care of him, while his parents went away for holiday. In a conversation with the pastor, he mentioned that he was quite comfortable with the arrangement. He was glad because they could get away and his staying in the clinic was his contribution to return gratitude and release them for a period from the burden and responsibility of caregiving.

Sometimes, detachment and being separated, can become a quite constructive option. For example, after the funeral of their aged mother who lived in a frail care unit until her death, the two sons acknowledged that visiting their mother, helped them to discover a new dimension that they were never aware of[8]. Detachment can also become a source for healing and exponent of care.

---

8   See also Thans 1991:29.

The establishment of trustworthy relationships can take on many different modes. In this respect, pastoral care can help family members to convey appreciation and gratitude that otherwise would have been difficult to express. To express and convey appreciation (validation), is not about "positive labelling" but fortification: Support for the courage to be; it empowers the trustworthiness of the other (due crediting) (Nagy & Krasner BGT:59).

The praxis of pastoral engagement

The basic thesis is that the situation of the pastor is about a paradoxical complexity. To respond to the appeal of the other cannot by any means be formalised into a programmatic agenda for caregiving. The real test for the authenticity of the praxis of pastoral engagements is the following challenging question: In terms of proximity, did I really engage with the other, and meet the need for an intimate encounter (caring nearness)?

The question does not imply that pastoral goals and objectives can be captured and articulated as in a manual for reparation. One cannot "produce" and "achieve" change. Remorse and penitence cannot be managed by the pastor. The competency resides in the other (Levinas QLT:50-51). Responsibility is about the "personal secret of the other". To re-enter into the intimate space of him-/her self, is not the task of the pastor, it is the responsibility and prerogative of the other (Van Riessen 1991:248).

The continuous focus on the other in the praxis of caregiving, implies that even the professional capacity of the pastor is dependent on the appeal by the other for qualitative and specialised care. In pastoral care one cannot pressurise the other into caregiving. That will be an indication of power abuse and manipulative care. This top-down approach is in fact a violation of the principle: Being there for the other (responsibility); wait for the other (patience) and being available for the other (concern). What is most needed is an attitude of modesty and respectful humility. Renée van Riessen (1991:237-239) mentions that, besides inspiration and being non-indifferent, modesty is decisive for pastoral engagements and meaningful encounters.

A pastoral habitus is the art of being a host: Inviting the other into a space of care, comfort and compassion. To negate the need of the other, to ignore signs of asking, are cruel. The other should be received and embraced within the strange paradox: The other who makes "my" humanity possible, as disruption of the order. In this sense, the pastor needs the other and not being aware of this reality, is to harm the integrity and dignity of the other.

The art of becoming a host for the other is the question about becoming a fellow human being for the other. This radical change is described in Luke 10:25-37 in the parable of the Good Samaritan. On the question posed by the expert of the law: "And who is my neighbour?" (Luke 10:29), Jesus reveals the key secret of caregiving: To become a neighbour for the vulnerable and hurt other (Luke 10:36). In fact, the caring challenge is about: "The one who has mercy for him" (v 37). To become vulnerable for the vulnerability of the other, is the essence of merciful compassion in caregiving. This is not about a deposit of mercy, but on becoming a wounded healer. The humanity of the other human being brings about change and a radical "conversion". This is not about an artificial transformation from egoism into altruism. However, in the meantime, I merely want to maintain and proof myself (altruism as masked egoism). What Nagy had in mind when he referred to the art of giving to the other and the return of receiving (receiving the other as subject), was to promote humane humanity within the confines of trustworthy interactions. It is in this mutuality that the expert of the law in Luke 10:25-37 was challenged to face his own attempts of self-justification.

The test for the praxis of the pastoral engagement is not whether I am "good" or "bad", but whether I am *there for the other* (available and near). The test is not about achievement, but the quality of a pastoral proximity. In this sense, one cannot "organise pastoral care" and operate in terms of managerial and learned counselling skills. The encounter and engagement are about merciful vulnerability and the promotion of humane humanity. The quest is for justice. And in exercising justice, fairness and trustworthiness, the other is always the critical factor, because I need to face the visage of the other.

In such an unmasking encounter, even hospitality is not the last criterium. The encounter is not about hospitality in itself; it does not reside in the attempt to proof that I am in fact "good". The fundamental and decisive factor is the concrete appeal of the foreigner. In his/her relationship with me, the other, the foreigner, is the one without context; the one that establishes "humane humanity" and summons me to appropriate acts of caregiving.

The quest for methodology in pastoral engagements

A contextual approach to a pastoral engagement is not about a naive approach. Methodology is indeed at stake in order to maintain a qualitative and disciplinary involvement. The establishment of healing, the maintenance of justice and the constitution of accountability and responsibility are not chaotic. Care is about valid intervention and appropriate processes of knowing. Albeit, in a pastoral methodology and epistemology, more than faith and piety are needed.

It is quite remarkable that Levinas links peace to "eschatology". The implication, however, is not that eschatology should be embraced merely by "praise and worship". Faith is not enough. Knowledge within processes of knowing is paramount (Levinas TO:17; TI: xii).

Proximity and an intimate encounter cannot be managed in terms of skills and methodology. Nevertheless, the pastoral endeavour needs methodological directives. A scientific approach and accurate reflection are without any doubt applicable to any form of practical engagement in caregiving. Sensitivity and compassion are instigated by an uncomfortable unrest concerning the well-being of subjectivity (the other). In fact, subjectivity is driven by an empathetic unrest concerning the vulnerability, suffering and dying of the other. It is exactly this *caring unrest* that founds pastoral care and constitutes its mandate. But this mandate demands a professional approach and method-based skills, regarding social interaction and communication. The social context (sociality) is embedded in intersubjectivity and plurality. For a scientific approach to pastoral care, the caregiver must be professionally equipped.

Equipment encompasses thorough training in listening skills and focused attention. To attend to the other and to focus on the other's need, imply more than merely being aware of the other. It presupposes pondering and reflection. It is a sensitised reflection that starts with the other as the primary source of knowledge (*primum intelligible*). The particularity of being can only fall prey to the gluttony of totality due to the lack of wisdom and prudent, mindful reflection (Levinas TO:29)[9].

Prudent attention and mindful reflection correlate with "infinite responsibility". From this mindfulness one can never quit. However, when this

---

9   Bonhoeffer (1970:16-18) refers to ignorance and stupidity as a kind of sin within the realm of evil. There is a destructive interplay between stupidity and the abuse of power. The stupid one is enabled to practise different modes of evil without acknowledging stupidity as diabolic destruction.

attention does not start with the responsibility and presence of the other, it can easily degenerate into over self-estimation. It is the other that constitutes my humanity and cuts me back to size[10].

The epiphany of the other human being is an infringement that creates space and acute awareness; it creates a kind of "ethical rationality". This ethical rationality constitutes authentic freedom (Bonhoeffer 1970:18). And it is within this rationality, that pastoral care operates in a disciplined and methodological way. The *ethical rationality* functions also as framework and source for pastoral engagements and the establishment of true humanity in a diverse, plural society.

Methodology is also applicable to the pastoral conversation. It is paramount that the encounter is not exposed to the exploitation of "power language" and "artificial rhetoric" (see Levinas TO:76-78). Talking for the sake of talking, is a subtle mode of injustice. It runs the danger of objectifying the other. The further danger in artificial rhetoric, is the flattering charm and convincing power of a strict logical argument; rhetoric speech can become a subtle form of bribing, flattery, propaganda and cunning diplomacy. According to Levinas (TO:76), this kind of rhetoric violates the unassailable freedom of the other.

All forms of wording and articulation by means of language are exposed to abuse and manipulation. It was already argued how forgiveness and exoneration can become confused and be applied inappropriately. Many misunderstandings become in this way highjacked and abused in many power struggles.

A straightforward methodology in pastoral engagement is to approach the other directly in terms of *"multidirected partiality"*. Appropriate wording is directed by responsibility; caring accountability framed by calling (predestination). To be guided by the word, is to be reminded that the other rendered me the opportunity to care. This kind of caring is an expression of prophetic vigilance and an attempt to prevent and combat power abuse; it resists an authoritarian stance and the smothering of totalitarian overwhelming.

---

10 See Henning Luther (1992:172) on the notion of the fragmented character of an I-identity. Life is indeed limited, frail and not absolute. One needs to acknowledge the fullness in the unavoidable fragmentation of life (Bonhoeffer 1970:246); every mode of knowledge is relative; life is not one-dimensional.

Sheer ignorance and denial of subjectivity and intersubjectivity endanger pastoral integrity. If helping is about powerful subjugation (totality) (Tieleman 1995:165), it becomes sheer exploitation. And a professional approach should never be about the annihilation of independent, responsible and accountable freedom (humane autonomy). The latter is for example, a huge danger in the sociological phenomenon of "proto-professionalisation" (Brinkgreve 1984; Brinkgreve, Onland & De Swaan 1979:17-24; Achterhuis 1988:294). The danger in proto-professionalisation is that human problems are reduced to disciplinary classification under the label of one category. In classification there is the real danger of subjects becoming merely "clients" within the formal space of a counselling room, run by the so-called expert.

When caring is built upon the deficiency-model, and not on the notion of subjective accountability/responsibility as resource (as in the case of contextual therapy), there will be huge difference in terms of the eventual therapeutic outcomes. There is indeed a difference in an approach that operates with the presupposition of defects or problems that can be easily fixed by an expert (outside approach), and an ethical informed approach. The latter starts with the ability of the other as resource for change. This approach is underlined by Nagy & Krasner (BGT:402): "… the real sign of care is demonstrated in a therapist's ability to let clients go, free of dependence even on the therapeutic relationship."

Pastoral care should opt for a "resource-based" model and not for a pathological approach. Help is about active cooperation from the other within the paradigm of responsibility. This approach does not mean to cast a blind eye for the shortcomings of the other. The other is indeed vulnerable. But vulnerability is not an infringement on accountability. The other is always other within intersubjectivity.

The following directives indicate the confines of methodology in pastoral caregiving:

(a) The group (social entity, family) is personified in separate dyadic relationships. In interactional networking, many others appear in the horizon of intersubjectivity (the third-factor). Differentiation is framed by plurality. The relationship between two, three, four people is diachronic. One should always reckon with the dialectics of equal – unequal; comparable – incomparable; diversity – plurality. The pastor is constantly challenged to deal with these paradoxes within the

complexity of networking and co-existence. In this dialectic a cause-effect methodology in order to synchronise and create a united totality, is not appropriate.
(b) In terms of the earning of entitlement, it is important to detect the potential in everybody involved. In this regard, the application of a (socio-)genogram in family care, can be most effective.
(c) An assessment has to be made how to address concerned issues in the family (group) in terms of relationality. The challenge is to invite others (brothers, sisters, important others) into the space of conversation and the networking encounter. To cooperate with all people involved, is to establish fairness.
(d) The person involved should be challenged to start redefining the context from an ethical perspective. As pastor must reckon with the abilities of people to re-*spond* in a responsible and appropriate way. From the pastor caring interventions require trustworthiness and a lot of patience.

The method of multidirected partiality: Conditional accountable regard

Contextuality implies an attitude and approach that deal with different people involved, even people that the pastor has not even yet met or encountered with before. With reference to the notion of multidirected partiality, the pastor is responsible for every person affected by the pastoral intervention. This is different from empathetic listening skills. Contexual caregiving is also not instigated and motivated by psychological acknowledgement. As pastor I am the covenantal partner for everybody involved within the existential networking of the other. Multidirected partiality is inclusive and intends to support and to help all others.

In multidirected partiality, the order is not to start with the I (of the pastor), and then afterwards to start thinking also about the third. The starting point is the opposite: In multidirected partiality, the pastor is converted to understand that the other is also dependent on all others involved. This insight is also applicable to all the neighbours involved within the existential horizon of the other. "The reversal has to start in the therapist's own mind."

Multidirected partiality is established as attitude of a pastor, when he/she is focused on the fact that everybody lives in more than one relationship (multilaterality) simultaneously. It is then my task to promote justice within multirelationality.

But is it possible to maintain a multilateral position when one is also subjectively speaking in fact merely partial and exposed to aberration and evil?

The presupposition is that for adopting an attitude of multilaterality, one needs to incorporate dialectical thinking within a contextual approach. It is about a different mindset; that is, to start thinking in terms of "and-and" (it is not about the exclusivity of an "or-or"). This approach can be linked to the anthropological starting point: A human being is structured by inter-subjectivity and endowed with a pre-knowledge regarding the difference between good and evil and to accept the responsibility for ethical responses. A human being can therefore indeed be rendered as guilty. Guilt should, thus, not be ignored in pastoral care.

This assumption has got theological implications. From the perspective of faith, one can emphatically state that God's mercy is all-inclusive. The more a human being becomes guilty, the more God's mercy is growing and expanding. More guilt does not diminish amazing grace.

The anthropological fact that human beings are gifted with the ability to discern between good and evil, implies that good and evil are not two equivalent magnitudes. Evil is not the opposite of good. It is a category sui generis and therefore penetrates and perforates good. Evil is a non-volatile (unwanted) responsibility and indication of refusal of all forms of responsibility (negligence). It is not about a reaction over against the good, because it operates on a level lower than good (Levinas HAM:124). Evil only pretends that it operates on the same level of good as a kind of twin-brother of good. However, this is according to Levinas an "indisputable lie" (Levinas HAM:124). Due to this subordinate position of evil, there is the possibility of change and transformation.

Ethics releases one from the natural disposition into the freedom of responsibility. This is not about a once and for all situation, but about a continual repetition in every situation; it is like a Kairos-moment that should be grasped immediately. It is intermittent and an infringement on Being. The implication is that there exists always the option to do good in terms of the preliminary state of original responsibility. But at the same time, it could indeed be rejected, and, therefore, the notion of guilt (displaced responsibility).

A contextual approach should always deal with the dialectical tension: *and-and*. There exists, for example, simultaneously the right to give, as well as the right to receive. The application of dialectics in contextual therapy does not imply that the dynamics of thesis – antithesis produced automatically the unity of a synthesis. The interplay between force and counter-force should be interpreted in terms of an ethical perspective: It is about a dialogistic approach. Essentially it is about the consequences of the art of giving-receiving within the mutuality of intersubjective relational networking. In this mutuality there is always a deficit. Thus, the importance of a dialogue, as well as the dynamics of self-delineation and self-validation. As pastor one will often be present (available) in order to validate the contribution of the other and to invite people to partake in the process.

In BGT, Nagy and Krasner differentiate between "multidirected partiality" and Carl Rogers' "*unconditional positive regard*". Their plea is for the paradigm of "*conditional accountable regard*". The validation is dependent on the credibility of everybody's willingness to take up responsibility for the care of the other (Nagy & Krasner BGT:281). They write: "… it is questionable to presume that therapists are privy to such vast supplies of reserves of empathetic giving, nurturing attitudes and offerings" (Nagy & Krasner BGT:380).

The relational reality within a contextual perspective is much more complicated than in the psychological reality as projected by Rogers. For Rogers, the whole of the relational dynamics is compiled by the client. Due to the goal of therapeutical engagement, namely empathetic listening, the therapist is easily becoming depersonalised as the alter-ego of the client (see Pfeiffer 1991:3). Later on, under the influence of Martin Buber, Rogers started to put both the person of the client and the therapist in the centre of the mutual encounter. But even then, it is still a question to what extent the dialogue has only merit as means for self-realisation. (Friedman 1992b:168).

Rogers refers to acceptance of the client by the therapist. "I'm willing for him to possess the feelings he possesses, to hold the attitudes he holds, to be the person he is … I am able to sense with a good deal of clarity the way the experience seems to him, really viewing it from within him, and yet without losing my own personhood, or separateness in that … there is a real, experiential meeting of persons in which each of us is changed" (cited in BGT:404; also in De Bruin 1983:243). But from a contextual approach, that is not the moment of healing. "The healing moment incorporates a transcendence of the therapist-client dialogue for the sake of involvement in a more fully responsible dialogue between the client and his family members" (Nagy & Krasner BGT:404).

From a contextual perspective, the component of healing does not reside in the client-therapist dialogue or an intrapsychic relation but in the dialogue between the client and his/her neighbours (the proximity of the other/others). Furthermore, the contextual approach is characterised by a "future-oriented inclusiveness" (Nagy & Krasner BGT:331). Applied to the context of pastoral care, it means that the pastor must be aware of the other's responsibility for the loyalty and solidarity of the other towards his/her neighbour (the others).

Solidarity and partiality do not mean that the pastor approves the wrong and offence in the family. Even the relationship of the pastor with every member is determined by the ethical endeavour of solidarity. Solidarity and partiality are always ethically qualified. The focus and scope of the pastor should always be the humanity of each other, and not in the first place the pathology and wrongdoing or shortcoming of the other. Multidirected partiality is focused on the dynamics of the "humane humanity" of the other human being. It is focused on the dialogue between the person being supported by the pastor and the others involved in helping and caring (relational resources of caregiving). In each case, differentiation is pychologically important, between "me" (the pastor) and the other, and between the other and his/her others. This is also an ethical concern.

There are always the pitfalls of identification and transference (whether positive or negative), but the notions of differentiation and partiality should function therapeutically within the dynamics of the other's relational networking; these notions are then monitored by the ethical concern. In combination, partiality and ethical concern help the pastor to measure his/her success in terms of own capacity and amount of input. But, if pastoral caregiving is merely about personal input and expectations, the pastor could become easily exposed to the threat of burnout due to constant negative feedback and personal disappointment (I am a failure). However, if the scope is the promotion of the relational reality of the other, and the question what has been done by others to the other, burnout can be prevented.

Multidirected partiality is indeed complex and always a challenge. However, the advantage is that it warns beforehand against possible pitfalls and promote incentives that help to combat stagnation. It relativises the position of the pastor and prevents that he/she needs to always have the last word. Multidirected partiality warns against the therapeutic temptation to come up with an instant solution (playing God). Multidirected partiality dismantles authoritative approaches (demanding modes of speech) and requires patience. The patience introduces resilience and flexibility in the pastoral approach and attitude with the message: There is always the perspective of change. In any case, pastoral caregiving operates within the unpredictable realm of the good (graceful well-being).

Patience is not about tolerance. The danger in toleration is that it degrades the other to the level of a victim. To be engaged in family conflicts can indeed become stressful. To avoid stress, the pastor can easily try to avoid conflict and opt for premature compromises. But this kind of compromise can be rendered as a form of betrayal. A premature compromise is not the same as premature exoneration. In premature compromise it is an attempt from the side of the pastor to settle the issue. At the background of premature exoneration, is the connection between the pastor and his/her neighbour, based on an ethical concern wherein one should keep in mind the danger of coming up with instant solutions and the artificiality of generous forgiving.

A very acute question surfaces when one wants to apply multidirected partiality to the spiritual realm of life: What is the impact of multidirected partiality on the relationship between faith and God, especially when one reckons with the fact that God is unequivocally partial; partial with vulnerable victims and exploited human beings?

The Bible maintains the dialectical tension between the first and the last; the rich and the poor; the fertile and the infertile, natural expectations and spiritual expectations. Within this stressful tension, the Bible always points in the direction of transformation and conversion – options for all human beings. It brings about timidity and modesty. One's attitude is framed by fragmentation and the provisional character of engagements and pastoral approaches. Eventually, pastoral intentions and incentives are directed towards the ultimate as eschatological promise.

Multidirected partiality is not built on feelings. It is founded by trustworthiness. When the pastor's intention is to care and to help people not to collapse under the heavy burden of his/her relational reality, the attitude of multidirected partiality is meant to support and to help carrying the relational burden. At the same time, it wants to divide the burden based on fairness so that others can become supportive as well.

Caregiving is not easy, in a contextual approach. The pastor has to reckon with the fact that one embarks on a route that stretches from the known into the unknown. The known refers to the identified care and specific desires. The unknown refers to the specific meaning of care within different relationships. For example, experiences of burnout and cases of complaint. The challenge to the pastor is not to act like a referee, because the undergirding intentions in the relationship are difficult for the pastor to detect. The undergirding motivational factor is rather to promote trustworthy relationships and justice.

Justice as frame of reference in contextual pastoral care

One of the fundamental issues in contextual pastoral care is the concern for the ethical dimension of relational networking. The challenge is to boil down to the core factor that determines the trustworthiness and fairness of encounters, namely the notion of justice. In order to probe into this basic order of justice, the counselling skills of back-track-hearing (reverse listening) and the art of connecting questioning (questions that establish trust and concern) are most helpful.

Back-track-hearing (listening in reverse; listening backwards)

Counselling within the tradition of Carl Rogers became associated with the notion of empathy. In the same way, one can say that one of the basic skills in pastoral care is the ability to listen empathetically. This is exactly the case with pastoral care in a contextual perspective. However, caring has to probe deeper than the level of the affective. It must listen back into the dynamics of intergenerational interaction. Required is the listening skill of back-tracking (reverse listening).

With back-tracking is meant to boil down to the basic dialectics of justice-injustice. One wants to listen to the notion of justice that comes into play when one listens through a "judicial ear" to narratives regarding the hurt of human beings. What one wants to pick up, is the level of sensitivity to what is fair or unfair in relational cases and concrete relationships. In other words, it is a listening on the level of "balances of fairness". This basic sensitivity is not primarily on the level of the affective, but about an intensified attention to the undergirding intrigue that shaped the ethical trajectories in life.

In the parable of the Good Samaritan, Jesus deflects the question of the expert in the law by means of listening back to the core issue at stake. The question is not who is my neighbour, but am I a neighbour to the other? Then follows the command: "Go and do likewise" (Luke 10:37). Jesus' appeal is an instruction on how to trace back in reverse listening to the basic challenge of justice and the injust violation of human beings: Go and exhibit justice and fairness.

In pastoral listening the challenge is to listen to basic issues concerning fairness and the failure of trustworthiness. The challenge is to boil down to issues and experiences that are often harmful due to a shortcoming of fairness and the violation of justice. Listening back is not to reveal or to unmask. The intention is to make an appeal, and to listen to what is not said, what is suppressed and concealed.

Connecting questions and connecting language ("rejunction")

Connecting language and questions are derived from *"rejunction"* (putting and coming together) (Nagy & Krasner TGN:481; BGT:420); "... estranged family members benefit from rejoining each other in responsible dialogue". Its aim is to restore and promote responsible dialogue between people that become estranged from one another and are not anymore able to bridge the gap.

The restoration of significant connections can be risky. It can lead to enforced unifications and the impression that reparation is always possible (Kern 1989:33). This is not the intention of contextual therapy. The focus is rather to address the disturbed "balance of justice" that caused mutual suffering.

Re-connecting language is not about reconciliation between estranged members. The pastor rather tries to listen and to articulate so that the person him/herself can start to re-establish harmed connections. The intention is to listen in such a way that a just relationship can be re-established within the relational context. These attempts can indeed lead to meaningful acts of reconciliation, even without the implication of permanent future coexistence and long-term sustainability. The point is: Contact is established with people who were initially excluded.

To apply the principle of connecting speech, is to oppose isolating and rejecting modes of conversing with one another. It wants to promote the goals of multidirected partiality. The challenge is to use as consequently as possible, words, images and interventions that can connect and overcome hurting schisms. To achieve this goal, it will be imperative to articulate and name the differences. It is about the pastoral challenge to pose questions that will help people to describe the conflicting areas in language that can bridge the gaps. Questions can be quite direct; however, they must not cause unnecessary anxiety (Nagy & Krasner TGN:351-352).

The intention in connecting questions is to make an appeal to the otherness of the other, and not merely to the subjectivity of the I. Its goal is to appeal to responsibility and bring an awareness of real partiality. It wants to establish connections with the relational reality of the other/others (the parents in cases of parent-child schisms). For example: "When you were the same age of your daughter/son, how did you find ways to help your mother/father?" "How did your mother/father express their appreciation?"

There are indeed many examples. However, at stake is the principle of partiality towards each person involved, especially the people with whom there were close existential connections.

Knowing one's own relational reality and awareness about possible pitfalls

An important condition for listening and conversing within the framework of justice, is that the pastor should know and accept his/her own context (people with whom I am connected existentially). This knowing and acknowledgment imply an awareness regarding pitfalls and obstacles. A contextual perspective in pastoral care is the willingness of the pastor to ponder on his/her own life story and how it is enmeshed with one's own family of origin. One's life story is inevitably connected to one's own future and ethical entanglements. This is the reason why the pastor needs to differentiate carefully between his/her own space and territory and the realm of the other.

One has the responsibility to respect limitations and personal, subjective boarders. The pastor must not transfer his/her personal dialectics between visible and invisible loyalty due to past experiences with his/her parents (or others/neighbours) to the reality of the other. One, thus, runs the danger of limiting pastoral caregiving to the other. Therefore, great concern needs to be taken not to use his/her own experiences as proto-type (better alternative) to the predicament of the other. The proto-type can lead to destructive modes of transfer and eventually be classified as "distrustful behaviour". Nagy writes: "… that positive transference to the therapist can itself amount to intrinsic disloyalty to the rejected parent and, naturally, amount to negative transference" (Nagy IL:20). In many cases, the therapist runs the danger to be rejected. What has been meant as support, can contribute to failure of the other and be viewed as an infringement on the life of the other.

What one needs to be aware of, is to give account of the pitfall of making the conversational partner very critical and even disloyal towards his/her context. Blaming the parents of the other can be "my" way (subconsciously) of being (invisible) loyal to my own parents. It is, therefore, imperative to acknowledge the border between own subjective experiences and the unique setting of the other. The pastor should always maintain the principle of non-indifference in all circumstances while taking at the same time own infringements seriously without projecting them onto the other.

The application of a genogram

A genogram is a graphic depiction of the family constellation over a certain amount of generations (Simon & Stierlin 1992:125)[11]. It is used by professionals in systems theories, as well as in family therapy.

The depiction is designed like a family tree with different symbols and connection lines. A small circle is used for the woman and a rectangular for the male. Different lines represent different modes of connections with different persons involved in the family history of the people involved. In the genogram, information about biographic data over at least three generations, is used to indicate important events like baptism, birth, marriage and date of death. The focus is on the intergenerational networking, starting with the youngest generation and the current relationship between individuals and the spouses.

The advantage of such an approach for a contextual model, is that facts, indicating important transitions, are depicted within the familial framework of data concerning the dynamics of interrelational connections. It is a very appropriate instrument in pastoral care, because it relates the positioning of members in the family to memories that influenced responses of individuals.

---

11 For more detail, see Giat Roberto 1992:107-120.

It gives an indication of the value of associations and its impact on responsible behaviour. For example, spouses or parents are asked to complete the genogram at home, and then to come back for conversation on what they felt and discovered by mentioning specific data and by drawing possible associations and connections.

The genogram is not so much about the depiction of emotions or associations of different interactions. But in the process of marking the events, the recorded facts (Nagy's first dimension of relational reality) are not merely an attempt to objectify associations, but also to detect the emotional value of interactions within an ethical perspective. In this respect, the genogram is a very handy resource.

The term "genogram" can give the impression that the information is only focused on relatives in the family history. The researchers suggest that one uses the term "*socio-genogram*", because it can also be used to refer to important friends, or other role models that played a decisive role in the lives of the people involved. It can revive memories regarding the impact of others on his/her life and stimulates pleasant associations. It can also bring back very painful events as well. The point is, it can help to link events with the ethical dimension of loyalty, fairness, trustworthiness and justice. Even shortcomings, hampering factors, modes of disassociation and subjective hurt can be brought back into the realm of accountability and responsibility. Photos or other important memorabilia could be linked to memorable events and help to strengthen the associative data and relational ties. In this regard, the genogram can promote re-connection and new modes of bonding within the intergenerational dynamics.

Another advantage of a genogram is that it brings under attention specific gaps in the history of the associations without making necessarily a final value assessment regarding the persons themselves. The information is not used to explain within a cause-and-effect series of connections. However, it can help to shed new light on established connections over a period. Just to talk with one another about the data, associations and connections, can stimulate interrelational and intergenerational dialogue. It can even create avenues for a new, fresh dialogue.

The making and design of the genogram help to dwell on gender issues and complex gender orientations. It probes into the legacy of intergenerational connections and could, thus, stir anger and unfinished business regarding the revolving slate. Even sexual issues could penetrate the intergenerational dialogue and then need attention. Other issues like the absent father or mother can also come into play in detecting the dialectical value of events.

The fact that attention is given to gender issues in the other's legacy can help to reflect on specific convictions, life views, belief systems and modes of loyalty or disloyalty. Furthermore, it can touch on issues regarding intrapsychic conflicts and hampering factors influencing the quality of current connections and the value of existing partnerships. Furthermore, one must know throughout all the interpreted data, cultural and community issues like customs and habits play a very decisive role and should also be taken care of.

By asking questions about associations and the value of the different connections, an appeal can be made on the responsibility of the person for both the known and even unforeseen consequences of actions and decisions. Especially, how they impacted on the other in the intergenerational networking. Intergenerational questioning helps to probe into the dimension of relational resources such as levels of trustworthiness.

One can call a genogram an intergenerational *auto*-biography. It can be viewed as an attempt to come to terms with one's own life-story. It can even reveal the need to be forgiven or to give forgiveness.

In the event of memory as "*re*-membering", the revisiting of data can be described as "*re-biographing*" (M Rotenberg in Kepnes 1992:78-84). These events of *re-membering, re-visiting* and *re-biographing* can be called a probing into relational truths and intergenerational dynamics. This kind of probing stimulates the re-evaluation of personal narratives within the framework of relational-ethical dimensions (relational ethics) and the human order of justice. Its further advantage is that it is helpful in the formulation of connective questions in order to deal with "rejunction" and to make use of social relational resources. On behalf of the present and the future generations.

The spiritual dimension in a contextual approach

Words on connection and associations with justice remind one that the realm of meta-concerns (spirituality) does play a role in daily life events. If one wants to restore justice, it becomes imperative to enter the realm of actions that represents a dimension that supersedes the phenomenological realm of sensual observation, namely the realm of transcendence and spirituality. One does not "feel" spirituality, but rather acts and enacts spirituality as a kind of liturgy of authentic living. This is about the realm of probing the value of responsibility for meaningful existence and significant orientation in the trajectories of life. In this realm, justice is revealed as a soulful issue and not merely a factual judicial concern. Thus, the reason why it is really sad that the discourse on justice is mainly exercised by lawyers and judges and not by caregivers and pastoral helpers. The optic of ethics captures more "soul" than words, affects and scientific facts can do.

In this regard, it is appropriate to refer to the meta-dimension of context in contextual therapy. In fact, context is less about backward and sideward assessments. For Nagy context is open towards the future; towards the other in his/her relational reality of ethical entanglements. Contextual therapy deals with perspectives regarding the mutuality and dialectics of relational vulnerability; its therapeutic focus is on responsibility and accountability to the other/others. This focus should not be interpreted as "contextualism"; that is, the attempt to reduce or relativise the other to a mere product of culture and history.

To avoid the danger of "contextualism", one needs to move further than Nagy's terminology that refers to generalisations such as "human beings". The use of terminology like "*the* justice of *the* human order" without referring to sources and specific data, could indeed be questioned. There is a tendency in Nagy's writings not to identify what is meant in a descriptive sense, and what is meant in a prescriptive mode. One can become confused indeed. Nagy runs the danger and risk to detect and distract from description (people are loyal) ethical prescription – prescriptive directions and ethical obligations (people should be loyal). The further risk is to refer to context in general and becoming vague. Context becomes merely a vague abstract concept – significance without a specific local meaning (context without actual contextuality).

Enacting the context in public: Liturgical dynamics as significant context

Due to the risk of dealing with "*the insignificance of context*" and the danger of "*significance without contextuality*", it becomes paramount to refer to the strange operational dynamics of liturgy. Liturgy as worship refers literally to a kind of public acting out of a conviction of faith; a kind of service by means of public demonstration of the content of faith: "gossiping the gospel". In worshipping it is about a service with symbolic meaning; an act of justice that stretches over one's own death; a service without reward; it exceeds the time frame of the one who enacted so that the result cannot be assessed in terms of temporal limitations. The only secure significant issue at stake is the mode of patience (Levinas HAM:70-71).

When one applies the meaning of liturgy, and the significance of context ("context" as in the sense of Nagy) to the setting of worship in a congregational framework of reference, several aspects come into play.

Every member in the congregation is located within social units that present themselves as totalities without necessarily coinciding with it simultaneously. The discontinuity within such coincidences create unique spaces for creativity and human freedom. This is a freedom founded by original heteronomy. It is determined by a divine Logos pre-existent to the creation of the cosmos (John 16:21). This Logos could be linked to the wisdom (*chokma*) in Proverbs 8:30. The Jewish Midrash connects this *chokma* with the Torah, therefore with ethics (see Schooneveld 1990).

The Logos is about an ethics that cannot be interpreted from the culture and totality as such. It is about ethics as consciousness and subjectivity, as investiture of freedom within the epiphany of visage. It can never coincide with totality. Our freedom is founded by a heteronomy; it coincides with accountability and responsibility, and, thus, needs care. This care is about the comfort of the Word and profiles the identity of pastoral care. Due to the connection to ethics and the Torah, caregiving includes discipline and admonishment.

The discipline is connected to service and determined by the eschatology of the Messianic peace. Rites and liturgy operationalise within this eschatological perspective and are, thus, not about cult or religious enthusiasm. The emphasis in caregiving should become more and more a reaching out (*diakonia*) and discipline (order of justice). It should promote freedom and trustworthiness as expressed in prayer and praise (Ps 66:17).

In prayers of intercession, the vulnerability and hurt of the cosmos is expressed. The hurt is not about fate, but the yearning of human beings in their acknowledgement of pain and suffering. It is a yearning for mercy; it makes an appeal to the pity and compassion of God (*rachamim*). It is his pity that sets free in ourselves a resource of compassionate being-with the predicament of the other/others. It wants to re-establish justice within the context of relational and ethical dynamics. The eventual and ultimate peace of the messianic future becomes the measure and normative criterion for the present as expressed in the mode of praise and worship.

Due to multidirected partiality, the pastor becomes in the event of liturgical intercession aware of the need of people, whether they are victims or perpetrators. Differentiation in this regard, is unavoidable. However, the pastor never has to act like a judgemental referee.

As in this case of prayer and praise, proclamation does not focus in the first place on emotions as key factors for relevant exegesis and the hermeneutics of preaching. Even the making of homiletical choices, should be inferred by consciousness and a critical intra-dialogue with oneself due to the appeal of the other. In this regard, the discipline of a reading schedule is congruent with a contextual perspective. To proclaim the word according to a schedule, can become a very appropriate homiletical form of discipline. In fact, the Other addresses the preacher; the text is in fact a critique on the intentions of the pastor/minister.

Proclamation is indeed a mode of infringement. It penetrates all areas of life, and should address not only shortcomings, but also constructive possible contributions. In this sense, it is always an infringement. However, the intention is to establish trust and to promote acknowledgement and trustworthiness. The focal point is not to address the traditional classified status of a human being (whore or deceiver), but to promote the competence to give, to reach out, to receive without even knowing about it (Matt 21:28-32).

Due to the notion of giving and receiving, prayer as thanksgiving is important. It creates an opportunity to dwell and ponder on what has been given and received; it instigates a deep sense of gratitude. In this way intercession transforms the person who is praying for the other into a humane subject of care and compassion (Boendermaker 1978:67). By means of intercession, a humane mode of justice is established. This is what is established in the so-called event of naming during baptism. In the naming, the person or child is connected to The Name (as already connected with her/ him).[12]

The establishment of trustworthy connections can even be helpful in terminal care and be applied for processes of mourning, grieving and comfort at funerals. Caregiving reveals not only compassionate being-with, but also

---

12 For the practice of providing guarantees and the connection with baptism, see Oskamp 1988:127-128; also for the reference to Nagy and the notion of transgenerational solidarity.

promotes trustworthy associations, and memories that do justice to the beloved and deceased one. The focus is then not on the affective side of mourning, but to pay respect to the value and dignity of the other. Even here, ethics is prior.

Concluding remarks

One can conclude and say that according to Levinas, eschatology is about the possibility of significance or meaning without context. This formulation is quite exceptional. To refer to this very strange formulation of Levinas at the end of an outline that has dealt predominantly with pastoral care in a contextual perspective, needs some clarification.

What Levinas had in mind, is the Other. In fact, it is the face/visage of the Other that has significance. It is not a sign of some-*thing*, or somebody else. The other is in this sense unique. This unique significance is an appeal, a yearning, eventually without language (a voiceless voice, a silent sound), but with a clear articulation: "To whom it may concern" (Schneider in: Cahier de L'Herne 1991:506). In this yearning and appeal, there is a deep need for contextual listening.

The appeal to reverse listening and intergenerational sensitivity is always concretely situated and contextual. The context frames significance and constitutes the hermeneutical framework of intersubjective caregiving. The context creates the social fabric of relational networking. The context is a "living organism", consisting and representing living human beings. It encompasses historical events, social and cultural networks. Contexts determine directives, obligations, merit, guilt and indebtedness. Especially to human beings who are sensitive to the calling of visage. Within the framework of responsibility and subjectivity, Nagy calls this network: The ethical fabric of human existence.

According to Nagy, in all these processes of relational interaction and ethical dynamics, the core issues at stake are "concern" and "care". Care loses its impact when it is separated from ethics and the principle of justice in human encounters. "Giving and receiving"; "compassionate being-with" within the interconnectedness of intersubjectivity, are always exposed to moral issues within daily events.

The reference to "concern" and "care," is not about the abstract idealism of sheer functionalism. It is without any illusion an expression of hope!

Care will become an illusion if it is driven by a normative ideal of what a "good relationship" ought to be. It becomes an illusion when the reality of the people involved, become subjugated to the totalitarian power of an abstract value. It will become merely functional when the relationship is described from the perspective of the effectivity of functions: The prescribed significance of social role fulfilment; psychological needs and sheer complementary need-satisfaction.

Human beings are neither angels nor animals; they are merely vulnerable beings in their quest for significant, humane modes of existence. Therefore, pastoral care in a contextual perspective, is about a way and praxis that assist, support and guide human beings to create together a space for the regaining/reclaiming of humanity within the realm of suffering and vulnerability. Instead of using the concept "vulnerability", and the notion of being vulnerable to one another, one could say: To be constantly exposed to one another (the mutuality of openness and substitution or replacement). In this fundamental co-human exposure, the quest for what is just and fair within contexts, is expressed by means of sincere modes of humane co-existence.

Co-humanity creates space for the preliminary human competence to be more concerned about the vulnerability and dying of the other than about own fears and concerns (consciousness and the investiture of "my" freedom). For appropriate caregiving it is posited that a "contextual perspective" is the paradigmatic framework wherein human beings is viewed within the competence/ability of their irrevocable responsibility – responsibility characterised as election; a predestined kind of calling; a mode of an existential "birth right". According to Levinas, the curvature of the intersubjective space could perhaps be signified as a mode of "divine presence": "God in cognito".

This presence opens up the context for true contextuality: It signifies a situation wherein even "meaning without a context" becomes possible and feasible. This is what pastoral care wants to promote: Humane encounters within the vulnerable and frail space of the other; the establishment of trustworthy interactions in society and the public space of communities.

Bibliography

Publications by Nagy, Spark, Krasner and co-authors

Boszormenyi-Nagy, Ivan & J.L. Framo eds., 1965. *Intensive family therapy*, New York: Brunner & Mazel. Also included in this publication:
Boszormenyi-Nagy, Ivan, 1965(a). *A theory of relationships: Experience and transaction* (pp. 33-86).
Dez. 1965(b). *Intensive family therapy as process* (pp. 87-143).

IL – Boszormenyi-Nagy, Ivan & Geraldine M. Spark, 1973. *Invisible Loyalties*, New York, NY: Harper & Row.

Boszormenyi-Nagy, Ivan, 1977. Mann und Frau – Verdienstkonten in den Geslechtsrollen, in: *Familiendynamik – Interdisziplinare Zeitschrift fur Praxis und Forschung* 2/1, pp. 1-10.

DB – Boszormenyi-Nagy, Ivan, 1975. Dialektische Betrachtung der Intergenerationen Familientherapie, in: *Ehe* 1975/3+4, pp. 117-131.

BGT- Boszormenyi-Nagy, Ivan & Barbara R. Krasner, 1986. *Between Give and Take – a Clinical Guide to Contextual Therapy*, New York, NY: Brunner & Mazel.

F – Boszormenyi-Nagy, Ivan, 1987. *Foundations of Contextual Therapy (Collected Papers)*, New York, NY: Brunner & Mazel.

Boszormenyi-Nagy, Ivan, 1995-1996. The Field of Family Therapy: Review and Mandate, in: *AFTA Newsletter*, Winter 1995-96, pp. 32-36.

Boszormenyi-Nagy, Ivan & D. Ulrich, 1981. Contextual Therapy, in: A.S. Gurman en D.P. Kniskern eds. *Handbook of Family Therapy*, pp. 159-186. New York, NY: Brunner & Mazel.

Krasner, Barbara R., Questing for Trustworthy Existence, 1986. in: *The Journal of Christian Healing* 8/2, pp. 11-17.

Krasner, Barbara R., 1991. *Adult Children, Adult Parents: Key to Direct Address*. Paper presented on a conference to honour the legacy of Martin Buber. San Diego, California. (12 pp.)

Krasner. Barbara R. & Austin J Joyce, 1991. *Ethical Imagination – Repairing the Breach*. Paper presented on a conference to honour the legacy of Martin Buber. San Diego, California. (11 pp.)

Krasner, Barbara R. & Austin J. Joyce, 1989. Male Invisibility: Breaking the Silence, in: *The Journal of Christian Healing* 11/1, pp. l6-21.

Interview with Ivan Nagy (VR/MK), on *20-1-1995 (*Not published*)*. The manuscript refers to the original English text. In the text there will be one citate from the Dutch text by authors (VR/MK). The text from an Interview on 20/1/1992 is not published officially. There is no hard copy, only field notes taken by the researchers. This text is differentiated from the 20/1/1992 text by its date:20/1/1995.

Citated translations

TGN – Boszormenyi-Nagy, Ivan & Barbara R. Krasner, 1994. *Tussen geven en nemen – over contextuele therapie*, Haarlem: De Toorts. Original title: *Between Give and Take*. Translation: Nelly Bakhuizen.

Publications by Buber

-, 1962. *Werke I – Schriften zur Philosophie,* München: Kösel/Heidelberg: Lambert Schneider.

SuSg – *Schuld und Schuldgefühle,* in: Werke I, München 1962(a) pp. 475-502. Also published in: *Psychiatry* 20, 1957, pp. 114-129, under the following title: *Guilt and Guilt feelings.* Original as presentation at the *Washington School for Psychiatry,* April 1957.

Logos – Zwei Reden, Heidelberg 1962(b). (Containing: *Das Wort, das gesprochen wird. Dem gemeinschaftlichen Folgen.*)

-, 1965. *Das dialogische Prinzip.* Heidelberg: Lambert Schneider. Including: *Ich und Du* (Also: Nachwort), *Zweisprache, Die Frage an den Einzelnen, Elemente des Zwischenmenslichen.*

-, 1965(a)/1988. *The Knowledge of Man – a Philosophy of the Interhuman, Selected essays,* London: Allen & Unwin /Atlantic Highlands, NJ: Humanities Press international. Translated by: Maurice Friedman and Ronald Gregor Smith. Including an introductory essay by Maurice Friedman. In the new edition is included an introduction by Alan Udorff. The latter is often cited by Friedman. See also in bibliography of **IL** as well as in **BGT**. The publication contains English translations from the following German essays:

Urdistanz und Beziehung; Elemente des Zwischenmenslichen; Dem gemeinschaftlichen Folgen; Das Wort, das gesprochen wird; Schuld und Schuldgefühle; Der Mensch und sein Gebild. Also the text of the dialogue between Buber and Carl Rogers from 1957 (University of Michigan).

Cited translations

-, 1966. Genezing door ontmoeting, in: Martin Buber, 1966. *Sluitsteen,* Rotterdam: Lemniscaat, pp. 134-139. Original title: *Heilung aus der Begegnung.* See also: Hans Trüb. Orginal title: *Nachlese.* Translation: M.M. van Hengel-Baauw (prose) & Sunya F. des Tombe (poetry).

SeSg – *Schuld en schuldgevoelens.* in: Tom de Bruin red., 1983. *Adam waar ben je?* Hilversum: B.Folkertsma Stichting voor Talmudica, pp. 207-236. Translation: H. de Bie.

Publications by Levinas

EE – 1986. *De l'existence a l'existant,* Paris: Vrin. (1947: Fontaine)
TA – 1979. *Le temps et l'autre,* Montpellier: Fata Morgana. (First publ. 1947)
MT – 1954. *Le Moi et la Totalité.* In: EN, pp. 25-52.
RA – 1958. *Une réligion d'adultes.* In: DL, pp. 24-41.
TI – 1968(3) (1961). *Totalité et Infini. Essai sur l'extériorité,* La Haye: Martinus Nijhoff.
DL – 1963. *Difficile liberté, Essais sur le judaisme,* Paris: Éditions Albin Michel.
EDHH – 1967 (2). *En découvrant l'existence avec Husserl et Heidegger,* Paris: Vrin.
QLT - 1968. *Quatre lectures talmudiques,* Paris: Les Éditions de Minuit.
HAH – 1972. *Humanisme de l'autre homme,* Montpellier: Fata Morgana.
AE – 1974. *Autrement qu'être ou au delà de l' essence,* La Haye: Martinus Nijhoff.
NP – 1976. *Noms propres,* Montpellier: Fata Morgana.
SaS – 1977. *Du sacré au saint,* Paris: Les Éditions de Minuit.
DQVI – 1982. *De Dieu qui vient à l'idee,* Paris: Vrin.
- *Dieu et la Philosophie.* Article in: DQVI. pp. 94-127.
AV – 1982. *L 'Au-Dela du verset – Lectures et discours talmudiques,* Paris: Les Éditions de Minuit.
EI – 1982. *Ethique et Infini. Dialogues avec Philippe Nemo,* Paris: Fayard.

TrI – 1984. *Transcendance et intelligibilité*, Geneve: Labor et Fides.
HS – 1987. *Hors sujet*, Montpellier: Fata Morgana.
- 1989. *Répondre d'autrui – Emmannuel Levinas (autour d'un entretien avec Emmanuel Lévinas)*, Aeschlimann, J. éd., Boudry-Neuchâtel: Baconnière.
EN – 1991. *Entre nous, essais sur le penser-à-l'autre*, Paris: Bernard Grasset.
- 1991. *Cahier de l'Herne. Emmanuel Levinas*, Catherine Chalier & Miguel Abensour dir., Paris: Éditions de l'Herne. (Articles by Levinas and other authors on Levinas; inter alia one by M. Schneider.)
- 1994. *Les Imprévues de l'Histoire*, Préface de Pierre Hayat, Paris: Fata Morgana. (Including: *Quelques réflexions sur la philosophie de l'hitlérisme* from 1934.)
- 1989. *Écriture et Sainteté*, in: Fr. Kaplan & J.L. Vieillard-Baron éds., *Introduction à la Philosophie de la Religion*, Paris: Le Cerf, pp. 353-362. Translation: Ab Kalshoven: *Schrift en Heiligheid* (1997, unpublished).

Other consulted Levinas translations (into Dutch)

ZZ – 1988. *Van het zijn naar de zijnde*, Baarn: Ambo. Translation: Ab Kalshoven. Preface: Theo de Boer.
DTA – 1989. *De tijd en de ander*, Baarn: Ambo. Translation: Ab Kalshoven.
TO – 1987. *De totaliteit en het Oneindige*, Baarn: Ambo. Translation: Theo de Boer & Chris Bremmers. Notes: Theo de Boer.
HAM – 1990. *Humanisme van de andere mens*, Kampen: Kok. Introduction and translation with notes: A. Th. Peperzak.
PV – 1989. *De plaatsvervanging*, Baarn: Ambo. Introducton and translation with notes: Theo de Boer.
AZ – 1991. *Anders dan zijn of het wezen voorbij*, Baarn: Ambo. Translation: Ab Kalshoven.
MG – 1978 (4). *Het menselijk gelaat*, Baarn: Ambo. Selection and introduction: Ad Peperzak. Translation: O. de Nobel & A. Peperzak.
AV – 1989. *Aan gene zijde van het vers – Talmoedische studies en essays*, Hilversum: Gooi en Sticht. Translation: Jan Engelen and Hub Nauts.
VTL – 1990. *Vier Talmoed Lessen*, Hilversum: Gooi en Sticht. Translation: C. Quené.
- 1990. *God en de filosofie*. 's-Gravenhage: Meinema. Translation, introduction and notes: Th. de Boer. (Original texts also in DQVI.)
EO – 1987. *Ethisch en oneindig – Gesprekken met Philippe Nemo*, Kampen: Kok. Introduction: R. Bakker. Translation: C. J. Huizinga.
To – 1994. *Tussen ons*, Baarn: Ambo. Translation: Ab Kalshoven.
- See also under: *IKON-Interview*.

General bibliography

ACEBT = *Amsterdamse Cahiers voor Exegese en Bijbelse Theologie*. Amsterdam: Societas Hebraïca Amstelodamensis.
Achterhuis, Hans, 1988. *Het rijk van de schaarste – van Thomas Hobbes tot Michel Foucault*, Utrecht: Ambo/Anthos.
Augsburger, David W., 1986. *Pastoral Counseling Across Cultures*. Philadelphia, PA: Westminster.
Baakman. Bernard H., 1990. *Van je familie moet je het hebben!* Den Haag: Boekencentrum (*Toerusting*).
Badinter, Elisabeth, 1989 (3). *De mythe van de moederliefde*, Amsterdam: Muntinga. Translation: Veronique Huijbregts & Marie Luyten.

Bamberger, Dr. S. (Translat.), 1981. *Pirke Awoth, Die Sprüche der Väter*, Basel: Morascha.
Banon, David, 1987. *La lecture infini*, Paris: Seuil.
Banon, Dewora, 1965. Scheiding, in: *Meesters der Hebreeuwse vertelkunst*. Amsterdam: J.M. Meulenhoff, pp. 65-71. Translation: J. Melkman.
Bauman, Zygmunt, 1995. *Life in Fragments – Essays in Postmodern Morality*, Oxford/Cambridge: Blackwell.
Bateson, Gregory, 1972. *Steps to an Ecology of Mind*, New York: Ballantine. (Including: Gregory Bateson, Don D. Jackson, Jay Haley & John H. Weakland, Toward a Theory of Schizofrenia. Published before in: *Behavioral Science* 1, 4, 1956).
Bateson, Gregory, 1980. *Mind and Nature*, Toronto/New York/London: Bantam Books. Translation in Dutch: Evelien Tonkens, Paul Sandwijk & Ton Maas, 1984. *Het verbindend patroon*, Amsterdam: Bert Bakker.
Benthem van den Bergh, G., 1978. De schuldvraag als orientatiemiddel, in: *De Gids* 144, no. 9/10, Amsterdam.
Bernasconi, Robert & Simon Critchley eds., 1991. *Re-reading Levinas*, Bloomington/Indianapolis, ID: Indiana University Press. (Essays regarding the discourse between Levinas en Derrida by other researchers. The discussion is inter alia about Levinas' view on femininity. See the critique by Luce Irigaray.)
Bernasconi, Robert & David Wood eds., 1988. *The Provocation of Levinas*, London/New York, NY: Routledge.
Bergson, H., 1924. *Essai sur les données immédiates de conscience*, Paris: Felix Alcan.
Berns, Egide, Samuel IJsseling & Paul Moyaert, red.,1979. *Denken in Parijs-Taal en Lacan, Foucault, Althusser, Derrida*, Alphen aan de Rijn/Brussel: Samsom.
Bettelheim, Bruno, 1991 (1956). *Freud's Vienna and Other Essays*, New York, NY: Vintage Books.
Blanchot, Maurice, 1942. *Aminadab*, Paris: Gallimard.
Bloch, Jochanan, 1977. *Die Aporie des Du – Probleme der Dialogik Martin Bubers*, Heidelberg: Lambert Schneider.
Boendermaker, J.P., 1978. Liturgie als epicentrum van pastoraat, in: Maarten B. Blom e.a. red., *Gestalten van pastoraat. Opstellen aangeboden aan Dr. W. Zijlstra*, Amsterdam: P.E.T., pp. 63-69.
Boer, Theo de, 1976. *Tussen filosofie en profetie – De wijsbegeerte van Emmanuel Levinas*, Baarn: Ambo.
Boer, Theo de, 1980. *Grondslagen van een kritische psychologie*, Baarn: Ambo.
Boer, Theo de, 1989. *De God van de filosofen en de God van Pascal – Op het grensgebied van filosofie en theologie*, 's-Gravenhage: Meinema.
Boer, Theo de, 1991. Ten overstaan van mijzelf – De plaats van de rationaliteit in de ethiek in: Herman Bleijendaal, Johan Goud & Eleen van Hove, red., *Emmanuel Levinas over psyche, kunst en moraal*, Baarn: Ambo, pp.131-137.
Boer, Theo de, 1993. *Awater en andere verhalen over subjectiviteit*, Amsterdam: Boom.
Bonhoeffer, Dietrich, 1970. *Widerstand und Ergebung – Briefe und Aufzeichnungen aus der Haft*, München: Christian Kaiser Verlag.
Bons-Storm, M., 1984. *Kritisch bezig zijn met pastoraat – Een verkenning van de interdisciplinaire implicaties van de practische theologie*, 's-Gravenhage: Boekencentrum.
Breukelman, F.H., 1989. *Gesprekken met Frans Breukelman*, red. Ype Bekker. Dussie Hofstra, Chris Mataheru & Annette Melzer, 's Gravenhage: Meinema.
Breukelman, F.H., 1992. *Bijbelse theologie – Het eerstelingschap van Israël* (1,2), Kampen: Kok.
Brinkgreve, Christien, 1984. *Psychoanalyse in Nederland – Een vestigingsstrijd*, Amsterdam: UvA. (Dissertation)

Brinkgreve, Christien, J.H. Onland & A. de Swaan, 1979. *De opkomst van het psychotherapeutisch bedrijf,* Utrecht/ Antwerpen: Spectrum.
Browning, Don S., Thomas Jobe & Ian S. Evinson, eds., 1990. *Religious and Ethical Factors in Psychiatric Practice,* Chicago, IL: Nelson-Hall.
Burggraeve, R., 1987. *Van zelfontplooiing naar verantwoordelijkheid- een ethische lezing van het verlangen: ontmoeting tussen psychoanalyse en Levinas,* Leuven/Amersfoort: Acco.
Burggraeve, R., 1991. *De bijbel geeft te denken,* Leuven/Amersfoort: Acco.
Brüggeman-Kruijff, Atie Th., 1993. *Bij de gratie van de transcendentie – In gesprek met Levinas over het vrouwelijke,* Amsterdam: VU Press. (Dissertation)
De Bruin, Tom red., 1983. *Adam waar ben je? – De betekenis van het mensbeeld in de Joodse traditie en in de psychotherapie,* Hilversum: B. Folkertsma Stichting voor Talmudica.
Canetti, Elias, 1981. *De behouden tong – geschiedenis van een jeugd,* Amsterdam: Arbeiderspers. Translation: Theodor Duquesnoy.
Cassuto, U., 1961. *A Commentary on the Book of Genesis,* Jerusalem: Magnes Press.
Chalier, Catherine, 1982. *Figures du Feminin – Lecture d'Emmanuel Lévinas,* Paris: La Nuit surveillée.
Chapman, A. H., 1976. *Harry Stack Sullivan – His life and his work,* New York, NY: Putnam.
Cohen, A., ed., 1979. *The Soncino Chumash – The Five Books of Moses with Haphtaroth,* London/ Jerusalem: Soncino Press.
Cohen, Richard A., 1994. *Elevations – The Height of the Good in Rosenzweig and Levinas,* Chicago, IL: The University of Chicago Press.
Contextuele Berichten, Tijdschrift van de Stichting Contextueel Pastoraat in Nederland, verschijnt sinds 1995 viermaal per jaar. www.contextueelpastoraat.nl
Cotroneo, Margaret, 1986. Families and Abuse: A Contextual Approach, in: Mark A. Karpel ed., *Family Resources,* New York/London: Guilford Press, pp. 413-437.
Cox, Murray & Alice Theilgaard, 1994. *Shakespeare as Prompter – The Amending Imagination and the Therapeutic Process,* London: J. Kingsley.
Cullberg, Johan, 1990. *Moderne psychiatrie, een psychodynamische benadering,* Baarn: Ambo. Translation from the original Swedish text: Petra Broomans & Wiveca Jongeneel.
Deurloo, K. A., 1967. *Kaïn en Abel,* Amsterdam: W. ten Have.
Devereux, George, 1978. *Ethnopsychoanalysis,* Berkeley, CA: University of California Press.
Doorn, Nel van: zie onder Luteyn- van Doorn
Dostojewski, F., 1981. *De gebroeders Karamazow,* Utrecht/Antwerpen: Veen. Translation: Marko Fondse.
Ducommun-Nagy, Catherine & Linda Schwoeri, 1995. *Contextual Therapy in the 1990's.* (Pre-publication copy, 35 pp.)
Ducommun-Nagy, C., 2008. Van onzichtbare naar bevrijdende loyaliteit. Leuven: Acco. Translated from French: May Michielsen.
Den Dulk, M., 1992. Contextuality: A Theological Paradigm, in: Otto Stange ed., *Pastoral Care and Context,* Amsterdam: VU Press, pp. 31-44.
Den Dulk, M., 1994. Nagy tegen de rest van de wereld – Klytaemnestra, Karel de Grote en Kaïn, *Lustrumconferentie VO-Contextueel Pastoraat okt.1994,* pp. 11-24. www.contextueelpastoraat.nl
Den Dulk, M., 1995. Die pastorale Dynamik der Rechtfertigungslehre Karl Barths, in: *Zeitschrift für dialektische Theologie,* 1995(11)/1, pp. 29-42.
Den Dulk, M., 1996. *Heren van de praxis,* Zoetermeer: Boekencentrum.
Duyndam, J., 1984. *De meervoudigheid van de mens als voorwaarde van ethiek,* Delft: Eburon.

Bibliography

Duyndam, J., 1994. Zorg en generositeit, in: Henk Manschot & Marian Verkerk red., *Ethiek van de zorg – een discussie*, Amsterdam: Boom, pp. 119-148.
Eliot, T.S., 1950. *The Cocktail Party*, London: Faber & Faber.
Epstein. A. L., 1978. *Ethos and Identity*, London: Tavistock.
Epstein, Helen, 1988. *Children of the Holocaust – Conversations with Sons and Daughters*, New York/London: Penguin.
Erikson, E. H., 1959. Problem of Ego Identity, *Psychological Issues* 1,1, New York: International Universities Press.
Fairbairn, W. R. D., 1992 (1952). *Psychoanalytic Studies of the Personality*, London: Routledge.
Finkielkraut, Alain, 1984. *La sagesse de l'amour*, Paris: Gallimard.
Foudraine, Jan, 1971. *Wie is van hout? Een gang door de psychiatrie*, Bilthoven: Ambo.
Frankl, Viktor, 1970. *Psychotherapy and Existentialism*, London: Souvenir Press.
Freire, Paulo, 1972. *Pedagogie van de onderdukten*, Baarn: In den Toren. Translation: J. E. A. Andriessen-van der Zande & J. P. de Vries.
Freud, Anna, 1973. *Het Ik en de afweermechanismen*, Bilthoven: Ambo. Translation: Elien Romme-Branbergen.
Freud, Sigmund, 1988. *Ziektegeschiedenissen*, deel 2, Meppel/Amsterdam: Boom. Translation: Adriaan Morriën & Henk Mulder.
Freud Loewenstein, Sophie, 1981. Mother and Daughter – an Epitaph, in: *Family Process* 1981 /3, pp. 3-10.
Friedman, Edwin H., 1985. *Generation to generation – Family process in church and synagogue*, New York, NY: Guilford Press.
Friedman, Maurice, 1976. *Martin Buber, the Life of Dialogue*, Chicago, IL: University of Chicago Press.
Friedman, Maurice, 1989. Martin Buber and Ivan Boszormenyi-Nagy: The Role of Dialogue in Contextual Therapy, *Psychotherapy* 26, 1989/3.
Friedman, Maurice, 1992 (a). *Dialogue and the Human Image*, Newbury Park, CA: Sage Publications.
Friedman, Maurice, 1992 (b). *Religion and Psychology*, New York, NY: Paragon House.
Friedman, Maurice, 1993. Dialogue, Speech, Nature, and Creation. Franz Rosenzweig's Critique of Buber's "I and Thou", *Modern Judaism* 13, pp. 109-118.
Friedman, Maurice, see also under: Schilpp.
Van Galen Last, H., 1975. *Van Nietzsche tot nu*, Groningen: J.B. Wolters Noordhoff.
Galle-van Luttikhuizen, Annelies, 1995. Opening in het levenslang van de misbruikte, in: *Praktische Theologie* 1995/1, pp. 36-46.
Van Gennep, F.O., 1989. *De terugkeer van de verloren Vader*, Baarn: Ten Have.
Gelinas, Denise, 1986. Unexpected Resources in treating Incest Families, in: Mark A. Karpel, ed., *Family Resources*, New York/ London: Guilford Press, pp. 327-358.
Giat Roberto, Laura, 1992. *Transgenerational Family Therapies*, New York, NY: Guilford Press.
Gibbs, Robert, 1992. *Correlations in Rosenzweig and Levinas*, Princeton, NJ: Princeton University Press.
Girard, René, 1961. *Mensonge Romantique – Vérité Romanesque*, Paris: Bernard Grasset.
Girard, René, 1972. *La Violence et le Sacré*, Paris: Bernard Grasset.
Girard, René, 1978. *Des choses cachées depuis la fondation du monde – Recherches avec J. M. Oughourlian et Guy Lefort*, Paris: Bernard Grasset.
Girard, René, 1982. *Le Bouc émissaire*, Paris: Bernard Grasset.
Glueck, Nelson, 1961. *Das Wort Hesed*, Berlin: Topelmann.
Goedhart, Sandor, (without year). *Reading the Ram* (unpublished paper, Syracuse USA).

Goedhart, Sandor, 1978. Oedipus and Laius" many murderers, in: *Diacritics,* March 1978.
Goud, Johan, 1992 (a). *Emmanuel Levinas und Karl Barth – Ein religionsphilosophischer und ethischer Vergleich,* Bonn/Berlin: Bouvier Verlag. (Dissertation 1984) Translation: Karin Gellinek.
Goud, Johan, 1992 (b). *God als raadsel,* Kampen: Kok Agora.
Graham, Larry K., 1992. *Care of Persons, Care of Worlds – A Psychosystems Approach to Pastoral Care and Counseling,* Nashville, TN: Abingdon Press.
Günther, Ralf, 1994-1995. *Straftat und Familienbindung – Wahrnehmungen und Aufgaben für die Seelsorge an Strafgefangenen,* Semesterarbeit Praktische Theologie, Universität Leipzig.
Hack, Christina, 1993. *Groter dan ons hart,* Zoetermeer: Boekencentrum. (Dissertation)
Hamel, Glikl, 1987. *De memoires van Glikl Hamel (1645-1724) – door haarzelf geschreven,* Amsterdam: Feministische Uitgeverij Sara. Translation from Jiddisch, introduction and remarks: Mira Rafalowicz.
Handelman, Susan A., 1991. *Fragments of Redemption – Jewish thought and literary theory in Benjamin, Sholem and Levinas,* Bloomington/ Indianapolis, ID: Indiana University Press.
Hannema, U.B., 1964. *De Hogerhuis-zaak,* Drachten: Laverman 1964. (Dissertation)
Hargrave, Terry D. & William T. Anderson, 1992. *Finishing well – Aging and Reparation in the Intergenerational Family,* New York, NY: Brunner & Mazel.
Hargrave, Terry D., 1994. *Families and Forgiveness – Healing Wounds in the Intergenerational Family,* New York, NY: Brunner & Mazel.
Havel, Vaclav, 1991 (1983). *Briefe an Olga – Betrachtungen aus dem Gefängnis,* Reinbek bei Hamburg: Rowohlt. Translation: Joachim Bruss.
Heins, Ronald, 1997. *Het had zo mooi kunnen zijn – over mogelijk contextueel pastoraat aan de handen van Ivan Boszormenyi-Nagy en Paul Tillich,* Amsterdam: scriptie Kerkelijke Opleiding UvA.
Heitink, Gerben, 1993. *Praktische theologie – geschiedenis, theorie, handelingsvelden,* Kampen: Kok.
Van Hekken, S.M.J. & J. Melse red., 1990. *Ernstig verwaarloosd – Hulpverlening aan kinderen en hun ouders naar de ideeën van Ivan Boszormenyi-Nagy,* Amsterdam/Lisse: Swets & Zeitlinger.
Helmers-van Tricht, Anne, 1992. *Lang zul je leven – Een onderzoek naar het verband tussen het bijbels gebod "eer uw vader en uw moeder" en het gedachtengoed van Ivan Boszormenyi-Nagy,* Amsterdam: scriptie Kerkelijke Opleiding UvA.
Herzberg, Abel, 1950. *Kroniek der jodenvervolging,* Arnhem/Amsterdam: Van Loghum Slaterus Meulenhoff.
Van Heusden, Ammy, 1983. In het voetspoor van Nagy, in: *Tijdschrift voor Psychotherapie* 1983(9) /3, pp. 140-144. Also in: Schlüter 1990.
Van Heusden, Ammy & ElseMarie van den Eerenbeemt, 1992. *Balans in beweging – Ivan Boszormenyi-Nagy en zijn visie op individuele en gezinstherapie,* Haarlem: De Toorts.
Hoensch, Jörg K., 1989. *A History of Modern Hungary 1867-1986,* London/New York: Longman.
Huizinga, Carl Jan, 1986. *Het goede onderricht,* Hengelo: published by author. (Dissertation)
Hutschemaekers, Giel, 1996. Hoe cliëntgericht is Cliëntgerichte Psychotherapie? Kanttekeningen bij een naamsverandering, in: *Tijdschrift voor Clientgerichte Psychotherapie,* 1996/2, pp. 14-27.
IKON-interview (Levinas), 1986. *Jij die mij aanziet.* Interviewer: France Guwy.

IKON-interview (Nagy), 1986. *Erven van toekomst.* Interviewer: ElseMarie van den Eerenbeemt. Text also in: Schlüter 1990.
Imbens, A. & I. Jonker, 1985. *Godsdienst en incest,* Amersfoort: De Horstink.
Irigaray, Luce, 1990. Questions à Emmanuel Lévinas, in: *Critique,* Nov. 1990, pp. 911-920.
Isaiah, A.B. a.o., 1949. *The Pentateuch and Rashi's Commentary,* Brooklyn: SS&R.
Jong, A.F de, 1971. Is het Gij in Bubers "Ich und Du" niet essentieel? in: *Nederlands Theologisch Tijdschrift,* januari 1971.
Jong, A.F. de, 1980. Emmanuel Levinas, Denker in twee dimensies, in: *Wending,* april 1980, pp. 278-287.
Jong, A.F. de, 1981. *Lossen en binden,* Amsterdam (Inaugural Lecture Universiteit van Amsterdam).
Jong, A.F. de, 1984. Enkele opmerkingen over het belang van Levinas voor het pastoraat, in: Joop Boendermaker e.a. red., *Doen wat er te doen staat – Denken over pastoraat, Opstellen aangeboden aan Prof. Dr. C. H. Lindijer* 's-Gravenhage: Boekencentrum, pp. 121-129.
Jong, A.F. de, 1989. Talen naar vrede, in: A.Lambo red., *Oecumennisme. Opstellen aangeboden aan Henk B. Kossen ter gelegenheid van zijn afscheid als kerkelijk hoogleraar,* Amsterdam: Algemene Doopsgezinde Sociëteit, pp. 109-120.
Josuttis, Manfred, 1988 (1974). *Praxis des Evangeliums zwischen Politik und Religion – Grundprobleme der praktischen Theologie,* München: Chr. Kaiser Verlag.
Kafka, Franz, 1982. *Het proces,* Amsterdam: Querido. Original title: "Der Prozess" (1925). Translation: Ruth Wolf.
Kafka, Franz, 1969. *Brief aan zijn vader,* Amsterdam: Querido. Original title: "Brief an den Vater" (1919). Translation: Nini Brunt.
Kaptein, R. & P. Tijmes, 1986. *De ander als model en obstakel,* Kampen: Kok Agora.
Kassai, Melinda, 1991. Hongarije, in: Jacques Neeven, Harm Ramkema & Erik van Schaik, red., *Van Tallin tot Tirana – Oost-Europa tijdens het Interbellum,* Utrecht: Werkgroep Oost Europa projecten, pp. 61-74.
Keij, Jan, 1992. *De struktuur van Levinas' denken.* Kampen: Kok Agora. (Dissertation)
Kepnes, S., 1992. *The Text as Thou: Martin Buber's Dialogical Hermeneutics and Narrative Theology,* Bloomington, IN: Indiana University Press.
Kern. R.G., 1989. Contextuele therapie – ervaringen en overwegingen, in: *Tijdschrift voor Psychotherapie* 15 /1, pp. 31-37.
Van Keulen, Ineke, 1995. De ene context is de andere niet, in: *Ophef, Tijdschrift voor hartstochtelijke theologie,* 2/2-3, pp. 8-11.
Kierkegaard, Soren, 1983. *Vrees en beven,* Baarn: Ten Have (1843). Original title: "Frygt og Bæven" (1843). Translation and introduction: W. R. Scholtens.
Kirk, G.S. & J. E. Raven, 1982. *The Pre-socratic Philosophers – A Critical History With a Selection of Texts,* Cambridge: Cambridge University Press.
Kohn, Hans, 1979 (1930). *Martin Buber,* Wiesbaden: Fourier Verlag.
Koopman, Thalien, 1995. De Kananese vrouw, in: *Contextuele Berichten,* (1)/1, pp. 9-16.
Korf, Jan, 1975. *Monumentenzorg en leven.* Zutphen: Walburg Pers.
Kosian, Marthe, 1994. Over macht en liefde. Een kritiek op Nagy vanuit het vrouwen pastoraat, MARA, (7) /2, pp. 45-52.
Krall, Hanna, 1993. *Tanz auf fremder Hochzeit,* Frankfurt am Main: Neue Kritik. Translation from Polish: Hubert Schumann.
Kroon, D. red., 1981. *Nooit zag ik Awater van zo nabij,* 's-Gravenhage: Bzztôh.
Kuiper, Frits, 1958. *Leven uit de hoop,* Amsterdam: H.J. Paris.
Lascaris, André, 1987. *Advocaat van de zondebok – Het werk van René Girard en het evangelie van Jezus,* Hilversum: Gooi en Sticht.

Lascaris, André, 1993. *Het soevereine slachtoffer – Een theologisch essay over geweld en onderdrukking.* Baarn: Ten Have.
Leeuw, Mechteld de & Wytske Strikwerda, 1995. *Over vreugde en verantwoordelijkheid. – De kwaliteit van de ouder-kind relatie geïnterpreteerd vauit de filosofie van Emmanuel Levinas,* Masterthesis orthopedagogiek, Katholieke Universiteit Nijmegen.
Leeuw, E.J. van der, 1991. *Schuld en schuldgevoelens en hun relationele belekenis voor verzetsslachtoffers,* thesis Masterclass contextuele therapie, Hogeschool van Amsterdam.
Leeuwen, A.Th. van, 1966. *Het Christendom in de wereld geschiedenis,* Amsterdam: Ten Have.
"Leidse Cursus" – Training van gezinstherapeuten 1967. *Verslag,* Leiden: Nederlands Instituut voor Praeventieve Geneeskunde TNO.
Lescourret, Marie-Anne, 1994. *Emmanuel Levinas,* Paris: Flammarion.
Levita, D. J. de, 1994. De behandeling van oorlogsgetraumatiseerde kinderen in ex Joegoslavië; een onderzoeks- en scholingsproject in Slovenië, in: *ICODO INFO* 94-2, Utrecht: Stichting ICODO, pp. 14-30.
Liedboek voor de Kerken, 1984. 's Gravenhage: Boekencentrum.
Lindijer, Coert H., 1984. *Pastor en therapeut,* 's-Gravenhage: Boekencentrum.
Lindijer, Coert H., 1995. *Tasten naar schaamte,* Kampen: Kok.
Lindt, Martijn, 1993. *Als je wortels taboe zijn – verwerking van levensproblemen bij kinderen van Nederlandse nationaal-socialisten,* Kampen: Kok. (Dissertation)
Lowe, Malcolm ed., 1990. *The New Testament and Christian-Jewish Dialogue – Studies in Honour of David Flusser,* Jerusalem: Ecumenical Theological Research Fraternity in Israël.
Luteyn-van Doorn, Nel, 1996. *Morgen begint gisteren – Een onderzoek naar het contextueel pastoraat zoals dat is voortgevloeid uit het ethisch-relationele gedachtengoed van Ivan Boszormenyi-Nagy in verbinding met exegetische verkenningen rondom het vijfde woord uit de decaloog,* Brussel: Licentiaats-verhandeling (Masterthesis, nr.167) Universitaire Faculteit voor Protestantse Godgeleerdheid.
Luteyn-van Doorn, Nel, 1996. *Legaat als opdracht van de gemeente of wettelijke aansprakelijkheid – Over bewaren van erfgoed aan de hand van de betekenis van het grondwoord sj"m"r en de contextuele visie van Ivan Boszormenyi-Nagy,* Amsterdam: scriptie Kerkelijke Opleiding UvA.
Luther, Henning, 1992. *Religion und Alltag – Bausteine zu einer Praktischen Theologie des Subjekts,* Stuttgart: Radius.
Maturana H. F. & F. Varela, 1980. *Autopoiesis and Cognition,* Dordrecht/Boston/London: Kluwer/Reidel.
McCreary, Alf, ed., 1981. *Profiles of Hope,* Belfast: Christian Journals Ltd.
Metz, Anne Marie, 1987. *Nooit meer gewoon,* Amsterdam: Balans.
Meulink-Korf, Hanneke, 1994. *Incest – Onontkoombaar en onverbrekelijk? Lesmateriaal voor VO-Contextueel Pastoraat,* Amsterdam: UvA/HvA, unpublished course materials.
Meulink-Korf, Hanneke & Aat van Rhijn, 1990. De ethische dimensie: een kleine antropologische verkenning, in: Dick Schlüter red., *In het voetspoor van Ivan Nagy,* Amsterdam: Voortgezette Opleidingen, pp. 143-151.
Meulink-Korf, Hanneke & Aat van Rhijn, 1991. Kontekstuele therapie en Kontekstueel pastoraat, in: *Praktische theologie* 1991/1, pp. 3-15.
Meulink-Korf, Hanneke & Aat van Rhijn, 1995. De andere context is de ene niet, een reactie, in: *Ophef, Tijdschrift voor hartstochtelijke theologie* (2)/5, pp. 41-43.
Meulink-Korf, Hanneke & Aat van Rhijn, 1996. Afscheid nemen – voor ieder mens anders, in: *De Open Poort. Belgisch Protestants maandblad voor geloof en samenleving* 1996/1, pp. 7-9.

Michielsen, May, 1992. *Het zelf-in-relatie en contextuele therapie,* thesis Masterclass contextuele therapie, Amsterdam: HvA.
Midrash Rabba, H. Freedman & Maurice Simon transl. and eds., 1951. London: Soncino Press.
Miller, Alice, 1979. *Das Drama des begabten Kindes – und die Suche nach dem wahren Selbst,* Frankfurt am Main: Suhrkamp. Translated by H. & H. Hannum as:
Miller, Alice, 1984. *Thou shalt not be aware,* New York, NY: Macmillan.
Mindszenty, József, 1974. *Erinnerungen,* Berlin: Propyläen.
Minnema, Attie, 1989. *Tot in het derde en vierde geslacht. Over de betekenis van de contextuele benadering van Ivan Boszormenyi-Nagy voor het pastoraal handelen,* Kampen: masterthesis Theologische Universiteit Kampen.
Minuchin, Salvador, 1974. *Families and Family Therapy, a Structural Approach,* Cambridge, MA: Harvard University Press. Also as: -, 1977. *Gezinstherapie,* Utrecht: Spectrum. Translation: M.A. Lombaers.
Miskotte, H.H., 1991. *Pastoraat en profetie,* Amsterdam (Inaugural Lecture Universiteit van Amsterdam).
Miskotte, H.H., 1992. *Pastor en profeet – over de andere kant van pastoraat,* Baarn: Ten Have.
Miskotte, K.H., 1932. *Het Wezen der Joodsche Religie,* Amsterdam: H.J. Paris. (Dissertation)
Miskotte, H.H., 1963. *Wenn die Götter schweigen,* München: Chr. Kaiser Verlag. Translation: H. Stoevesandt. For the German translation is the original text reviewed and extended by the author. Original title: -, 1956. *Als de goden zwijgen,* Amsterdam: Uitg. Holland.
Mitscherlich, Alexander & Margarete, 1967. *Die Unfähigkeit zu trauern – Grundlagen kollektiven Verhaltens,* München: Piper Verlag.
Mönnich, C. W., 1967. *Geding der vrijheid – De betrekkingen der oosterse en westerse kerken tot de val van Constantinopel (1453),* Zwolle: W.E.J. Tjeenk Willink.
Mooij, Antoine, 1977. *Taal en verlangen – Lacans theorie van de psychoanalyse,* Meppel: Boom.
Moore, T. 1992. *Care of the Soul. How to Add Depth and Meaning to your Everyday Life.* London: Piatkus.
Nauer, D. 2010. *Seelsorge. Sorge um die Seele.* Stuttgart: Kohlhammer.
Neeleman, Albert, 1995. In: *Systeemtherapie, tijdschrift voor systeemtheoretische psychotherapie,* 1995/2, p. 108.
Neher, André, 1970. *L'Exil de la Parole – du silence biblique au silence d'Auschwitz,* Paris: Seuil. Translation by J. Faber, as: Neher, André, 1992. *De ballingschap van het Woord,* Baarn: Gooi en Sticht.
Nicolai. N. J., 1991. Incest als trauma: Implicaties en consequenties voor de behandeling, in: *Tijdschrift voor Psychotherapie* 17 /1, pp. 12-30.
Nieskens, Els, 1995. Ervaringen met contextuele hulpverlening; een kind kan uit het gezin geplaats worden, het gezin nooit uit een kind, in: Herman Baartman red., *Op gebaande paden? Ontwikkelingen in diagnostiek, hulpverlening en preventie met betrekking tot seksueel misbruik van kinderen,* Utrecht: SWP, pp. 131-144.
Nijhoff, Martinus, 1964. *Verzamelde Gedichten,* Den Haag: Bert Bakker/ Daamen.
Nijk, A. J., 1962. Meditatie van een lezer, in: Het bittere raadsel van de goede schepping, *Wending,* juli/augustus 1962, pp. 374-390.
Nijk, A.J., 1978. *De mythe van de zelfontplooiing,* Meppel: Boom.
O'Connor, Noreen, The Personal is Political: Discursive Practice of the Face-to-Face, in: Robert Bernasconi & David Wood eds., 1988. *The Provocation of Levinas – Rethinking the Other,* London: Routledge, pp. 57-69.

Oele, Bastiaan, 1989, De praktijk van de contextuele therapie van Ivan Boszormenyi-Nagy: het verdienen van vrijheid, in: J. Hendrickx e.a. red, *Handboek Gezinstherapie 10*, Deventer: Van Loghum Slaterus, pp. 1-20 (C.1).

Onderwaater, Annelies, 1986. *De onverbrekelijke band tussen ouders en kinderen*, Lisse: Swets & Zeitlinger. (Fourth edition: 1995. *De theorie van Nagy*. Lisse: Swets & Zeitlinger.)

Oskamp, Paul, 1988. *Doopborgen – profile en profijt*, 's-Gravenhage: Boekencentrum. (Dissertation)

Oughourlian, Jean-Michel, 1982. *Un mime nommé désir*, Paris: Grasset.

Pas, Alice van der, 1982. De humane verdeelsleutel – Dr. Ivan Boszormenyi-Nagy over het begrip gerechtigdheid, interview met Nagy in: *Tijdschrift voor Maatschappelijk Werk* Kwartaal 36 (1982) /4, pp. 29-34.

Pasveer, Joh., 1992. *De gemeente tussen openheid en identiteit – Een open-systeemtheorie als model voor de gemeente ten dienste van haar opbouw*, Gorinchem: Narratio. (Dissertation)

Patton, John, 1985. *Is Human Forgiveness Possible? – A Pastoral Care Perspective*, Nashville, TN: Abingdon Press.

Patton, John, 1987. Generationsübergreifende Gesichtspunkte in der Seelsorge, in: *Wege zur Menschen* 39, pp. 181-192.

Peperzak, Adriaan T. ed., 1995. *Ethics as First Philosophy – The Significance of Emmanuel Levinas for Philosophy, Literature and Religion*, New York/London: Routledge.

Pfeifer, Samuel Hrsg., 1991. *Seelsorge und Psychotherapie – Chancen und Grenzen der Integration*, Moers: Brendow.

Pfeiffer, Wolfgang M., 1996. De relatie: de belangrijkste werkzame factor in de gesprekspsychotherapie, in: *Tijdschrift voor cliëntgerichte psychotherapie* 34 (1996)/1, pp. 3-14.

Pizzey, Erin & Jeff Shapiro, 1982. *Prone to Violence*, Feltham Middlesex: Hamlyn.

Pirke Awoth. See: Bamberger.

Plantier, Edith, 1994. Nagy en vader-dochter incest. Kritiek vanuit de vrouwenhulpverlening, *MARA, tijdschrift voor feminisme en theologie* 1 /2, pp. 52-57.

Plantier, Edith, 1995-1996. Nagy en de vrouwen, *Contexuele Berichten* 1 /3, pp. 9-12.

Poorthuis, Marcel, 1992. *Het gelaat van de Messias*, Hilversum/ Zoetermeer: Boekencentrum.

Poorthuis, Marcel, 1995. Buber and Levinas. From dialogue to substition, in: *Mededelingen – Levinas-Studiekring* 1/1, pp. 11-26. (Originally in: Annales de Philosophie 15- 1994.)

Pot, Anne Margriet, 1996. *Caregiver's Perspectives – A Longitudinal Study on the Psychological Distress of lnformal Caregivers of Demented Elderly*, Amsterdam: VU Press. (Dissertation)

PSVG-infomap, 1993. Herma Tigchelaar en Ineke van Keulen red., *Loyaliteit – steen des aanstoots? Nagy en feministische partijdigheid in vrouwenhulpverlening en vrouwenpastoraat*, Den Haag: Protestantse Stichting voor Voorlichting en Vorming omtrent Relaties en Seksualiteit.

Renes, Petra N., 1994. *Exoneration in het werk van Nagy en Krasner en vergeving in het Onze Vader*, Amsterdam: scriptie Kerkelijke Opleiding UvA, Amsterdam.

Rhijn, Aat van, 1992. *Door de hemel uit de droom geholpen – over de betekenis van het werk van Levinas voor de contextuele benadering, Afscheidscollege*. Amsterdam: HvA.

Rhijn, Aat van, 1994. *Levinas en Buber: een mislukte dialoog of een tegoed?* Amsterdam: masterthesis UvA.

Rhijn, Aat van, 1995-1996. Met al uw "kracht" (Deut.6:5); Duber en Levinas in gesprek, in: *Om het levende woord* 1995/5, Kampen: Kok, pp. 133-139.

Rhijn, Aat van & André Lascaris, 1981. Going Dutch, in: Alf McCreary, ed., *Profiles of hope*, Belfast: Christian Journals Ltd., pp. 73-83.
Rhijn, Aat van, See also: Meulink-Korf. Also, under: Wit.
Ricoeur, Paul, 1965. *De l'interprétation – Essai sur Freud*, Paris: Seuil.
Ricoeur, Paul, 1985. *Temps et Récit*, tome 3, Paris: Seuil.
Riessen, Renee van, 1991. *Erotiek en dood – met het oog op transcendentie in de filosofie van Levinas*, Kampen: Kok Agora. (Dissertation)
Rogers, Carl R., 1961. *On Becoming a Person – a Therapist's View of Psychotherapy*, Boston, MA: Houghton Mifflin.
Rosenzweig, Franz, 1954 (1921). *Der Stern der Erlösung*, Heidelberg: Lambert Schneider.
Rosenzweig, Rachel, 1978. *Solidarität mit den Leidenden im Judentum*, Berlin/New York, NY: De Gruyter.
Rouppe van der Voort, F.J.M., 1990. *Doorlichting van de psychotherapeutische relatie vanuit de ethische stellingname van Emmanuel Levinas*, Delft: Eburon.
Rouppe van der Voort, F.J.M., 1991. *Intersubjectiviteit – wederzijdse begrenzing van de psychoanalyse en de fenomenologie van Levinas*, Delft: Eburon. (Dissertation)
Rutter, Virginia, 1992. Ivan Boszormenyi-Nagy receives AAMFT's highest honor, *Family Therapy News*, June 1992. Alexandria, VA: American Association for Marriage and Family Therapy.
Safranski, Rudiger, 1994. *Ein Meister aus Deutschland – Heidegger und seine Zeit*, München/Wien: Carl Hanser.
Satir, Virginia, 1976. Gezinstherapie, Deventer: Van Loghum Slaterus. Original title: *Conjoint Family Therapy*. Translation: G. van Kooten.
Schilpp, Paul Arthur & Maurice Friedman, eds., 1967. *The Philosophy of Martin Buber* (The Library of Living Philosophers, volume XII), La Salle: Open Court. German edition: P.A. Schilpp & M. Friedman, hrsg., 1963. *Martin Buber*, Stuttgart: Kohlhammer.
Schipani, D. S. & L. D. Bueckert. 2009. Epilogue. Growing in Wisdom as Spiritual caregivers. In: D. S. Schipani, L. D. Bueckert (eds.), *Interfaith Spiritual Care. Understanding and Practices*. Kitchener: Pandora Press, 1-7.
Schlüter, Dick, red., 1990. *In het voetspoor van Ivan Nagy – Opstellen over kenmerken en toepassingsgebieden van de intergenerationele familietherapie: de contextuele therapie*, Amsterdam: Voortgezette Opleidingen.
Schneider, Monique, 1991. La proximite chez Levinas et le "Nebenmensch" freudien, in: *Cahier de l'Herne – Emmanuel Levinas*. (See under: Levinas.)
Scholem, Gershom, 1982. *Van Berlijn naar Jeruzalem*, Amstelveen: Amphora Books. Original title: *Von Berlin nach Jeruzalem, Jugenderinnerungen*. Translation: Yge Foppema.
Schooneveld, J., 1990. Thora in the flesh, see in: Lowe, Malcolm, ed., pp. 77-94.
Shakespeare, William, 1987 (1623). *The Tempest*, London: Wordsworth.
Simon. Fritz B. & Helm Stierlin, 1992. *Die Sprache der Familientherapie – Ein Vokabular*, Stuttgart: Klett-Cotta.
Skynner, A.C. Robin, 1979. *One Flesh: Seperate Persons – Principles of Family and Marital Psychotherapy*, London: Constable.
Sleurink, Hans & Johan Frieswijk, 1985. *De zaak Hogerhuis*, Leeuwarden: Friese Pers.
Smelik,E.L., 1943. *Vergelden en vergeven*, 's Gravenhage: D.A. Daamen.
Stierlin, Helm, 1969. *Conflict and reconciliation, A Study in Human Relations and Schizophrenia*, New York: Anchor Books.
Stierlin, Helm, 1980. *Eltern und Kinder – Das Drama von Trennung und Versöhnung im Jugendalter*, Frankfurt am Main: Suhrkamp.

Stierlin, Helm, Ingeborg Rilcker-Emden, Norbert Wetzel & Michael Wirsching, 1985. *Das erste Familiengespräch – Theorie-Praxis-Beispiele*, Stuttgart: Klett-Cotta.
Storm, Marianne, 1996. *Verantwoordelijkheid*, Amsterdam: scriptie Kerkelijke Opleiding UvA.
Strack, H.L. & P. Billerbeck, 1994 (1926). *Kommentar zum Neuen Testament aus Talmud und Midrasch*, München: C.H. Beck.
Strijd, Krijn, 1978. Pastoraat – in dienst waarvan? in: Maarten B. Blom e.a. red., *Gestalten van postoraat – Opstellen aangeboden aan Dr. W. Zijlstra,* Amsterdam: P.E.T., pp.1-9.
Thans, Marianne, 1991. Kontekstueel pastoraat in het verpleeghuis, in: *Praktische theologie* 1991/1, pp. 16-30.
TRE = *Theologische Realenzyklopädie*, Band Xl, 1983. Berlin/New York: De Gruyter.
Thurneysen, Eduard, 1948. *Die Lehre von der Seelsorge*, München: Christian Kaiser Verlag.
Tieleman, Dick, 1995. *Geloofscrisis als gezichtsbedrog – spiritualiteit en pastoraat in een postmoderne cultuur*, Kampen: Kok.
Tillo, G.P.P. van, 1989. *Godsdienst- en pastoraalsociologie aan een Universiteit voor Theologie en Pastoraat – Een visie en een programma*, Heerlen: UTP. (Inaugural Lecture Universiteit voor Theologie en Pastoraat)
Trüb, Hans, 1971 (1951). *Heilung aus der Begegnung*, Stuttgart: Ernst Klett. After the death of Trüb published by E. Michel & A. Soborowitz. Preface by Martin Buber.
Veltkamp, H.J., 1989. *Pastoraat als gelijkenis – De gelijkenis als model voor pastoraal handelen*, Kampen: Kok Ten Have. (Dissertation)
Verbeek, Th., 1977. *Inleiding tot de geschiedenis van de psychologie*, Utrecht/Antwerpen: Spectrum.
Vogels, Frida, 1992. *De harde kern* (I en II). Amsterdam: Muntinga.
Watzlawick, Paul, Janet Helmick Beavin & Don D. Jackson, 1974 (4). *De pragmatische aspecten van de menselijke communicatie,* Deventer: Bohn Stafleu van Loghum. Original title: *Pragmatics of Human Communications*. Translation: G.R. de Bruin.
Westermann, Claus, 1981. *Genesis,* Neukirchen: Neukirchener Verlag. (Serie: Biblisches Kommentar Altes Testament.)
Wiesel, Elie, 1994. *Tous les fleuves vont á la mer – Memoires*, Paris: Seuil.
Wit, Jan, 1982. *Terwijl ik wacht wat mij de wereld doet*. Baarn: Bosch & Keuning.
Wit, Jan & Aat van Rhijn, 1958. *Kracht van gewijsde*, Utrecht: Vrijzinnig Christelijke Jeugd Centrale.
Zeldin, Theodore, 1994. *An Intimate History of Humanity*, London: Minerva.
Zijlstra, W., 1989. *Op zoek naar een nieuwe horizon – Handboek voor klinische pastorale vorming*, Nijkerk: G.F. Callenbach.
Zuidema, Willem e.a., *Isaäk wordt weer geofferd*, Baarn: Ten Have.
Zweerman, Theo, 1992. Wagen en wonen – Over een tekst van Franciscus van Assisi, in: Koen Boey e.a. red., *Om de waarheid te zeggen, opstellen over filosofie en literatuur, aangeboden aan Ad Peperzak*, Kampen: Kok Agora, pp. 227-242.

Glossarial explanation of core concepts

(See also the Glossary in Nagy & Krasner BGT:413-422)

Context: Interrelational web of trustworthy networking and interdependent mutuality, established by people involved (other/others) within the concrete setting of dynamic interaction. Context is determined by the dual exchange of giving and receiving. It describes the ethical dynamics of relational interaction, indicating the quality of intersubjectivity. With personal context (subjective dynamics) is meant: The current relational networking of a person, including both past relationships, as well as future relationships.

Exposition: One can say that *"contextual" is about the dynamics of relational ethics and the factor of ethical entanglements in the mutuality of human encounters.* As such, "contextual" is merely a concept. In combination with ethics, contextuality can be redefined as *the ethical dynamics of relational interaction, indicating the quality of intersubjectivity.* The advantage of such a definition is that the therapist should not anymore be concerned about a "trick" or "skill" how to manage the situation therapeutically. In the encounter it is rather straightforward and (seemingly) quite simple: Just "plant seeds" that invite the other into the dialogue and summon human beings to responsible and re-*spond*-able responses to difficult life challenges (Nagy & Krasner TGN:321; BGT: 277).

The endeavour of an ethical redefinition is not about an attempt by the therapist to redefine the "relational context". The redefinition is about a process wherein all significant members, belonging to somebody's relational reality, are involved as persons or individuals within the mutual dynamics of relationships. According to the intersubjective order of being, all people involved are subjects of the ethical redefinition of the relational context. "Contextual therapy aims at the goal of *eliciting* trust resources of close relationships" (Nagy F:191; italics VR/MK). What the therapist should do is to evoke "trust resources". For this new approach, a radical mindset is most needed: "Reversal has to start in the therapist's own mind" (Nagy & Spark IL:374).

The terms "contextual" and "contextual therapy" should thus be understood as a *process of ethical redefinition of relationships* and not as a diagnostic endeavour.

Destructive entitlement: In cases where a child is deprived from his/her right on trust (to receive care, to be treated in terms of trustworthiness, fairness, loyalty), "overentitlement" sets in. Nagy refers to the fact that it can be justified that a child (even later in years) starts to view the realm of adulthood (parents and/or others) as debtors, and responds, thus, accordingly. Due to indebtedness and merit, the child's claim becomes justified. However, it can also cause destructive behaviour with possible consequences for new forms of injustice. When freedom is deprived from investiture, or in cases of a lack of investiture, a situation is established with possible negative/destructive consequences for the interactional dynamics of relationships.

Dialogue: Mutual interaction directed and founded by accountability and qualified by re-*spond*-ability. The dialogue is not symmetric, homoeomorphic, but heteronomous and diachronic. When a person, for example, in cases of substance abuse, stops using drugs, due to concern for genetic consequences, this decision can be viewed as an investment to the intergenerational dynamics. It could be that in terms of short or even long-term benefits there could be virtually no direct form of repayment. The most rewarding repayment will perhaps be, when the offspring will keep this investment (contribution to familial, intergenerational dynamics) in mind when dealing with the sequence of coming, future generations (See Nagy & Krasner TGN:474; BGT:415).

The starting point in the dialogue is not the eventual mutuality as demand for justice as in many cases, but the quality of the responsibility and the respect for the unique separate value of the other/others.

Dimension: Reference is to the "four dimensions of the relational reality". These dimensions refer to clusters of multi-factors that determine human behaviour. These four dimensions are: Facts of life (existential happenstances); psychological factors; transactional patterns in relational interaction, and relational ethics. They influence one another and should be viewed as an interconnected web of human, relational networking. (Later Nagy and

Ducommun-Nagy added some notes concerning a fifth dimension, of ontic dependence.)

Ethical dimension *(the dimension of ethics, dimension of relational ethics, the ethic of due consideration, merited trust)*: It refers to fairness in the distribution of credits/assets (surplus) and loads/burdens/demands between all partners involved (multidirected partiality). One needs to reckon with everyone affected by eventual possible consequences inflicted by the acts/behaviour of the other within a specific context. (See also under: multidirected partiality.)

The ethical dimension is not about a very specific demarcated field or setting; it is always existent and, in all situations, applicable. Ethical concern is not an adiaphoron – indifference to the vicissitudes of life. It is in fact a viewpoint and fundamental perspective. (Nagy often uses the term of viewpoint/perspective in his writings; see for example TGN:203.) In terms of Levinas: Ethics is about optics.

Entitlement: The fundamental right to trustworthy care, nurture and education; that is, to be born in a humane space and environment of safety. Entitlement refers to respect guaranteed by responsible upbringing. In fact, it is about the just demand that a human being earns due to righteous acts and trustworthy modes of care (earning of entitlement). It is not always possible to transfer merit from one situation to another. However, the expectation is that a person with "entitlement" will act in other relationships also with a growing sense of trustworthiness, freedom and responsibility. Merit will become a cornerstone for a sustainable mode of care (constructive entitlement).

In one's existential capacity and competence, one can develop a sense of trustworthiness (personal trust). It can be viewed as a mode of investiture; it represents the power and spirit of subjectivity and does not reflect in the first instance ego-strength.

Exoneration: It is about an action that grants the exonerator his/her freedom; that is, to restore the freedom of the exonerator. It is about a kind of reaching out to the fate of the parent by means of a passive mode. This sensitivity for the predicament (fate) of the parent, operates from a future mode of being, that is in fact not yet the time of the parent. This reaching out from the future to the past of the parent, can serve as a kind of trace (even guide) for the restoring of relationships (relational healing).

Ledger: It refers to a ledger of merit; a kind of bookkeeping regarding the balance between merit and indebtedness of two interrelated persons. A family consists of more than one person; a person lives within a multitude of relationships. The ledger (or ledgers) function as a kind of systemic, familial memory regarding give-and-take in all particular relationships. In order to detect whether the relationship was fair or not, an important criterion will be whether the relationship was symmetric or asymmetric. The parent-child relationship is asymmetric. The relationship between siblings, spouses and friends can be rendered as symmetric (but not in a totalitarian sense).

The family ledger consists of different forms of balances that cannot be compared, and, thus, be outbalanced. On the other hand, a separate balance cannot end with a zero balance. For example: My guilt towards the other cannot be balanced out by the guilt of the other's guilt towards me. Irrespective of the question whether the relationships are intergenerational or "horizontal", relationships are embedded in asymmetric and symmetric mutuality.

Legacy: It is about the ethical imperative to existing current generations; to scrutinise the heritage of ancestors in order to decide what should be handed over to the next generation that will be beneficiary for human well-being. In this process of scrutiny, the notion of gender-orientation deserves attention.

Loyalty: Vertical: It is about the specific character of intergenerational connectedness. Horizontal: Sustainable and continuous connectedness with a relational partner (friend, spouse). Loyalty always implies the character of preference and functions according to a triadic structure: I am loyal towards the other (the preferred one) in front of a possible third (the one who is not preferred). This kind of connectedness implies "loyalty conflicts". A very intriguing form of loyalty to deal with in dialoguing, is "split loyalty" (loyalty to one parent is becoming difficult to maintain due to infringement by the other). In such a setting of split loyalty, the child becomes exposed to "parentification". Loyalty that is forbidden in a specific relational setting (invisible loyalty), is in fact an obstacle for personal individuation, as well as for commitments to the other/others. It refers furthermore to trustworthy deeds that can only be exercised by this very particular human being.

Multidirected partiality: It is about the challenge in therapy to side with every particular person involved in the interrelational networking of systems. It can indeed be the case that the therapist cannot credit a person for current behaviour due to his/her wrongdoing (for example: child abuse). However, it does not exclude the option that the therapist can acknowledge to the guilty, his/her suffering from hurt or forms of being victimised during his/her youth. Multidirected partiality presupposes that the therapist is personally responsible and accountable for the impact of therapeutic interventions of each person involved. The therapist must even reckon with implications on people not directly involved – the invisible other. Multidirected partiality focuses on the multirelational networking of everybody involved (directly or indirectly). It is sensitive for the particularity of each person as individual; it establishes a kind of feedback about personal engagement; – with acknowledgement for the vulnerability of the client for the sake of the vulnerability of his/ her other(s).

Parentification: Literally it refers to the process of making somebody (a child) a parent (on becoming a parent). The child is "forced" to take on more than age appropriate responsibility for a relationship. In cases of temporal role-shifting within severe stressful settings, parentification is not necessarily destructive. It can be a child's appropriate adaptation to temporary family strain. The younger person is, thus, exposed to an opportunity to learn in a very early stage in life what responsible caring is about.

Parentification becomes destructive when parents abuse the dedication and commitments of their children (Nagy: innate loyalty) and when it happens without acknowledgement from the parent for the contributions of the child. Being too generous and permissive towards children, can also be a mode of parentification. It is indeed a quite unique ability of a child to hand over and pledge his/her autonomy (that the child cannot manage yet) to somebody else. It is in fact a kind of risk, a mode of sacrifice.

Explanation: Parentification should be read and understood in connection with the art of giving. The notion of "*parentification*" in the process of guiding children into adulthood, is not per se about a destructive process (a pathological mode of parenthood) but can be a constructive investment in the developmental growth into maturity. However, in this process of becoming a parent and guiding of children into the responsibility of being an adult, Nagy also warned against the possible dangers of destructive modes of parenting (Nagy & Krasner BGT:65). He refers to "destructive idealising"; that is, the danger that parents work with inappropriate images (distorted perceptions) that do not fit the reality and personality of the child.

Rejunction: The establishment of renewed connections by means of responsible dialogue with family members, or any other important person from whom one has become estranged. It is about a personal choice to earn entitlement by means of constructive self-validation.

Resources (relational resources): Relational resources can be rendered as the fuel that establishes fairness. Contextual therapy is an endeavour to mobilise these relational sources for helping and support. It does not focus so much on the removal of pathological symptoms; the focus is rather on prevention and the promotion of relational healing and helping (enrichment of relational resources and authentic responsibility).

Revolving slate: A new victim is established because a person with an unpaid debt, transfers the "guilt" and hurt to another relation, other than the one where the debt has been caused. The other (or other group) is then been treated in an unfair way, rather than to focus on the guilty one. It is about a kind of transmission of injustice; that is, a mode of relational consequence wherein restorative revenge eventually creates "new victims". However, the problem is that innocent victims could be treated in the long run as original and causal culprits. In intergenerational terminology, the "revolving slate" implies that the children inherit an outstanding account about something that was unsettled between the parents and their ancestors. The outstanding guilt of pre-generations now becomes the responsibility of possible "innocent children" (Nagy & Spark IL:65).

Self-delineation: It refers to the ability within relationships to demarcate one's own individual borders, specifically regarding my need and right to give and to receive. The degree to which a self can be delineated is co-determined by former relationships (formative dynamics).

Self-validation: It is about the capacity to earn credit for relational integrity. This process implies that one should reckon with the self-delineation of the other. In order to earn entitlement, concern for the self-delineation of the other, is decisive.

Transgenerational solidarity: Responsible engagement regarding the quality of life for future and coming generations. With reference to the notion of a "transgenerational tribunal", the "future other/others", become an "invisible third". Contrary to the notion of loyalty with its structure of mutuality (especially in horizontal loyalty), transgenerational solidarity is not determined by mutuality, and, thus, about a one-sided influence. The future generation makes an appeal on personal accountability. Personal accountability becomes a future investment without any form of direct reward or any form of repayment.

The giving child: Caring behaviour of children; the contribution of giving: Children as resources for healing. Their contribution is about a passive competence, preceding even subjective freedom.

Tribunal: It is about the intrinsic ethical character and structure of relational dynamics; that is, the interactional dynamics becomes in itself a judging factor. The therapist can reckon with the intrinsic tribunal within the networking dynamics in order to support them in their quest for justice and fairness. It releases the therapist from the burden to act as judge in destructive human interaction.

Summary

The background of the publication is a joint study, as outcome from teaching experience, the practice of pastoral caregiving and psychotherapeutic endeavours. The original impetus for the research project was the disciplinary tension between the foundations and theory of contextual therapy as introduced by Ivan Boszormenyi-Nagy, and Emmanuel Levinas' radical philosophy of ethics and metaphysical thinking.

The further intention was to provide sound theory formation within the field and practice of contextual therapy. Thus, the focus on conceptualisation and the concern for paradigmatic reflection on the notion of intergenerational connectedness. The latter is about an interactional dynamic of intersubjectivity wherein every person is viewed as a loyal and contributing subject. Due to the paradigmatic framework of ethics and the quest for a human order of justice, every subject involved is endowed with indebtedness and merit. Indebtedness as key factor in an ethical approach refers to both past and coming generations.

To embark on an investigation of the mandate for pastoral encounters within the vulnerable space of the other, the *undergirding hypothesis* of the research project is the following: Nagy's reflection on justice, and its ethical implication for a transgenerational model, shape a kind of "operational anthropology" wherein accountability and responsibility are predetermined by the problematic dilemma of freedom and the predicament of not being free. This is the reason why a rereading of Nagy within the framework of Levinas' philosophy can help psychotherapy to undergo a paradigm switch from intrapsychic inclusiveness to relational networking and contextual interaction. Therefore, in terms of Levinas' terminology, responsibility does not emanate from a totalitarian, dominating structure (manipulative power play). One mode of totalitarian manipulation is morality based upon the abuse of power. Another mode is general ideas extrapolated into ideology. Ideas then become an ideological force that is compulsory for every concrete human situation. In the same way, the notion of "intergenerational structures" and "family systems" have been abused by many ideological views on family care.

Summary

Significant for the work of Levinas is his defense of the unique subjectivity. Due to the mysterious "*désir métaphysique*", subjectivity is shaped by the presence and visage of the other – the irrefutable responsibility for the other. The other in his/her otherness cannot be subordinated to any context.

Nagy and Levinas neither met, nor knew one another's work. Between them there is a world of differences. Nevertheless, the basic assumption is that there are points where their approaches intersect, especially with regard to the realm of ethics, the individual sphere of being a subject and the dynamics of interactive subjectivity.

A key point is the fact that Nagy underpins his theory by the dialogical philosophy of Martin Buber. Although criticised by Levinas, the advantage of a reciprocal approach is the emphasis on the unique ontological identity of the "I" within Buber's "dialogical model".

Chapter I is about an exposition of some of the main and specific theoretic concepts in the work of Nagy that portrays his paradigmatic framework of thinking. Attention is given to: Indebtedness and merit between the generations; guilt and accountability; loyalty and justice, as well as the "need" for giving as an "entitlement" within relational interaction.

The assumption is that many of the paradigmatic issues addressed and discussed by Nagy, are indeed applicable to pastoral theology and the ministerial field of pastoral care (see Chapter VI). In this regard, it is decisive to deal with concepts operating in psychotherapy. Immediately anthropology and the significance of the destiny of our being human come into play. Despite the more general or scientific context, important perspectives are addressed that can contribute to a theological reflection on the practice of caregiving.

Methodologically speaking, the theoretic outline tried to incorporate exegetical material from biblical exegesis and the Jewish background of Christian reflection. This has been done in order to come up with an integral approach in caregiving. In the original Dutch document biblical perspectives were discussed under different exegetical appendixes called "Sidelights"; that is, Jonathan's love for David (1 Sam 17:1–18:1); "With all your means" (Deut 6:5); Abraham's plea and intercession for Sodom (Gen 18); The binding of Isaac (Gen 22); The labourers in the vineyard (Matt 19:27–20:16). These sections are concerned about loyalty and subjectivity, about creation and re-creation, continuity and discontinuity. The intention was that each of these exegetical notes should be read in connection with the undergirding argument of the research project, namely, to reread Nagy within the framework of Levinas' philosophy in order to enhance the quality of pastoral engagement and the practice of caregiving. Thus, the decision to incorporate into the core text with new headings in the English version, these previously mentioned exegetical interludes.

Chapter II is about the basic viewpoints of Nagy's "contextual model" within the confines of helping and healing. First attention is given to biographical notes including some background details about the history of important developments in Nagy's thinking. Two important influential factors for the understanding of Nagy's theoretical reflecting are discussed: (a) the "internal object-relations-theory" (advocated by Ronald Fairbairn), and (b) the application of system-theory in family care (advocated by Gregory Bateson). Fairbairn, a structural Neo-Freudian, viewed the human mind as embedded in social relational networking. According to Nagy this framework has an analogy with Buber's I-Thou-dialogue "as foundation of being and becoming" (BGT:26). This parallel served as an early foundation for a contextual approach (BGT:26). However, Fairbairn remained mainly interested in the structures of the intrapsychic. Bateson, starting from system theory, interpreted phenomena that were traditionally diagnosed as schizophrenic, as behavioural dysfunctions within the social context of communication. Thus, the importance of the dynamic field of human interactions. The work of Bateson and his colleagues on double-binding and communication within families, contributed to a deepened understanding of psychotic confusion. The presupposition is that seriously confusing and personal disorientation should be assessed within the communication patterns of the familial system. In this regard, rigid patterns of communication tend to contribute to personal disintegration.

Nagy searched with "dogged perseverance" for an epistemological model that could integrate the psychological individual viewpoints with the premises of systems theory. "Transactional patterning remains a formal and shallow therapeutic framework if it fails to allow for the simultaneous coexistence of several individuals' rights and motives" (BGT:32). Such a new "nosology" requires terms that transcend the limitations of each of these frameworks.

For the work of Nagy in this field, the study refers to the term "operational anthropology". In this regard, one must reckon with the fact that Nagy is neither an anthropologist nor a philosopher. As a therapist he tries to find anthropological notions in order to help people who are suffering, as well as their family members and significant others (including those not yet born), to cope with the demands of life and hurt within the interrelation dynamics of human coexistence. The focus on Nagy's anthropological position and theoretical postulation, attends to the following: Loyalty, justice and social dynamics, as well as the dialectical theory on relationships. In this regard, the paradigm shift from dialectics to dialogistic is discussed.

It is important to take into consideration that Nagy is in the first place not concerned with the dialogue between the client(s) and the therapist. However, he does emphasise the dialogue between the client and his/her significant others (also the coming generation): Dialogue as reciprocity of care and a requirement of genuine equitability, becomes especially important in asymmetrical relationships.

Chapter III focuses on Nagy's concern for the interplay between "context" and "ethical dimension". It deals inter alia with the question: What is the meaning of a contextual approach in human well-being? Could Martin Buber's "I-Thou" approach be incorporated in theory formation for an intergenerational model in family care?

"Context" is viewed not as an explanatory principle but as a process of redefinition of intersubjective relationships in terms of fairness or unfairness. In this process each person (family member) is subject of the redefinition, so that everyone can be or become a relational trust-resource for every other significant other. The redefinition of the context is relationally and ethically qualified.

Nagy never strictly defined the meaning of "ethics" in his work. The research project tried to unearth the meaning and describe three main aspects: (a) Human existence as intrinsically ethical. (b) The thesis that there is a very special "ability" available in every human being to contribute to therapeutic change. An example is the notion of the "giving child" and his/her ability to surrender her/his autonomy. This contribution is being called: a passive ability. The contribution and ability are not in the first place about pathology, but about a very human capacity and competence to care for others, even when such a challenge runs against one's self-interest. It is in this regard, why it is apparently not fair, to reduce the child's acts of giving (contributing) to merely the realm of "psychological needs". (c) The juridical language of Nagy. It appears that juridical terminology serves to map the psychological and interactional reality from an ethical viewpoint. This is consistent with Nagy's point of departure, namely, how to do and operate justice.

Ethics in Nagy's work is not about a super- or under-structure of "being". Ethics represents the dynamic perspective of fair relating.

Nagy found in Buber's writings a model that can be described as "two or more individuals in a personally engaged relationship" (F:241). The implication is that therapy should deal with the notion of multi-partiality within coexisting multi-personal criteria (BGT:30). For Nagy, Buber's I-Thou model became his paradigmatic framework for the basic hermeneutics of interactive human encounters. In this regard, Maurice Friedman's emphasis on the notion of responsibility in mutuality and dialogue, plays an influential role.

References were made to the following writings of Buber: *Ich und Du* ("I and Thou"); the short text *Healing through Meeting*, and the lecture *Guilt and Guilt feeling*. Attention is also paid to a related article of Buber: *What is Common to All*.

The undergirding critical argument is that Buber's basic ontological structure is not appropriate for Nagy's attempt to base the relational dynamics of human encounters in ethics. An ontological foundation threatens the separate value of the relational bipolarities. Buber's "realm of the between" should thus be directed by the basic principle of "justice". Thus, Buber's notion of the "justice of the human order" which is indeed regarded as most helpful. The basic argument is that justice does not begin with reciprocity. Thus, the following vital questions: What can found subjectivity? How is it possible to deal with subjectivity and the notions of accountability and responsibility without running into the danger of a totalising objectification?

Chapter IV describes Levinas' thinking. Simultaneously it deals with Nagy's contention about the unique quality of "subject" and "subjectivity". The title of this chapter refers to Nagy's connection between "the context of the human order of justice" and the role of the so called "silent partner" within the dynamics of intergenerational relationships. The outline deals with Levinas' idea of "truth manifesting itself in humility" (EN:71-72; TO:80-81). In this regard, the biblical expression of "The voice of fragile silence" (1 Kings 19:12-13) is quite illuminating. Nagy refers to "this voice" as "a silent partner" (BGT:98). In Levinas' work this "truth" (the voice of fragile silence) becomes anchored in the totalising "subject" which is transformed into "subjectivity"; in French: *Avatar de son subjectivité*.

Summary

After a short outline on Levinas' biography, the outlines concerning his philosophy, in which "subjectivity" and "non-indifference" for the other as "stranger, widow and orphan" are the crucial points, are sketched. After arguing that the other is to be rendered as always "first" (prior), attention is given to detecting traces of "subjectivity" (Levinas) in the work of Nagy. The question is posed: How could Nagy's ethical dimension, and his use of the terms "accountability" and "responsibility", could have made any sense, if there is no "*avatar*" (transformation) into "subjectivity"? It is due to this question that Nagy turns to Levinas' notion of the "other/Other" rather than the emphasis on intrapsychic dynamics as in psychotherapy. The other renders subjectivity the possibility to express responsibility. Entitlement, within a relational dynamic of intersubjectivity, establishes realised responsibility.

Chapter V turns to the quest for freedom and deliverance. Especially, how to deal with relational hurt and harm. In this respect, the notion of exoneration and its link with forgiveness turns up. Thus, the discussion on Levinas' notion of "*le pardon*", and his objections against a flat horizontal dual structure. Here the notion of *L'un pour l'autre* (the one-for-the-other), which is always realised in a triadic situation, comes into play. In forgiveness a third factor is present. Real forgiveness is not a continuous process within the interplay between "guilt" and pardoning (not guilty). Forgiveness demands a new creation.

The chapter deals inter alia with Nagy's concept of "exoneration". Nagy emphatically distinguishes exoneration from forgiveness. Nagy clearly opts for exoneration due to his fear that forgiveness is too closely associated with a general romantic understanding of generosity. Exoneration should be linked to retribution. Thus, the importance to introduce a juridical term. With the concept "exoneration", Nagy appears to be seeking conditions which can transform fatal intergenerational transmissions. For Nagy, exoneration should be linked to fairness and loyalty in order to contribute to renewed relationship and the possibility of transformation; that is, the making of a total new start. Exoneration is fundamentally about a reassessment which has the features of "*tesjoewa*" (changeover, an existential reversal).

"Destructive entitlement" should be changed from a deadly dazzling grief into a sorrowful "conversion" that will inevitably lead to life (the duality of giving and receiving) within the conscience of the so-called destructively entitled person. This means a radical renewal of "my" companionship with the other.

Summary

Chapter VI is about pastoral care and pastoral theology from a contextual perspective. As argued in the previous chapters, pastoral care is defined as a defence of subjectivity. The church or the parish primarily consists of different persons, not of congenials. The argument is that it is the pastor's mandate to understand personal entanglements as ethical entanglements. Therefore, multidirected partiality plays a decisive role in "contextual healing and helping". It is embedded in ethics and directed by the moral principle of *L'un pour l'autre*: the other person is also the neighbour of another other. That is the meaning of: "To keep to the Word" (see Martin Luther's pious slogan: *Erhalt uns, Herr, bei deinem Wort*). Personal accountability cannot be reduced to the result of any totality. Thus, neither to "church" nor to "family" as objectified abstractions. A contextual perspective means a view on families and family-life that is not mythical, but de-totalising. It is eventually the lasting accountability that qualifies relating persons as "family".

Several concluding statements about pastoral care have been made. The importance of "re-hearing" in pastoral encounters has been underlined. What should be addressed is a specific desire: The desire for making peace with the other(s), and the spiritual need to be received in peace. The more I hear in what the other tells me, the more the desire for trustworthiness (despite the fear to be become abused by related others) is promoted. Furthermore, the more the other is freed from the urge to protect his/her others against the "I" (me), the better one is enabled to deal with human vulnerability within the confines of our human quest for dignity.

The emphasis on ethics in multi-directed partiality enables the multi-laterality of the person. The contextual approach is therefore not to be interpreted as sheer moralism. The intention is to instil trustworthiness and to establish the status of ethics as primordial in human encounters.

Reference has been made to the importance of "rejunctive" language in pastoral care. The pitfall of making the other seemingly disloyal, is discussed. The importance of using a socio-genogram (a special graphic depiction of interrelational associations – a kind of systemic map) in processes of caring has been pointed out.

The following concluding remarks are applicable to a therapeutic approach in caregiving: The meaning of the other is not reducible; the appeal of the other is situated in a context; helping is not founded in the affective (emotional dimension); transformation and change are embedded in the "ethical fabric" (Nagy) of relationships and the notion of interactional indebtedness. Each person has an irrefutable responsibility, which is a unique election (a kind of "right of primogeniture"). In line with Levinas, this calling could be called "the curve of the intersubjective space – perhaps the presence of God". This makes the context open to the awe of unpredictability and the surprise of sustainable "peace"; it helps one to deal in significant encounters with another possible meta-dimension and eschatological option: "meaning without context". In a nutshell, the mandate for the practice of pastoral care should be linked to the disturbing factor of the other. A theological perspective resides in the biblical principle of merciful grace, pity and compassion (*hèsèd*), as enfleshed in the dynamics of human relationships.

CPSIA information can be obtained
at www.ICGtesting.com
Printed in the USA
BVHW011653240220
573143BV00009BA/338